MECHANISMS IN THE
PATHOGENESIS OF
ENTERIC DISEASES 2

ADVANCES IN EXPERIMENTAL MEDICINE AND BIOLOGY

A Continuation Order Plan is available for this series. A continuation order will bring delivery of each new volume immediately upon publication. Volumes are billed only upon actual shipment. For further information please contact the publisher.

MECHANISMS IN THE PATHOGENESIS OF ENTERIC DISEASES 2

Edited by

Prem S. Paul

Iowa State University
Ames, Iowa

and

David H. Francis

South Dakota State University
Brookings, South Dakota

KLUWER ACADEMIC / PLENUM PUBLISHERS
NEW YORK, BOSTON, DORDRECHT, LONDON, MOSCOW

Library of Congress Cataloging-in-Publication Data

Mechanisms in the pathogenesis of enteric diseases 2/edited by Prem S. Paul and David
H. Francis.
     p. ; cm. — (Advances in experimental medicine and biology; v. 473)
     Includes bibliographic references and index.
     ISBN 0-306-46214-1
     1. Intestines—Infections—Pathophysiology—Congresses. I. Paul, Prem S. II. Francis,
David H. III. International Rushmore Conference on Mechanisms in the Pathogenesis of
Enteric Diseases (2nd: 1998: Rapid City, S.D.) IV. Series.
     [DNLM: 1. Gastrointestinal Diseases—microbiology—Congresses. 2. Gastrointestinal
Diseases—pathophysiology—Congresses. WI 140 M486 1999]
RC862.E47 M43 1999
616.3′407—dc21

                                                  99-048628

ISSN 0065-2598

Proceedings of the Second International Rushmore Conference on Mechanisms in the Pathogenesis of Enteric
Diseases, held September 30–October 3, 1998, in Rapid City, South Dakota

ISBN 0-306-46214-1

©1999 Kluwer Academic / Plenum Publishers, New York
233 Spring Street, New York, N.Y. 10013

10 9 8 7 6 5 4 3 2 1

A C.I.P. record for this book is available from the Library of Congress

PREFACE

This book, *Mechanisms in the Pathogenesis of Enteric Diseases 2*, is an outcome of the Second International Rushmore Conference on Mechanisms in the Pathogenesis of Enteric Diseases, held September 30–October 3, 1998 in Rapid City, South Dakota, USA. Its chapters represent many of the reviews and papers presented at the conference. The meeting was organized by members of the North-Central Regional Research Committee "NC-62", a consortium of researchers of bovine and swine enteric diseases from land-grant institutions supported by the United States Department of Agriculture. The Rushmore Conferences were conceived as a forum for an interdisciplinary discussion of mechanisms of infectious enteric diseases. It was intended that such a discussion would stimulate cross-pollination of ideas, and nurture synergistic collaborations among scientists who might otherwise not interact. Enteric diseases are caused by widely divergent pathogens and parasites in broadly different settings, and affect multiple organ systems. Some enteric diseases affect a single species, while others may affect multiple species, perhaps including human beings. Some enteric diseases were present in antiquity, while others have recently emerged. Knowledge regarding a particular disease or pathogen has frequently proven useful in understanding another disease or pathogen, because common themes in pathogenesis exist. As this knowledge base grows, strategies in the prevention and control of various enteric diseases often converge. Cross-disciplinary discussions and collaborations facilitate growth of this knowledge base, as well as development of tools for disease interdiction. It is hoped that the Second International Rushmore conference has had such a facilitating effect.

Participants in the conference came from 13 countries in the continents of North and South America, Europe, and Asia. They represented institutions of higher learning, government agencies, and private industry. Participants brought expertise from many disciplines in both human and veterinary medicine. These multiple perspectives, and an informal atmosphere, provided an environment for lively and thought-provoking discussions. Conference topics included: Pathobiology of Gastroenteric Diseases; Mechanisms of Identity and Interaction between Host and Pathogen; Effector Mechanisms in, and Regulation of, Pathogenic Activity; Epidemiology; and Novel Approaches to Prevention and Therapy. These topics were addressed by ten keynote, and six additional invited speakers. Oral and poster presentations were presented by other conference participants. Keynote speakers included Drs. Richard Guerrant, University of Virginia School of Medicine; Fergus Shanahan, National University of Ireland; Rodney Berg, Louisiana State University; Marian Horzinek, Utrecht University; Mary Estes, Baylor College of Medicine (Houston); Virginia Miller, Washington University (St. Louis); James Slauch, University of Illinois; Roger Glass, Centers for Disease Control (Atlanta); Lucía Cárdenas-Freytag, Tulane University School of Medicine (New Orleans); and Luis Enjuanes, Antonomous University (Madrid). Invited presentations were given by Drs. Linda Saif, Ohio State University; Rodney Moxley, University of Nebraska; David Francis, South Dakota State University; Michael Konkel, Washington State University; Andreas Bäumler, Texas A & M University; and Richard Isaacson, University of Illinois.

Members of the conference organizing committee were Drs. David Francis and David Benfield, South Dakota State University; Richard Isaacson, University of Illinois; Lynn Joens, University of Arizona; Rodney Moxley, University of Nebraska; Prem Paul and Mike Wannemuehlar, Iowa State University; and Linda Saif, Ohio State University. Drs. Francis and Benfield were the conference hosts. The conference organizing committee expresses sincere thanks to all who presented speeches or papers at the Second International Rushmore Conference, joined in discussions, and provided an enthusiastic environment for presentations and discussions, as well as vendors whose services made conference attendance enjoyable. The committee expresses special gratitude to organizations whose financial support made the conference possible. Financial contributors included: South Dakota/NSF EPSCoR (conference support grant EPS-9720642); USDA-NRICGP (conference support grant No. 9802205); Bayer—Agriculture Division, Shawnee Mission, Kansas; Pfizer-Central Research Division, Lincoln, Nebraska; Boehringer Ingelheim Animal Health, Saint Joseph, Missouri; Grand Laboratories, Inc., Freeman, South Dakota; Eli Lilly and Company Foundation, Indianapolis, Indiana; and Wyeth-Lederle Vaccines and Pediatrics (Wyeth-Ayerst Laboratories), Pearl River, NY.

Prem S. Paul
David H. Francis

CONTENTS

INTESTINAL LYMPHOEPITHELIAL COMMUNICATION

Fergus Shanahan

Department of Medicine
National University of Ireland
Cork, Ireland

1. SUMMARY

The close anatomic juxtaposition of epithelial cells with lymphocytes lining the intestinal tract facilitates communication between the two cell types. This intercellular dialogue is important for mucosal development and has a conditioning effect on mucosal structure, function, and response to tissue injury. Lymphoepithelial communication is bi-directional, and mediated in large part, by shared ligands and receptors. The chemical messengers involved include cytokines, growth factors, local hormones, and products of arachidonate metabolism. The interdependency between the epithelium and adjacent lymphoid cells is such that the epithelium is considered to have a central role in the mucosal immune system and is an active participant in both the afferent and efferent limbs of the mucosal immune response. The molecular crosstalk between the epithelium and adjacent lymphocytes is just one aspect of a more complex network of intercellular signalling within the intestinal mucosa and upon which the integrity of the mucosa is dependent. Thus, there are extensive interactions between nerve and immune cells and between the enteric flora and the epithelium and amongst intestinal mesenchymal cells including fibroblasts and vascular endothelial cells. Disruption of any aspect of the mucosal microenvironment, as has been achieved with selective genetically engineered murine models, is associated with impaired mucosal defence and inflammation.

Mailing Address: Dr. F. Shanahan, Department of Medicine, Cork University Hospital, Cork, Ireland, Tel: 353-21-901226; Fax: 353-21-345300; e-mail: Fshanahan@ucc.ie

Mechanisms in the Pathogenesis of Enteric Diseases 2, edited by Paul and Francis.
Kluwer Academic / Plenum Publishers, New York, 1999.

2. INTRODUCTION

The notion that different cell-types juxtaposed within a specialised tissue might communicate with one another seems intuitively self-evident, but the extent of lymphoepithelial interactions within the gastrointestinal mucosa has only recently become apparent. The purpose of this brief overview is to present a perspective on integrative immunoepithelial physiology in health and disease. Recent reports are emphasised; more comprehensive analysis including details of earlier studies have been reviewed elsewhere (Castro, 1982; Befus, 1990; Castro and Arntzen, 1993; Perdue and McKay, 1994; Shanahan, 1994; Stenson and Alpers, 1994).

The intestinal epithelium in health and disease is engaged in continual dialogue with neighbouring lymphoid cells both above and below the basement membrane. Only a single layer of cells above the basement membrane separates the external environment (enteric lumen) from the internal milieu. Within this layer, the intraepithelial lymphocytes (IELs) account for approximately ten percent of the cells and collectively represent a significant lymphoid mass, which in aggregate, would approximate to the size of the spleen (Brandtzaeg et al., 1989). These cells are functionally and phenotypically distinct from peripheral lymphocytes and from lymphocytes below the epithelial basement membrane within the lamina propria of the gut. The IELs are comprised of two sub-populations, one dependent on the thymic microenvironment for differentiation and the other being thymus independent. It appears that the gastrointestinal epithelium can substitute for the thymic epithelial microenvironment and promote self-nonself education and T cell differentiation for the thymus independent subset of IELs (Lefrançois and Puddington, 1995; Klein, 1996; Saito et al., 1998). In this way, the mucosal intestinal epithelium is considered to be a primary lymphoid organ.

Beneath the basement membrane within the lamina propria is a diversity of immunoinflammatory effector cells of all types including T and B lymphocytes, plasma cells, phagocytes, and dendritic cells, representing a state of "controlled" inflammation primed for host defence (Shanahan, 1994). The existence of this physiologic controlled inflammatory infiltrate is a defining feature of mucosal tissues. Although the close anatomic juxtaposition of epithelial and immune cells is particularly suited to intercellular communication, each of the cellular components within the mucosal microenvironment transmits and receives regulatory signals from adjacent cells, and this molecular cross-talk has a conditioning effect on mucosal structure and function (Shanahan, 1994). Indeed, genetically engineered disruption of any component of the mucosal microenvironment, including the epithelium, mucosal T cells, cytokines or the enteric glial cells, as has been achieved with several murine models, is associated with impaired mucosal defence and uncontrolled inflammation (Shanahan, 1994b; Bush et al., 1998; Shanahan and O'Sullivan, 1999).

3. THE SYNTAX OF IMMUNOEPITHELIAL COMMUNICATION

Communication between the epithelium and the mucosal immune system is bi-directional. Epithelial cells and lymphocytes share several ligands and receptors that provide mutual reciprocal regulatory signals. Both cell-types can elaborate cytokines in response to tissue injury and both express functional cytokine receptors (Reinecker and Podolsky, 1995; Reinecker, et al., 1996). However, lymphoepithelial interactions are tissue-specific. Thus, the immune system is regionally specialized and compartmentalised depending on the local microenvironment. An example of tissue-specific control of immunity is epithelial-derived stem cell factor (SCF) which regulated IEL maturation by acting on specific receptors on IELs that are absent from the most lymphocytes outside the epithelium (Puddington et al., 1994).

Bi-directional lymphoepithelial communication is also mediated by non-cytokines such as prostaglandins and neuropeptides (Phipps et al., 1991; Shanahan and Anton, 1994; Shanahan, 1997). Prostaglandins such as PGE-2 are produced by colonic epithelial cells in response to tumor necrosis factor (TNF-a) and interleukin-1 (IL-1), but production of these proinflammatory cytokines is inhibited by PGE-2, representing a negative feedback loop (Vidrich et al., 1998).

Another intriguing example of mucosal cross-talk mediated by non-cytokines is the paracrine network involving thyrotropin releasing hormone (TRH). This has been shown to act on murine epithelial cells through specific receptors (TRH-R), eliciting local release of thyrotropin-stimulating hormone (TSH), which exerts a receptor-mediated (TSH-R) regulatory influence on adjacent IELs. The central role of TSH and the tissue specificity of this paracrine regulatory network was confirmed by the finding of selective impairment of IEL development in mice that have a mutant TSH receptor (Wang et al., 1997).

Immunoepithelial paracrine networks may include signals from additional cell-types including local fibroblasts (Berschneider and Powell, 1992; Fritsch et al., 1997) and neurons (Nagura et al., 1996). The neuropeptide substance P has been shown to have immunomodulatory properties and can trigger pro-inflammatory cytokine production by mononuclear cells. We have mapped the distribution of substance P receptors within the intestine and have shown that the substance P (NK-1) receptor is expressed by all subsets of mucosal lymphocytes but not by peripheral blood lymphocytes (Goode et al., 1998a). The receptor is also expressed by epithelial cells and this expression is regulated by pro-inflammatory cytokines from activated lymphocytes (Goode et al., 1998b). One of the direct functional effects of substance P on epithelium is proliferation and this may have particular significance in response to epithelial injury. Thus, substance P may mediate a tricellular network in which local release of the neuropeptide by mucosal neurons in response to tissue injury stimulates a cytokine response by lymphocytes which upregulate the expression of the substance P receptor on the epithelium, thereby promoting epithelial proliferation and healing.

4. LYMPHOEPITHELIAL INTERDEPENDENCY FOR GROWTH AND DEVELOPMENT

Several lines of evidence indicate that lymphoepithelial communication is central to the optimal development of both enterocytes and IELs. The production of growth factors and cytokines such as interleukin 7 by the epithelium are required for normal development of intra-epithelial lymphocytes (Watanabe et al., 1995). Mice lacking the gene for the interleukin 7 receptor, normally present on IELs, also lack the subpopulation of IELs within the gut epithelium which express the gamma-delta ($\gamma\delta$) T cell receptor, whereas other T cell populations (alpha-beta receptor-bearing IELs) are preserved (Williams, 1998). The requirement of lympho-epithelial interaction for mucosal growth and development is reciprocal; mice lacking gamma-delta IELs have severely impaired development of intestinal epithelium (Boismenu and Havran, 1994; Komano et al., 1995).

In addition to normal enterocyte development, epithelial differentiation from enterocyte to the antigen transport or M cell phenotype is conditioned by mucosal lymphocytes from Peyer's patches. Thus, when mucosal lymphocytes isolated from aggregates of intestinal lymphoid follicles (Peyer's patches) are co-cultured with differentiated enterocytes, the enterocytes assume the characteristics of M cells (Kernéis et al., 1997).

5. THE EPITHELIUM AS A COMPONENT OF MUCOSAL IMMUNITY

It has been known for decades that epithelia at mucosal surfaces transport polymeric immunoglobulin A into external secretions. When dimeric IgA binds to its receptor (secretory component) at the basolateral surface of the enterocyte, it is transported across the enterocyte and released into the external lumen still bound to secretory component which renders the immunoglobulin resistant to proteolytic cleavage by intestinal enzymes (Braendtzaeg et al., 1989). Secretory component is, therefore, referred to as the sacrificial receptor. More recently, it has become evident that the enterocyte has a more versatile contribution to mucosal immunity and participates in the humoral and cellular components of both the afferent and the efferent limbs of the mucosal immune response (Table 1).

Although the M cells (also known as follicle-associated epithelium) overlying Peyer's patches and individual lymphoid follicles are strategically placed and optimally designed for antigen sampling and transport to the underlying mucosal lymphoid tissue (Kraehenbuhl and Neutra, 1992), there is evidence that the fully differentiated surface enterocytes may also exhibit antigen uptake processing and presentation in association with Class 1 and Class 2 MHC molecules (Mayer and Shlien, 1987; Hershberg et al., 1997). This process is likely to be less efficient than that which occurs with the professional antigen presenting cells, such as dendritic cells and macrophages within the lamina propria but quantitatively might be important given the relative abundance of enterocytes. In general, enterocytes tend to promote presentation to CD8[+] lymphocytes facilitating their proliferation with an associated suppressive effect on mucosal immunity. This pathway is thought to represent a homeostatic downregulatory process to avoid potentially harmful immunoinflammatory responses to otherwise innocuous enteric antigens. In the setting of chronic inflammatory bowel disease (Crohn's disease

Table 1. Participation of the intestinal epithelium in the afferent and efferent limbs of the mucosal immune response

Mucosal Immune Response	Enterocyte Involvement
Afferent or sensory limb	Antigen uptake
	Antigen presentation and processing
Efferent or effector limb	Immunoglobulin transport
	Cytokine production
	Growth factors
	Prostaglandins and other mediators
	Local "hormones"
	Complement factors

and ulcerative colitis), it has been suggested that this form of lymphoepithelial communication is defective. Instead of suppression, enterocytes from patients with inflammatory bowel disease have been reported to promote the proliferation of lymphocytes with a helper (CD4) phenotype, thereby favouring amplification of an established inflammatory disease process (Mayer et al., 1990).

At the efferent limb of the mucosal immune response, the epithelium not only transports immunoglobulin A but can also generate cytokines and is a source of other factors that contribute to or modify immunoinflammatory reactions. These include prostaglandins and other arachidonate metabolites (Shannon et al., 1993; Vidrich et al., 1998), growth factors (Podolsky, 1993), complement factors (Andoh et al., 1996), and nitric oxide synthase (Singer et al., 1996). Perhaps the clearest evidence for an epithelial contribution to the immunoinflammatory response is in defence against invasive bacteria. In this context, there is compelling evidence that epithelial cells act as sensors for microbial infection. Through the medium of proinflammatory cytokines and other proinflammatory factors, they transduce the infectious signal into an active recruitment of the mucosal immunoinflammatory response (Kagnoff and Eckmann, 1997).

An additional emerging theme is the co-ordinate role of enterocytes and intra-epithelial γδ IEL in linking innate or natural intestinal defence with acquired immunity. The innate immune response is rapid and non-specific; it is composed of phagocytes and interferons which limit the spread of infection. In contrast, the acquired response has slower humoral and cellular limbs which specifically recognise pathogens and develop memory cells. The γδ subset of IEL may co-ordinate the interplay between the innate and acquired immune response. γδ-IEL recognise stress-associated antigens and are activated by injured epithelium. In response to this, they elaborate a series of factors including epithelial growth factors which promote epithelial healing, chemokines which recruit inflammatory cells to the injured site, and regulatory cytokines which activate the humoral and cellular limbs of the slower but more specific acquired immune response (Mak and Ferrick, 1998).

6. IMMUNOLOGICAL MODULATION OF EPITHELIAL FUNCTION

It is almost two decades since the concept of immunological regulation of intestinal epithelial cell function was first promoted (Castro, 1982). This was quickly supported by evidence from several investigators with early reports based mainly on the influence of mast cell products on ion transport (Baird et al., 1984; Baird et al., 1987; Crowe et al., 1990; Barrett, 1991). Subsequent studies extended the range of epithelial functions subject to immune regulation and broadened spectrum of immune-derived mediators involved to include prostaglandins, growth factors, neuropeptides, and cytokines (Bern et al., 1989; Befus, 1990; Perdue and McKay, 1994; Shanahan, 1994). Almost every aspect of epithelial physiology has been shown to be influenced by cytokines or other products of the mucosal immune system (Table 2). Since epithelial cells not only express receptors for several cytokines (Reinecker and Podolsky, 1995; Reinecker et al., 1996), but can also be induced to elaborate cytokines in response to infectious or other inflammatory stimuli, the potential for autocrine feedback regulation exists and has been demonstrated (Taylor et al., 1998).

Table 2. Representative epithelial functions that are influenced by cytokines and other immune-derived factors

Epithelial Function Regulated by Cytokines	References*
Ion transport	Perdue and McKay, 1994
Permeability	Madara and Stafford, 1989
Proliferation and Restitution	Dignass and Podolsky, 1993
Expression of surface molecules	Shanahan, 1994; Perdue and
— adhesion molecules	McKay, 1994
— secretory component	
— major histocompatibilty complex	
Metabolic activity	
— iNOS induction	Singer et al., 1996
— cytokine elaboration	Kagnoff and Eckmann, 1997
— complement factors	Andoh et al., 1996
— arachidonate metabolism	Shannon et al., 1993; Vidrich
	et al., 1998

*reference citations are representative not comprehensive.

7. LYMPHOEPITHELIAL AGGRESSION—THE FAS COUNTERATTACK!

Increasing evidence suggests that epithelial cells under certain circumstances may express the Fas ligand (FasL) which triggers cells to undergo receptor-mediated apoptosis using the Fas receptor (FasR, CD95). This confers a protective advantage against potentially harmful inflammatory reactions and is one of the mechanisms of immune privilege within the cornea and ocular epithelium (Griffith et al., 1997). Recently, we have shown that colonic epithelial carcinoma cell lines express FasL and can kill activated lymphocytes in vitro (O'Connell et al., 1996). This suggests that epithelial cancers of the gut can evade the immune system by making a pre-emptive strike against activated tumor-infiltrating lymphocytes (the "Fas counterattack"). The observation has been confirmed by others in several other cancers (Walker et al., 1998), and there is evidence that this counterattack mechanism may be operative in vivo (Bennett et al., 1998). To avoid autocrine cell suicide, the cancer cell must first disable its own Fas receptor-mediated pathway to apoptosis before it expresses Fas L; several molecular mechanisms appear to confer this resistance to apoptosis on the cancer cell (O'Connell et al., 1999).

Whether FasR-FasL interactions contribute to the normal crypt-to-surface cycle of gastrointestinal epithelial proliferation followed by apoptosis and shedding, is uncertain. Evidence for expression of Fas L by enterocytes, other than Paneth cells, has been controversial, but the co-expression of FasR and FasL by surface, but not crypt epithelia, could theoretically account for triggering apoptosis by autocrine suicide or paracrine fratricide at the end of the epithelial life span. We have recently reported evidence for the expression of Fas L at the mRNA and protein levels within the upper layers of the esophageal epithelium where it is co-expressed with Fas R thereby facilitating cellular suicide and fratricide (Bennett et al., 1999). In addition, epithelial expression of Fas L within the esophagus correlates with areas of exclusion of intraepithelial lymphocytes. This suggests that normal esophageal epithelium might be another site of immune privilege. This concept is consistent with the well recognised paucity of inflammatory cells within the esophageal epithelium in reflux esophagitis and may be one of the mechanisms by which the esophagus is protected from inflammatory reactions.

8. CONCLUSION

Regional specialization of the immune response and the conditioning influence of the local microenvironment within different tissues is well illustrated by lympho-epithelial communication within the intestine. Normal mucosal homeostasis is dependent on this bi-directional intercellular communication. The presence of local paracrine and juxtacrine immunoregulatory networks of chemical messengers within the intestine highlights the importance of studying the mucosal immune system in context, ie. within its natural environment.

ACKNOWLEDGMENTS

The author is supported, in part, by the Health Research Board of Ireland and by the Cork Cancer Research Center.

REFERENCES

Andoh, A., Fujiyama, Y., Sumiyoshi, K.-I., Sakumoto, H., and Bamba, T., 1996, Interleukin 4 acts as an inducer of decay-accelerating factor gene expression in human intestinal epithelial cells. Gastroenterology 111:911–918.

Baird, A.W., Coombs, R.R.A., McLaughlan, P., and Cuthbert, A.W., 1984, Immediate hypersensitivity reactions to cow milk proteins in isolated epithelium from ileum of milk-drinking guinea pigs: comparisons with colonic epithelia. Int. Arch. Allergy Appl. Immunol. 75:255–263.

Baird, A.W., Cuthbert, A.W., and MacVinish, L.J., 1987, Type 1 hypersensitivity reactions in reconstructed tissues using syngeneic cell types. Br. J. Pharmacol. 91:857–869.

Barrett, K.E., 1991, Immune-related intestinal chloride secretion. III. Acute and chronic effects of mast cell mediators on chloride secretion by a human colonic epithelial cell line. J. Immunol. 147:959–964.

Befus, A.D., 1990, Immunophysiology: influence of the mucosal immune system on intestinal function, In: Immunology and immunopathology of the liver and gastrointestinal tract., Targan, S.R. and Shanahan, F. (editors), Igaku-Shoin, New York, Tokyo, pp. 205–229.

Bennett, M.W., O'Connell, J., O'Sullivan, G.C., Brady, C., Roche, D., Collins, J.K., and Shanahan, F., 1998, The Fas counterattack in vivo: apoptotic depletion of tumor-infiltrating lymphocytes (TIL) associated with Fas ligand (FasL) expression by human esophageal carcinoma. J. Immunol. 160:5669–5675.

Bennett, M.W., O'Connell, J., O'Sullivan, G.C., Roche, R., Brady, C., Kelly, J., Collins, J.K., and Shanahan, F., 1999, Fas ligand and Fas receptor are coexpressed in normal human esophageal epithelium; a potential mechanism of apoptotic epithelial turnover. Diseases of the Esophagus (in press).

Bern, J.M., Sturbaum, C.W., Karayalcin, S.S., Berschneider, H.M., Wachsman, J.T., and Powell, D.W., 1989, Immune system control of rat and rabbit colonic electrolye transport. Role of prostaglandins and enteric nervous system. J. Clin. Invest. 83:1810–1820.

Boismenu, R. and Havran, W.L., 1994, Modulation of epithelial cell growth by intraepithelial $\gamma\delta$ T cells. Science 266:1253–1255.

Brandtzaeg, P., Halstensen, T.S., Kett, K., Karjci, P., Kvale, D., Rognum, T.O., Scott, H., and Sollid, L.M., 1989, Immunobiology and immunopathology of human gut mucosa: humoral immunity and intraepithelial lymphocytes. Gastroenterology 97:1562–84.

Bush, T.G., Savidge, T.C., Freeman, T.C., Cox, H.J., Campbell, E.A., Mucke, L., Johnson, M.H., and Sofroniew, M.V., 1998, Fulminant jejuno-ileitis following ablation of enteric glia in adult transgenic mice. Cell 93:189–21.

Castro, G.A., 1982, Immunological regulation of epithelial function. Am. J. Physiol. 243 (Gastrointest. Liver Physiol. 6):G321–G329.

Castro, G.A. and Arntzen, C.J., 1993, Immunophysiology of the gut: a research frontier for integrative studies of the common mucosal immune system, Am. J. Physiol. 265 (Gastrointest. Liver Physiol. 28):G599–G610.

Crowe, S.E., Sestini, P., and Perdue, M.H., 1990, Allergic reactions of rat jejunal mucosa. Ion transport responses to luminal antigenand inflammatory mediators. Gastroenterology 99:74–82.

Fritsch, C., Simon-Assmann, P., Kedinger, M., and Evans, G.S., 1997, Cytokines modulate fibroblast phenotype and epithelial-stroma interactions in rat intestine. Gastroenterology 112:826–838.

Goode, T., O'Connell, J., Sternini, C., Anton, P., O'Sullivan, G.C., Collins, J.K., and Shanahan, F., 1998a, Substance P (NK-1) receptor is a marker of human mucosal but not peripheral mononuclear cells: molecular quantitation and localization. J. Immunol.161::2232–2240.

Goode, T., O'Connell, J., O'Sullivan, G.C., Collins, J.K., and Shanahan, F., 1998b, Cytokine induced expression of substance P (NK-1) receptors in human colonic epithelial cells. Gastroenterology 114:A373.

Griffith, T.S. and Ferguson, T.A., 1997, The role of FasL-induced apoptosis in immune privilege. Immunol. Today 18:240–244.

Hershberg, R.M., Framson, P.E., Cho, D.H., Lee, L.Y., Kovats, S., Beitz, J., Blum, J.S., and Nepom, G.T., 1997, Intestinal epithelial cells use two distinct pathways for HLA class II antigen processing. J. Clin. Invest. 11:204–215.

Kagnoff, M.F. and Eckmann, L, 1997, Epithelial cells as sensors for microbial infection. J. Clin. Invest. 100:6–10.

Kernéis, S., Bogdanova, A., Kraehenbuhlm J.-P., and Pringault, E, 1997, Conversion by Peyer's Patch lymphocytes of human enterocytes into M cells that transport bacteria. Science 277:949–952.

Klein, J.R., 1996, Whence the intestinal intraepithelial lymphocyte? J. Exp. Med. 184:1203–1206.

Komano, H., Fujiura, Y., Kawaguchi, M, Matsumoto, S., Hashimoto, Y., Obano, S., Mombaerts, P., Tonegawa, S., Yamamoto, H., Itohara, S., Nanno, M., and Ishikawa, H., 1995, Homeostasis regulation of intestinal epithelia by intraepithelial γδ T-cells. Proc. Natl. Acad. Sci. USA 92:6147–6151.

Kraehenbuhl, J.-P. and Neutra, M.R., 1992, Molecular and cellular basis of immune protection at mucosal surfaces. Physiological Reviews 72:853–879.

Lefrançois, L. and Puddington, L., 1995, Extrathymic intestinal T-cell development: virtual reality? Immunol. Today 16:16–21.

Madara, J.L. and Stafford, J., 1989, Interferon-g directly affects barrier function of cultured intestinal epithelial monolayers. J. Clin. Invest. 83:724–727.

Mak, T.W. and Ferrick, D.A., 1998, The γδ T-cell bridge: linking innate and acquired immunity. Nature Medicine 4:764–765.

Mayer, L. and Shlien, R., 1987, Evidence for function of Ia molecules on gut epithelial cells in man. J. Exp. Med. 166:1471–1483.

Mayer, L. and Eisenhardt, D., 1990, Lack of induction of suppressor T cells by intestinal epithelial cells from patients with inflammatory bowel disease. J. Clin. Invest. 86:1255–1260.

Mostov, K.E., 1994, Transepithelial transport of immunoglobulins. Annu. Rev. Immunol. 12:63–84.

Nagura, H., Kubota, M., and Kimura, N., 1996, Neuroendocrine regulation of mucosal immune responses. In: Essentials of Mucosal Immunology, editors, Kagnoff, M.F. and Kiyono, H., Academic Press, San Diego, pp. 125–139.

O'Connell, J., O'Sullivan, G.C., Collins, J.K., and Shanahan, F., 1996, The Fas counter attack: Fas-mediated T cell killing by colon cancer cells expressing Fas ligand. J. Exp. Med. 184:1075–1082.

O'Connell, J., Bennett, M.W., O'Sullivan, G.C., Collins, J.K., and Shanahan, F., 1999, The Fas counterattack: cancer as a site of immune privilege. Immunol. Today 20:46–52.

Perdue, M.H. and McKay, D.M., 1994, Integrative immunophysiology in the intestinal mucosa. Am. J. Physiol. 267 (Gastrointest Liver Physiol. 30):G151–G165.

Phipps, R.P., Stein, S.H., and Roper, R.L., 1991, A new view of prostaglandin E regulation of the immune response. Immunol. Today 12:349–351.

Podolsky, D.K., 1993, Regulation of intestinal epithelial proliferation: a few answers, many questions. Am. J. Physiol. 264 (Gastrointest. Liver Physiol. 27):G179–G186.

Puddington, L., Olson, S., and Lefrançois, L., 1994, Interactions between stem cell factor and c-kit are required for intestinal immune system homeostasis. Immunity 1:733–739.

Reinecker, H.-C. and Podolsky, D.K., 1995, Human intestinal epithelial cells express functional cytokine receptors sharing the common γc chain of the interleukin-2 receptor. Proc. Natl. Acad. Sci. USA 92:8353–8357.

Reinecker, H.-C., MacDermott, R.P., Mirau, S., Dignass, A., and Podolsky, D.K., 1996, Intestinal epithelial cells both express and respond to interleukin 15. Gastroenterology 111:1706–1713.

Saito, H., Kanamori, Y., Takemori, T., Nariuchi, H., Kubota, E., Takahashi-Iwanaga, H., Iwanaga, T., and Ishikawa, H., 1998, Generation of intestinal T cells from progenitors residing in gut cryptopatches. Science 280:275–278.

Shanahan, F., 1994, The intestinal immune system. In: Physiology of the Gastrointestinal Tract, Editor, Johnson, L.R., Raven Press, New York, pp. 643–684.

Shanahan, F., 1994b, Gene-targeted immunologic knockouts: new models of inflammatory bowel disease. Gastroenterology 107:312–314.

Shanahan, F. and Anton, P., 1994, Role of peptides in the regulation of the mucosal immune and inflammatory response. In: Gut peptides: Biochemistry and Physiology, edited by Walsh, J.H. and Dockray, G.J., Raven Press, New York, pp. 851–867.

Shanahan, F., 1997, A gut reaction: lymphoepithelial communication in the intestine. Science 275:1897–1898.

Shanahan, F. and O'Sullivan, G.C., 1999, Glial cells, mucosal integrity, and inflammatory bowel disease. Gastroenterology (in press).

Shannon, V.R., Stenson, W.F., and Holtzman, M.J., 1993, Induction of epithelial arachidonate 12-lipoxygenase at active stites of inflammatory bowel disease. Am. J. Physiol. 264:G104–G111.

Singer, I.I., Kawka, D.W., Scott, S., Weidner, J.R., Mumford, R.A., Riehl, T.E., and Stenson, W.F., 1996, Expression of inducible nitric oxide synthase and nitrotyrosine in colonic epithelium in inflammatory bowel disease. Gastroenterology 111:871–885.

Stadnyk, A.W. and Waterhouse, C.M., 1997, Epithelial cytokines in intestinal inflammation and mucosal immunity. Curr. Opin. Gastroenterol 13:510–517.

Stenson, W.F. and Alpers, D.H., 1994, A parable on the dangers of overclassification: can an enterocyte assume immune functions? Curr. Opinion Gastroenterology 10:121–124.

Taylor, C.T., Dzus, A.L., and Colgan, S.P., 1998, Autocrine regulation of epithelial permeability by hypoxia: role of polarized release of tumor necrosis factor a. Gastroenterology 114:657–668.

Vidrich, A., Anton, P., and Shanahan, F., 1998, Immunoepithelial interactions: Cytokine modulation of colonic epithelial growth. In Vitro (in press Nov/Dec 1998).

Walker, P.R., Saas, P., and Dietrich, P.-Y., 1998, Tumor expression of Fas ligand (CD95L) and the consequences. Curr. Opin. Immunol. 10:564–572.

Wang, J., Whetsell, M., and Klein, J.R., 1997, Local hormone networks and intestinal T cell homeostasis. Science 275:1937–1939.

Watanabe, M., Ueno, Y., Yajima, T., Iwao, Y., Tsuchiya, M., Ishikawa, H., Aiso, S., Hibi, T., and Ishii, H., 1995, Interleukin 7 is produced by human intestinal epithelial cells and regulates the proliferation of intestinal mucosal lymphocytes. J. Clin. Invest. 95:2945–2953.

Williams, N., 1998, T cells on the mucosal frontline. Science 280:198–200.

2

BACTERIAL TRANSLOCATION FROM THE GASTROINTESTINAL TRACT

Rodney D. Berg

Department of Microbiology and Immunology
Louisiana State University Medical Center-Shreveport
Shreveport, Louisiana 71130

SUMMARY

Bacterial translocation is defined as the passage of viable bacteria from the gastrointestinal (GI) tract to extraintestinal sites, such as the mesenteric lymph node complex (MLN) , liver, spleen, kidney, and bloodstream. The three primary mechanisms promoting bacterial translocation in animal models are identified as: (a) disruption of the ecologic GI equilibrium to allow intestinal bacterial overgrowth, (b) increased permeability of the intestinal mucosal barrier, and (c) deficiencies in host immune defenses. These mechanisms can act in concert to promote synergistically the systemic spread of indigenous translocating bacteria to cause lethal sepsis. In animal models in which the intestinal barrier is not physically damaged, indigenous bacteria translocate by an intracellular route through the epithelial cells lining the intestines and then travel via the lymph to the MLN. In animal models exhibiting damage to the mucosal epithelium, indigenous bacteria translocate intercellularly between the epithelial cells to directly access the blood. Indigenous GI bacteria have been cultured directly from the MLN of various types of patients. Thus, evidence is accumulating that translocation of indigenous bacteria from the GI tract is an important early step in the pathogenesis of opportunistic infections originating from the GI tract.

1. INTRODUCTION

Bacterial translocation is defined as the passage of viable indigenous bacteria from the gastrointestinal (GI) tract to the mesenteric lymph node complex (MLN) and other extraintestinal sites, such as the spleen, liver, kidney, peritoneal cavity, and bloodstream (Berg and Garlington, 1979). Translocation is an appropriate term since it simply describes the relocation of bacteria from one site to another without implying the actual mechanisms. In the healthy adult host, various indigenous bacteria are continuously

Mechanisms in the Pathogenesis of Enteric Diseases 2, edited by Paul and Francis.
Kluwer Academic / Plenum Publishers, New York, 1999.

translocating across the intestinal mucosa at a very low rate (Berg, 1980b). These "spontaneously" translocating bacteria are normally killed by the innate host immune defenses during their transit through the intestinal lamina propria, in the draining lymph and *in situ* in reticuloendothelial organs, such as the MLN. Thus, only rarely are viable indigenous GI bacteria cultured from the MLN or other extraintestinal organs of normal adult mice or rats with an intact intestinal barrier and a competent immune system.

The major route of translocation of indigenous GI bacteria in hosts with an intact intestinal barrier is intracellularly through the intestinal epithelial cells (Berg, 1981a; Berg, 1983c; Berg, 1985). Intestinal epithelial cells can be thought of as "nonprofessional" phagocytes that readily take in any particle or bacterium that comes in close contact. Thus, translocating bacteria pass through the individual epithelial cells lining the GI tract and are transported via the lymphatics to the MLN. The translocating bacteria can then spread from the MLN to other extraintestinal sites, such as the liver, spleen, peritoneal cavity, and bloodstream. Indigenous GI bacteria readily translocate by this intracellular route in animal models exhibiting intestinal bacterial overgrowth (Berg, 1983c).

In models exhibiting increased intestinal permeability or actual mucosal damage, such as animals subjected to hemorrhagic or endotoxic shock, indigenous bacteria can translocate intercellularly between the intestinal epithelial cells or through ulcerations left by denuded epithelial cells (Berg, 1983c). Bacteria translocating by the intercellular route can bypass the lymph to reach the blood directly.

The various species of indigenous bacteria do not all translocate at the same rate from the GI tract. Gram-negative, facultatively anaerobic *Enterobacteriaceae*, such as *Escherichia coli, Klebsiella pneumoniae,* and *Proteus mirabilis*, translocate at a greater rate from the GI tract to the MLN than the other bacteria comprising the indigenous GI microflora (Steffen, Berg, and Deitch, 1988). These *Enterobacteriaceae* are the same bacterial types that most commonly cause septicemia in hospitalized patients, with *E. coli* being the most prominent (Donnenberg et al., 1994). Obligately anaerobic bacteria, such as *Bacteroides* and *Fusobacterium*, are the least efficient translocators. Interestingly, the indigenous obligate anaerobes are ineffective at translocating from the GI tract and yet they colonize at the highest population levels (e.g. 10^{10-11}/g cecum). Preliminary evidence suggests that sensitivity to oxygen may be one mechanism that inhibits obligate anaerobes from translocating from the GI tract at a greater rate (Berg and Itoh, 1986). The Gram-positive, oxygen-tolerant bacteria, such as *Staphylococcus epidermidis*, translocate at an intermediate rate between the *Enterobacteriaceae* and the obligate anaerobes.

We have identified three primary mechanisms that promote the translocation of indigenous bacteria from the GI tract: (a) intestinal overgrowth following disruption of the intestinal microecology, (b) increased intestinal permeability, and (c) host immunodeficiency (Berg, 1995; Berg, 1992a; Berg, 1992b; Berg, 1992c). In clinical situations, more than one mechanism often is operating to promote bacterial translocation from the GI tract.

2. PRIMARY MECHANISMS PROMOTING BACTERIAL TRANSLOCATION

2.1. Intestinal Bacterial Overgrowth

Intestinal bacterial overgrowth is the most effective of the three primary translocation promoting mechanisms in initiating bacterial translocation from the GI tract to the

MLN. That is, a greater percentage of MLN cultures are positive in animal models of intestinal bacterial overgrowth than in animal models exhibiting immunodeficiency or even physical damage to the intestinal mucosa (Berg, 1998). Immunodeficiency, however, is particularly effective in promoting the spread of translocating bacteria from the MLN to other organs because of decreased killing of the translocating bacteria.

Intestinal bacterial overgrowth is a common occurrence in patients receiving antibiotic therapy. Patients treated with oral antibiotics often exhibit the side effect of intestinal overgrowth by antibiotic-resistant indigenous bacteria or even colonization by antibiotic-resistant exogenous bacteria. To simulate this clinical condition in an animal model, mice were given for 4 days an oral antibiotic active against indigenous obligate anaerobes, i.e. penicillin, clindamycin or metronidazole. The antibiotic then was discontinued and the mice tested for bacterial translocation to the MLN at various time periods (Berg, 1981b). Within 2 days following the antibiotic, the numbers of indigenous obligate anaerobes in the cecum decreased 1000-fold whereas the numbers of indigenous *Enterobacteriaceae* increased 10,000-fold (10^4/g to 10^9/g cecum). Removal of the antagonistic obligate anaerobes by the antibiotic treatment allowed the indigenous *Enterobacteriaceae* to populate the GI tract at abnormally high levels, i.e. intestinal bacterial overgrowth. The *Enterobacteriaceae* translocated to the MLN concomitantly with their increase in population levels. *Enterobacteriaceae* cultured from the MLN in order of frequency were *Enterobacter cloacae, Enterobacter aerogenes, Klebsiella pneumoniae, E. coli, Proteus morganii*, and *P. mirabilis.*

The obligate anaerobe populations increased back to their normal high levels when the oral antibiotic was discontinued on day 4 and the indigenous *Enterobacteriaceae* were again antagonized to their normal levels of 10^4/g cecum. Surprisingly, the mice continued to exhibit *Enterobacteriaceae* translocation to their MLNs for the next 26 days. Thus, even though the oral antibiotic was given for only 4 days, intestinal bacterial overgrowth caused by the disruption of the normal GI microecology and the concomitant bacterial translocation continued for several days. These data in animal models suggest that patients receiving oral antibiotic therapy are at increased risk to bacterial translocation and the subsequent opportunistic infections originating from their GI tract for a period of time after their antibiotic therapy is discontinued.

There are other clinical situations, in addition to oral antibiotic therapy, that lead to intestinal bacterial overgrowth and promote bacterial translocation, such as parenteral alimentation, enteral alimentation, protein malnutrition, and endotoxic shock (Berg, 1985). The various animal models in which we have demonstrated intestinal bacterial overgrowth promoting bacterial translocation from the GI tract are listed in Table 1.

There is a direct "cause and effect" relationship between bacterial population levels in the GI tract and bacterial translocation from the GI tract to the MLN. When germfree mice are monoassociated with *E. coli*, the cecal populations of *E. coli* reach approximately 10^{10}/g and translocating *E. coli* are cultured from 100% of the MLNs tested. When these *E. coli*-monoassociated gnotobiotes are then inoculated with the whole cecal contents from conventional mice, *E. coli* cecal populations decrease 1000-fold within 48 hours due to antagonism by the obligate anaerobes and *E. coli* no longer can be cultured from the MLN (Berg and Owens, 1979). Since inoculation of these mice with heat-treated, formalin-treated, or filter-sterilized cecal contents has no effect, viable obligate anaerobes are required in the inoculum to antagonize the indigenous *E. coli* populations (Berg, 1980a).

This direct relationship between cecal bacterial population levels and bacterial translocation to the MLN is even more dramatically demonstrated by comparing the

Table 1. Animal models in which intestinal bacterial overgrowth promotes bacterial translocation

- Oral antibiotics
- Gnotobiotic mice
- Endotoxic shock
- Zymosan shock
- Starvation
- Protein malnutrition
- Parenteral (IV) alimentation
- Enteral (oral) alimentation
- Bowel obstruction
- Bile duct ligation
- Streptozotocin-induced diabetes

cecal populations of three different species of *Enterobacteriaceae* in triassociated gnotobiotic mice with the translocation rate of these three species to the MLN (Steffen and Berg, 1983). Germfree mice were triassociated with indigenous *E. coli*, *K. pneumoniae*, and *P. mirabilis* for 1, 3, 5, and 12 weeks. The proportion of each of the three bacterial species in the total cecal populations was compared to the proportion of each bacterial species translocating to the MLN. The mean percentages for each bacterial species in the cecum and the MLN for all four time points are presented in Fig. 1. *E. coli* comprised of 25% of the bacteria in the cecum of the triassociated gnotobiotes and 32% of the bacteria translocating to the MLN. Similarly, *K. pneumoniae* comprised 66% of the cecal bacteria compared with 54% bacteria isolated from the MLN and *P. mirabilis* comprised 10% of the cecal bacteria and 14% of the MLN bacteria. Thus, the proportion of each of the three bacterial species in the cecum is statistically the same as the proportion of each of the three bacterial species translocating to the MLN demonstrating a direct relationship between cecal population levels and translocation to the MLN.

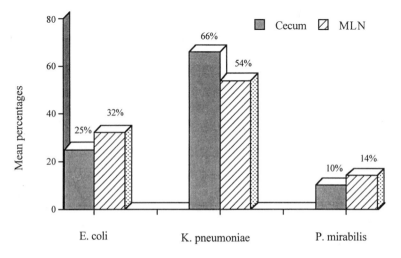

Figure 1. Proportion of bacteria in cecum directly relates to proportion of bacteria translocating to MLN.

The indigenous *Enterbacteriaceae* establish a "steady-state" pattern of translocation from the GI tract to the MLN. That is, the *Enterbacteriaceae* are continuously
translocating from the GI tract to the MLN. This is easily demonstrated in the *E. coli*
bacterial overgrowth model. The numbers of translocating *E. coli* cultured from the
MLN of *E. coli*-monoassociated gnotobiotic mice is the same after either 2 days or 100
days of monoassociation (Berg and Owens, 1979). *E. coli* maintains GI population
levels of 10^{9-10}/g intestinal contents throughout the entire 100 days. If these *E. coli*-
monoassociated gnotobiotes are treated with oral penicillin, the MLN cultures become
negative for translocating *E. coli* within 24 hours. Thus, translocating *E. coli* do not
establish a permanent "infection" in the MLN, but rather the *E. coli* in the GI tract
continuously "seed" the MLN to establish the "steady-state" pattern. It is interesting
that the host immune defenses do not over time become better able to eliminate the
translocating *E. coli*, even after 100 days of monoassociation. It also is interesting that
the *E. coli* do not overcome the host immune defenses and establish an infection in the
MLN. It must be noted that the indigenous *E. coli* strain tested in these experiments
is relatively nonpathogenic and the results would likely be different utilizing more
pathogenic bacterial strains.

The MLN complex collects lymph draining from various regions of the GI tract.
The small portion of the MLN complex that is seen separated from the main body of
the MLN drains lymph from the distal ileum, cecum, and ascending colon; the regions
of the GI tract containing the greatest populations of indigenous bacteria. In contrast,
the main body of the MLN complex drains lymph from the jejunum and proximal ileum
which harbor fewer numbers of indigenous bacteria. Interestingly, the portion of the
MLN complex draining lymph from GI regions containing the highest populations of
bacteria (i.e. the small MLN portion) also contains greater numbers of translocating
bacteria than the larger main MLN body (Gautreaux, Deitch, and Berg, 1994a). These
observations again illustrate that the higher the bacterial populations in the GI tract,
the greater the translocation from the GI tract to the MLN.

The intestinal bacterial overgrowth model has been used extensively in the study
of bacterial translocation and has several advantages over other translocation
models. It has already been mentioned that the indigenous GI bacteria translocate
initially to the MLN more efficiently in the intestinal overgrowth model than in the
other models of translocation. Intestinal bacterial overgrowth usually promotes
translocation to 100% of the MLNs tested. In healthy hosts, these translocating
bacteria are usually confined to the MLN and do not spread to other organs or sites.
Another advantage of the intestinal overgrowth model is that bacterial challenge is
by a "natural" oral route rather than by the "artificial" intravenous or intraperitoneal
injection often used in pathogenesis experiments. Bacterial translocation to the MLN
and other organs also is an extremely sensitive indicator of bacterial infection.
Translocation to the MLN thus demonstrates bacterial infection when other measure-
ments, such as blood cultures and clinical infection symptoms, are negative. Theoretically, a single translocating bacterium will produce a positive MLN culture. In fact,
MLN culturing has proved much more sensitive for detecting translocating bacteria
translocating than employing fluorescein-labeled or even radiolabeled challenge bacteria (Alexander, et al., 1990). Most importantly, promotion of bacterial translocation
in the intestinal overgrowth model is due directly to bacterial overgrowth and not con-
founded by variables, such as increased intestinal permeability or physical injury to the
intestinal epithelium; variables present in the more complex models of bacterial
translocation.

2.2. Increased Intestinal Permeability

In animal models exhibiting intestinal bacterial overgrowth, indigenous bacteria translocate across the intact undamaged intestinal mucosa to reach extraintestinal sites. In this case, the bacteria are engulfed by the intestinal epithelial cells and transported intracellularly across the intestinal barrier. Obviously, intestinal bacteria also can cross the epithelial barrier if there is physical damage to the intestinal mucosa or increased intestinal permeability (Table 2).

For example, ricinoleic acid (12-hydroxy-9-octadecenoic acid), the pharmacologically active constituent of castor oil, given once IG to mice severely damages the intestinal mucosa and readily promotes bacterial translocation (Morehouse et al., 1986). Massive exfoliation of columnar epithelial cells in the proximal small intestine occurs within 2 hours after ricinoleic acid administration and both facultative and obligate anaerobic bacteria translocate to the MLN, spleen, and liver. The incidence of bacterial translocation is greatest at 4 days following ricinoleic acid administration and ceases by 7 days when the mucosal epithelial barrier has regenerated.

Shock with ischemia/reperfusion injury to the intestinal mucosa also readily promotes bacterial translocation from the GI tract. For example, mice injected once IP with *E. coli* 026:B6 endotoxin exhibit ischemia/reperfusion injury and concomitant translocation of indigenous bacteria to their MLNs within 24 hr (Deitch and Berg, 1987). To determine which components of the endotoxin structure are involved in promoting bacterial translocation, mice were injected with endotoxin from six R-mutant strains of *Salmonella* all differing in their endotoxin composition (i.e. Ra, Rb, Rc, Rd, Re, or lipid A) (Deitch et al., 1989b). Injection of intact *Salmonella* whole endotoxin (wild type), the Ra endotoxin fragment, or the Rb endotoxin fragment increased bacterial translocation to the MLN. Injection of the smaller endotoxin fragments, Rc, Rd, Re, or lipid A alone did not promote bacterial translocation. Apparently, endotoxin must contain the terminal three sugars of the core polysaccharide in order to induce mucosal damage and promote bacterial translocation.

Endotoxin-challenged mice exhibit intestinal edema and separation of the epithelium from the lamina propria. Both endotoxin and lipid A produce their toxic manifestations by stimulating host cells, especially macrophages, to release mediator substances that then act as second messengers to disrupt various homeostatic systems. For example, oxygen-free radicals generated by xanthine oxidase are released during ischemia/reperfusion (Parks et al., 1982). Injection of the translocation-promoting Ra endotoxin fragment increased ileal xanthine oxidase and xanthine dehydrogenase activities, whereas injection of the nonpromoting Rc and Re endotoxin fragments did not increase these enzymatic activities. Consequently, intestinal damage and subse-

Table 2. Animal models in which increased intestinal permeability or mucosal damage promotes bacterial translocation

- Ricinoleic acid IG (castor oil)
- Gnotobiotic mice
- Endotoxic shock
- Zymosan (yeast polysaccharide) shock
- Thermal injury
- Hemorrhagic shock

quent bacterial translocation are reduced when the animals are pretreated with allopurinol, a xanthine oxidase inhibitor, dimethylsulfoxide, a hydroxyl scavenger, or deferoxamine, an iron chelator (Deitch et al., 1989a; Deitch et al., 1989b; Deitch et al., 1988). Intestinal mucosal damage and bacterial translocation also are inhibited in animals fed a tungsten-supplemented, molybdenum-free diet to deplete intestinal xanthine oxidase for 2 weeks prior to endotoxin challenge (Deitch et al., 1988). These studies demonstrate that xanthine-generated hydroxyl radicals are responsible, in part, for the intestinal mucosal damage and bacterial translocation occurring during endotoxic shock.

Only very small amounts of endotoxin are normally absorbed from the GI tract even though the intestines contain large populations of indigenous gram-negative bacteria and endotoxin is continuously released during their cell growth, and particularly during their death and lysis. The small amount of endotoxin that is normally absorbed is easily detoxified by liver Kuppfer cells (Nolan, 1981). However, in certain clinical situations, such as bacterial infection and hemorrhagic shock, intestinal permeability is increased and there is concomitant translocation of bacteria and bacterial endotoxin from the GI tract to the lymph and portal and systemic circulations. In these severely ill patients, bacteria and endotoxin readily cross the mucosal barrier to gain access to extraintestinal tissues and the bloodstream. The translocated endotoxin activates plasma protein cascades, resident macrophages, and circulating neutrophils to release monokines and proteins that, in turn, further increase gut mucosal permeability. Thus, a cycle is initiated with increased translocation of both bacteria and endotoxin and increased damage to the intestinal barrier.

Similar to endotoxic shock, hemorrhagic shock and the shock of thermal injury also induce intestinal mucosal damage and promote bacterial translocation from the GI tract (Baker et al., 1987; Baker et al., 1988; Maejima, Deitch, and Berg, 1984a; Maejima, Deitch, and Berg, 1984b). For example, rats submitted to hemorrhagic shock for 90 minutes exhibit ileal mucosa necrosis and increased bacterial translocation to their MLNs. The mucosal damage occurring in hemorrhagic shock and thermal injury also is due to oxidants generated by xanthine oxidase (Deitch et al., 1989a; Deitch et al., 1988). Oxygen-free radicals generated during the period of intestinal reperfusion are particularly important. Allopurinol administered orally prior to hemorrhagic shock reduces the mucosal damage and decreases bacterial translocation (Deitch et al., 1989a; Deitch et al., 1988). Rats fed the tungsten-supplemented, molybdenum-free diet to inactivate xanthine oxidase prior to hemorrhagic shock also exhibit reduced mucosal damage and decreased bacterial translocation as compared with control rats fed a regular diet (Deitch et al., 1989a; Deitch et al., 1988).

A relationship among endotoxemia, intestinal ischemia, and shock was first proposed by Ravin and Fine (Ravin and Fine, 1962). More recently, it is hypothesized that failure of the intestinal barrier in conjunction with hepatic dysfunction promotes or potentiates multiple organ failure syndrome (Carrico et al., 1986). Thus, bacterial translocation from the GI tract is possibly an early step in the multiple organ failure pathogenesis. Multiple organ failure is a common final pathway leading to death in a variety of hospitalized patients.

2.3. Host Immunodeficiency

The practical definition of bacterial translocation includes not only the physical passage of bacteria across the intestinal epithelial barrier but also the survivability of translocating bacteria in transit through the lamina propria and in situ in reticuloendothelial organs, such as the MLN. For example, if translocating bacteria are killed in route from the GI tract to extraintestinal sites or in situ in the MLN by resident macrophages, cultures of the MLN will be negative and by definition bacterial translocation will not have taken place even though indigenous bacteria physically crossed the intestinal epithelium and "migrated" to the MLN. Thus, the host immune defenses are integral components in the pathogenesis of bacterial translocation from the GI tract.

Mice injected once IP with one of the immunosuppressive agents, cyclophosphamide, prednisone, methotrexate, 5-fluorouracil, or cytosine arabinoside, exhibit translocation of various indigenous GI bacteria to their MLN, spleen, and liver (Berg, 1983a). Host immune deficiency also is responsible, in part, for the promotion of bacterial translocation in animal models of diabetes (Berg, 1985), leukemia (Penn, Maca, and Berg, 1986), endotoxemia (Deitch and Berg, 1987), thermal injury (Maejima, Deitch, and Berg, 1984b), and hemorrhagic shock (Baker et al., 1987) (Table 3). These complex animal models demonstrate the importance of host immune defenses in preventing bacterial translocation but do not delineate the relative roles of the major immune compartments or identify the immune mechanisms actually responsible for killing the translocating microorganisms.

2.3.1. Serum and Secretory Immunity. It is likely that anti-bacterial serum antibodies act as opsonins to enhance phagocytosis and killing of translocating bacteria by polymorphonuclear leukocytes and macrophages. *E. coli* translocation to the liver and spleen is decreased in *E. coli*-monoassociated SPF mice vaccinated IP with heat-killed *E. coli* to induce anti-*E. coli* IgG and IgM serum antibodies (Gautreaux, Deitch, and Berg, 1990). However, *E. coli* translocation to the MLN is not decreased in these mice vaccinated with *E. coli*. Serum immunity therefore does not appear to decrease the initial translocation of *E. coli* from the GI tract across the intestinal epithelium to the MLN, but is effective in reducing the systemic spread of translocating *E. coli* from the MLN to the other organs and sites. Serum immunity, however, has not been studied sufficiently to draw any firm conclusions concerning its exact role in the host defense against bacterial translocation.

It seems likely that specific anti-bacterial secretory IgA on intestinal mucosal surfaces is be a major factor in the defense against bacterial translocation. Indigenous bacteria must come in close contact with intestinal epithelial cells prior to their translo-

Table 3. Animal models in which host immunodeficiency promotes bacterial translocation

- Injection of immunosuppressive agents
- Genetically athymic (*nu/nu*) mice
- Beige/nude (*bg/bg;nu/nu*) mice
- Thymectomized (*nu/+*) mice
- T cell-depleted (anti-CD4/anti-CD8) mice
- Lymphoma
- Leukemia
- Streptozotocin-induced diabetes
- Thermal injury
- Endotoxic shock
- Hemorrhagic shock

cation across the intestinal mucosa. Secretory IgA has been shown to inhibit the association of *Vibrio cholerae* and *Salmonella typhimurium* with the intestinal epithelium (Michetti et al., 1992; Winner et al., 1991). In fact, "spontaneous" bacterial translocation from the GI tract to the MLN occurring in athymic nude mice may be due in part to lack of T cell-dependent IgA in the intestinal secretions (Owens and Berg, 1980). Again, this area has been little studied and there is no definitive information to date concerning the specific role of secretory IgA in the defense against bacterial translocation from the GI tract.

2.3.2. T Cell-Mediated Immunity. Thymectomy of neonatal mice promotes the translocation of indigenous bacteria from the GI tract to 46% of MLN, spleen, liver, and kidneys compared with only 5% positive organs in control sham-thymectomized mice (Owens and Berg, 1982). Athymic (*nu/nu*) mice exhibit "spontaneous" translocation of aerobic, facultative, and obligately anaerobic bacteria to 50% of their MLN, spleen, liver, and kidneys compared with 5% positive organs in control euthymic (*nu/+*) mice (Owens and Berg, 1980). Neonatal thymuses grafted from heterozygous donor (*nu/+*) mice to homozygous (*nu/nu*) recipients decreases bacterial translocation in the recipients from 58% to 8% of these organs. These experiments dramatically demonstrate that T cell-mediated immunity contributes to the host defense against bacterial translocation, and is especially effective in preventing the spread of translocating bacteria from the MLN to other extraintestinal sites, such as the spleen, liver, and kidney.

To further delineate the role of T cells in host defense against bacterial translocation, mice were depleted of CD4$^+$ and/or CD8$^+$ T cells via injections of specific anti-T cell monoclonal antibodies and tested for increased bacterial translocation (Gautreaux, Deitch, and Berg, 1993). Mice were depleted of CD4$^+$ T cells with two IP injections of monoclonal antibody GK1.5 (rat anti-mouse CD4) and/or depleted of CD8$^+$ T cells with two IP injections of monoclonal antibody 2.43 (rat anti-mouse CD8). Flow cytofluorometric analyses demonstrated 100% depletion of CD4$^+$ and CD8$^+$ T cells in the spleen, MLN, intestinal lamina propria, and intestinal epithelium. The T cell-depleted mice then were antibiotic-decontaminated with oral penicillin plus streptomycin and monoassociated with streptomycin-resistant *E. coli* C25. Neither antibiotic-decontamination or *E. coli* monoassociation changed the T cell phenotypic profiles in the spleen, MLN, intestinal lamina propria, or intestinal epithelium. *E. coli* translocation from the GI tract to the MLN was increased in these mice depleted of either CD4$^+$ T cells, CD8$^+$ T cells, or both CD4$^+$ and CD8$^+$ T cells. Depletion of CD4$^+$ and/or CD8$^+$ T cells also increased translocation to the MLN of indigenous GI bacteria in mice not antibiotic-decontaminated but harboring their full complement of indigenous GI bacteria. These results are in agreement with our previous studies with athymic *nu/nu* mice, thymus-grafted *nu/nu* mice, and thymectomized (*nu/+*) mice demonstrating the importance of T cell-mediated immunity in the host defense against bacterial translocation.

To further confirm the role of T cell-mediated immunity in the defense against bacterial translocation, CD4$^+$ and/or CD8$^+$ T cells harvested from donor mice were adoptively transferred to mice that had been depleted of T cells by thymectomy plus two IP injections of anti- CD4$^+$ and CD8$^+$ T cell monoclonal antibodies as described above (Gautreaux, Deitch, and Berg, 1994b). The thymectomized mice depleted of CD4$^+$ and/or CD8$^+$ T cells were antibiotic-decontaminated and monoassociated with *E. coli* as before. *E. coli* translocation to the MLN was increased in these T cell-depleted mice as in the earlier experiments and the adoptive transfer of CD4$^+$ and/or CD8$^+$ T cells from the MLN or spleens of donor mice reduced the *E. coli* translocation. The adoptive T cells migrated to the MLN and intestinal lamina propria of the recipients as demonstrated by the detection of Thy-1.1$^+$ donor T cells in the Thy-1.2$^+$ recipients.

Our observation that either CD4$^+$ or CD8$^+$ adoptively-transferred T cells reduces *E. coli* translocation suggests an effector function common to both subsets of T cells. Direct cytotoxicity by T cells as a defense against bacterial translocation is unlikely because both CD4$^+$ and CD8$^+$ T cells kill only MHC-restricted targets. It is possible, however, that viable translocating bacteria are contained within MHC I and II-expressing macrophages. In this case, both CD4$^+$ and CD8$^+$ T cell subsets could be functional. CD4$^+$ and CD8$^+$ T cells also secrete gamma interferon and granulocyte-/macrophage colony-stimulating factor, both of which activate phagocytic cells. Phagocytic cells, such as macrophages, are likely the ultimate immune effector cells in the defense against bacterial translocation. Quantitation of the types of cytokines produced by the adoptive CD4$^+$ or CD8$^+$ T cells in situ in the MLN, intestinal lamina propria, and intestinal epithelium of recipient mice will provide additional insights into the T cell-mediated mechanisms.

2.3.3. Macrophages. Translocating bacteria are always cultured from the MLN prior to their appearance in organs, such as the liver or spleen, in the various animal models examined to date (Berg, 1981a; Berg, 1983c; Berg, 1992c). Thus, resident macrophages are strategically located in the MLN; the route whereby indigenous bacteria usually translocate from the GI tract. Nonspecific activation of macrophages and polymorphonuclear leukocytes to more efficiently engulf and kill a variety of bacterial types would be a particularly effective defense measure since it cannot be predicted with certainty which of the many different bacterial species in the GI tract will translocate under various conditions. Three immunomodulators known to nonspecifically activate macrophages, namely yeast glucan, muramyl dipeptide, and formalin-killed *Propionibacterium acnes* (formerly classified as *Corynebacterium parvum*), were tested for their abilities to decrease bacterial translocation to the MLN (Fuller and Berg, 1985). Mice were antibiotic-decontaminated, monoassociated with indigenous *E. coli*, *P. mirabilis*, or *E. cloacae*, injected once IP with either of the immunomodulators, and tested 1 week later for bacterial translocation to the MLN. All three immunomodulators induced splenomegaly, a lymphoreticular response commonly reported to indicate macrophage activation. *P. acnes* but not glucan or muramyl dipeptide vaccination decreased bacterial translocation to the MLN. Plastic-adherent spleen or MLN cells (predominantly macrophages) from *P. acnes*-vaccinated mice adoptively- transferred to nonvaccinated recipients also inhibited bacterial translocation, whereas nonadherent control cells (predominantly lymphocytes) did not. (Gautreaux, Deitch, and Berg, 1990). These results suggest that macrophages are important effector cells in the host immune defense against bacterial translocation.

P. acnes vaccination readily reduces *E. coli* translocation to the MLN of antibiotic-decontaminated conventional mice monoassociated with *E. coli* (Fuller and Berg, 1985). Surprisingly, however, *P. acnes* vaccination does not reduce *E. coli* translocation to the MLN of gnotobiotic (ex-germfree) mice monoassociated with *E. coli*. The *E. coli*-monoassociated gnotobiotic mice were immunologically stimulated by *P. acnes* vaccination since they exhibited even greater splenomegaly than the *P. acnes*-vaccinated, antibiotic-decontaminated conventional mice. *E. coli* also populated the GI tracts of both *E. coli*-monoassociated gnotobiotic and *E. coli*-monoassociated conventional mice to the same high levels (e.g. 10^9/g cecum). Apparently the mouse immune system must be "primed" by antigens of the indigenous GI microflora before a second stimulation by *P. acnes* vaccination activates macrophages sufficiently to kill the translocating bacteria.

To test this hypothesis, adult germfree mice were colonized with the whole cecal microflora from conventional mice for 8 weeks to "prime" their immune system. Thus, the germfree mice received all 400–500 species of bacteria indigenous to the mouse GI tract. After 8 weeks, the associated gnotobiotes were decontaminated with oral antibiotics to remove the indigenous microflora, monoassociated with *E. coli*, and vaccinated with killed *P. acnes* similar to the experiments described above for conventional mice. Surprisingly, *P. acnes* vaccination still did not reduce *E. coli* translocation to the MLN in these adult gnotobiotes exposed to the entire indigenous GI microflora for 8 weeks (Berg and Itoh, 1986). Further experimentation revealed that germfree mice must be exposed to the whole indigenous GI microflora within 1 week after birth in order for *P. acnes* vaccination at 8 weeks of age to inhibit *E. coli* translocation to the MLN (Berg and Itoh, 1986). These experiments dramatically demonstrate the profound influence of the indigenous GI microflora on the immunologic development of the host (Berg, 1996; Berg, 1983b).

It has been suggested that in certain situations activated macrophages and/or polymorphonuclear leukocytes actually promote rather than inhibit bacterial translocation by engulfing and transporting translocating bacteria from the GI tract to extraintestinal sites (Wells, Maddus, and Simmons, 1987). For example, polymorphonuclear leukocytes appear to engulf indigenous bacteria in the GI tract and transport them to inflammatory abdominal abscesses (Wells, Maddus, and Simmons, 1987). On the other hand, bacterial translocation from the GI tract to the MLN and liver is neither increased nor decreased in *op/op* mice genetically deficient in CSF-1-dependent macrophage populations (Feltis et al., 1994). Only a few *op/op* mice were tested, however, so it is difficult to draw firm conclusions. Nonetheless, it is evident that more research is required to identify clinical situations in which macrophage activation might actually promote rather than prevent bacterial translocation from the GI tract.

Mucosal immunity (secretory IgA), cell-mediated immunity (macrophages and T cells), and serum immunity (IgG and IgM) are all likely involved in the host immune defense against bacterial translocation. However, the relative contributions of each of these immune compartments in the host defense against bacterial translocation or the immunologic mechanisms involved have not been elucidated. This information is required if we are to formulate immunologic strategies to prevent these opportunistic infections originating from the GI tract.

3. COMBINATION OF TRANSLOCATION PROMOTION MECHANISMS

In complex animal models of translocation, such as endotoxic shock, hemorrhagic shock, thermal injury, and streptozotocin-induced diabetes, more than one mechanism is operating to promote bacterial translocation (Berg, 1995; Berg, 1983c; Berg, 1992b). In fact, in some models the major promotion mechanisms can act synergistically to induce bacterial translocation and increase the systemic spread of translocating bacteria. This is easily demonstrated in mice given the combination of an oral antibiotic plus an immunosuppressive agent injected IP (Berg, Wommack, and Deitch, 1988) (Table 4). Oral

Table 4. Synergistic promotion of bacterial translocation to
the mesenteric lymph nodes (MLN) by intestinal bacterial
overgrowth plus immunosuppression

Oral antibiotic	Immunosuppressive agent	MLN cultures positive (%)	Peritoneal cavity cultures positive (%)
Penicillin	None	100	0
None	Cyclophosphamide	17	0
None	Prednisolone	46	0
Penicillin	Cyclophosphamide	39	80
Penicillin	Prednisolone	95	75

Penicillin given orally ad libitum for 7 days; cyclophosphamide given 4X IP at
100 mg/kg over 7 days; prednisolone given 4X IP at 100 mg/kg over 7 days. The
bacteria isolated from the MLN and peritoneal cavity cultures were identified as
Enterobacteriaceae.

penicillin disrupts the GI ecology and allows intestinal bacterial overgrowth by the
indigenous *Enterobacteriaceae* resistant to penicillin. Thus, oral penicillin alone promotes the translocation of *Enterobacteriaceae* to 100% of the MLN cultured. However,
the *Enterobacteriaceae* do not spread beyond the MLN since the peritoneal cavity cultures remain sterile. An immunosuppressive agent (e.g. cyclophosphamide or prednisolone) given alone also promotes *Enterobacteriaceae* translocation to the MLN but
not nearly as effectively as does oral penicillin. Again, the peritoneal cavity cultures
remain sterile. The combination of oral penicillin plus either cyclophosphamide IP or
prednisolone IP, however, synergistically promotes *Enterobacteriacea* translocation and
the *Enterobacteriaceae* spread systemically; 80% of the peritoneal cultures become positive with penicillin plus cyclophosphamide and 75% become positive with penicillin plus
prednisolone.

Treatment with the combination of an oral antibiotic plus an immunosuppressive
agent for longer than 7 days even produces lethal sepsis by the translocating bacteria.
For example, the combination of oral clindamycin plus IP prednisolone promotes the
systemic spread of translocating bacteria from the MLN to the peritoneal cavity and
bloodstream. In fact, mice given this combination of clindamycin plus prednisolone all
die of septicemia within 2 weeks. The indigenous bacteria causing lethal sepsis in these
mice were identified as *E. coli, K. pneumoniae, E. aerogenes*, and *P. mirabilis*. The antibi-
otic/immunosuppressive agent combination therefore synergistically promotes bacterial translocation from the GI tract and, particularly, allows the translocating bacteria
to spread systemically to cause lethal infection.

The synergistic promotion of bacterial translocation by multiple mechanisms
also has been demonstrated in other animal models. For example, protein malnutrition
alone produces histologic atrophy of the mucosa of the small bowel and cecum but
the mucosal barrier remains intact and translocation is not increased (Deitch,
Winterton, and Berg, 1987). The combination of protein malnutrition plus one IP
injection of endotoxin, however, produces intestinal ulcerations with concomitant bacterial translocation from the GI tract (Ma et al., 1989). Similarly, a 30% total body
surface area burn plus one IP injection with endotoxin causes intestinal mucosal
damage and synergistically promotes bacterial translocation from the GI tract (Deitch
and Berg, 1987).

4. OTHER FACTORS INFLUENCING BACTERIAL TRANSLOCATION

It seems possible that various strains of mice might exhibit different patterns of bacterial translocation since host immune competence is a major determining factor in the pathogenesis of bacterial translocation. It is well-known that different strains of mice vary in their immune response to various infectious agents and these immune reactions are genetically determined. Consequently, translocation of indigenous bacteria from the GI tract to the MLN was tested in fourteen inbred mouse strains (Maejima, Shimoda, and Berg, 1984). Only two of these fourteen strains exhibited "spontaneous" translocation of indigenous GI bacteria. The numbers of translocating bacteria were so low, however, that spontaneous translocation was no different statistically from the strains not exhibiting translocation.

To further examine a possible role for host genetics in the promotion of bacterial translocation, ten inbred mouse strains were antibiotic-decontaminated with oral penicillin plus streptomycin, monoassociated with streptomycin-resistant *E. coli* C25, and tested 2 days later for *E. coli* C25 translocation to the MLN (Maejima, Shimoda, and Berg, 1984). In this model, *E. coli* C25 intestinal overgrowth promotes *E. coli* C25 translocation to the MLN. Any influence of host genetics on *E. coli* C25 translocation will be recognized by an increase in the numbers of *E. coli* C25 translocating to the MLN. As expected, *E. coli* C25 maintained similar high cecal populations in all ten mouse strains and translocated to 100% of the MLNs cultured. However, there were no significant differences among mouse strains as to the either the incidence of *E. coli* C25 translocation to the MLN or the numbers of translocating *E. coli* C25 per MLN, suggesting that host genetics do not appreciably influence the rate of *E. coli* translocation from the GI tract.

Virulence determinants have been identified and characterized for nonindigenous pathogenic bacteria, such as *Shigella* and *Salmonella*, that promote their passage from the GI lumen into host tissues. It is not known whether indigenous GI bacteria possess virulence determinants than promote their translocation from the GI tract. Comparisons of *E. coli* isolates possessing virulence determinants have been made between indigenous *E. coli* strains isolated from the feces of healthy adults with *E. coli* strains causing extraintestinal infection in patients (Table 5). Even though a higher percentage of *E. coli* isolates from extraintestinal sites of patients compared with isolates from feces of healthy subjects exhibit the putative virulence determinants listed in Table 5, these differences are not statistically significant. Thus, there is no clear association of one or even a set of *E. coli* virulence determinants with any extraintestinal infection caused by *E. coli* originating from the GI tract, even for *E. coli* septicemia.

To examine this question further, the translocation of known pathogenic *E. coli* strains, supposedly possessing potent virulence determinants, was compared to the translocation of various *E. coli* strains indigenous to the mouse GI tract (Berg, Berg, and Block, 1996) (Table 6). Conventional mice were antibiotic-decontaminated and monoassociated for 4 days with *E. coli* strains indigenous to mice, *E. coli* strains pathogenic to mice, or *E. coli* strains pathogenic to humans. All the *E. coli* strains readily colonized the antibiotic-decontaminated mice at similar high population levels. As expected, the *E. coli* strains indigenous to mice (*E. coli* C25, *E. coli* M14, *E. coli* M21) translocated at only low numbers to the MLN. *E. coli* 1925–86 isolated from a domestic cat at autopsy and *E. coli* 1109–92 isolated from a rat at autopsy also translocated

Table 5. Percentages of *E. coli* isolates exhibiting particular virulence determinants from hospitalized patients compared with healthy subjects

Putative virulence determinant	*E. coli* isolates from extraintestinal sites of patients (%)	*E. coli* isolates from feces of healthy subjects (%)	References
Hemolysin	35–59	5–18	Smith, 1963 Cooke, 1968 Minshew *et al.*, 1978 Johnson, 1991 Siitonen, 1992
Aerobactin	69	34	Carbonetti *et al.*, 1986
Colicin V	12–18	0	Minshew *et al.*, 1978 Smith, 1963
P fimbriae	59	11–15	Minshew *et al.*, 1978 Siitonen, 1992
Adhesin operon (*pap, sfa, afa, hly*)	69 (exhibit at least one operon)	ND	Maslow *et al.*, 1993

ND denotes not done.

at only low numbers to the MLN. Surprisingly, *E. coli* O18, a common cause of human neonatal meningitis/septicemia, translocated to the MLN at similar low numbers. Even more surprisingly, *E. coli* 2348/69, a prototype human enteropathogenic strain (EPEC) and *E. coli* EI-37, a prototype human enteroinvasive strain (EIEC) translocated to the MLN at levels 10-fold lower than that of any of the indigenous *E. coli* strains tested. Thus, enteropathogenic and enteroinvasive *E. coli* strains known to possess multiple virulence determinants do not translocate from the GI tract to the MLN of mice at a

Table 6. Comparison of translocation to MLN of various indigenous and nonindigenous *E. coli* strains at 4 days following challenge

Challenge *E. coli* strain	Translocation to MLN at 4 days		Cecal population Mean CFU per gram cecum
	Mean CFU per whole MLN (positive/total)	Mean CFU per gram MLN	
Indigenous strains			
E. coli C25	30	297	4.00×10^{10}
E. coli M14	12	237	1.27×10^{10}
E. coli M21	27	502	1.89×10^{10}
Nonindigenous pathogenic strains			
E. coli 1925–86	60	551	1.41×10^{10}
E. coli 1109–92	73	926	3.99×10^{10}
E. coli O18	39	377	4.38×10^{10}
E. coli EI-37	1.6	14.6	9.39×10^{9}
E. coli 2348/69	1.5	16.9	1.28×10^{10}

SPF mice antibiotic-decontaminated with penicillin plus streptomycin and then monoassociated with each of the *E. coli* strains; tested for *E. coli* translocation to MLN at 4 days.
E. coli C25 obtained from Dr. Rolf Freter, University of Michigan; *E. coli* M14 and M21 obtained from Dr. Carol Wells, University of Minnesota; *E. coli* 1925–86 and 1109–92 obtained from Dr. Earl Steffen, University of Missouri; *E. coli* O18 obtained from ATCC; *E. coli* EI-37 and 2348/69 obtained from Dr. James Kaper, University of Maryland.

rate higher than the relatively nonpathogenic *E. coli* strains indigenous to the mouse GI tract.

Since specific adhesins or other bacterial virulence determinants do not appear to be essential in the translocation of indigenous or even pathogenic strains of *E. coli*, we also tested whether nonviable plastic particles (i.e. latex beads) completely lacking virulence factors also might translocate from the GI tract (Berg et al., 1996). Normal and antibiotic-decontaminated mice were inoculated IG three times per day with 2.8 × 10^7 fluorescein-labeled latex beads 1.0μ or 5.0μ in size. The latex particles were detected microscopically in the MLN as early as 24 hrs following IG inoculation and peak latex translocation occurred at 4 days. Latex particles (1μ in size) translocated to the MLN at a higher rate in this model than either indigenous or pathogenic *E. coli* strains (1μ in size). This was the case even though the latex particle challenge (10^7) is at least 1000-fold less than the population levels reached by *E. coli* in the monoassoci- ated mice (10^{10}/g cecum). Furthermore, the concentration of latex particles in the GI lumen begins to decrease immediately following IG inoculation of the latex particles due to normal intestinal peristalsis. Thus, challenge latex particles are continuously eliminated from the GI tract without resupply, whereas the challenge *E. coli* multiplies in the GI tract and maintains extremely high population levels (10^{10}/g cecum). On the other hand, translocating *E. coli* are likely killed in route to the MLN and in situ in the MLN and the number of viable *E. coli* cultured from the MLN represent the number of *E. coli* crossing the intestinal epithelium minus the number of killed *E. coli* en route. Conversely, latex particles are not "killed" by the host immune system and phagocytic cells may actually promote latex particle translocation by engulf latex particles and transporting them to the MLN.

Latex particles translocated at the same rate to the MLN in mice harboring their entire complement of indigenous GI bacteria (400–500 species) as in antibiotic- decontaminated mice with a drastically reduced indigenous GI microflora. Thus, the enormous numbers of indigenous obligately anaerobic bacteria normally layered on the intestinal mucosa does not appear to physically hinder the passage of latex parti- cles across the mucosal barrier.

There is not as yet enough information to conclude whether virulence determi- nants promote the initial translocation of indigenous bacteria across the intestinal barrier and/or protect the translocating bacteria in the hostile environment of extrain- testinal sites. These preliminary results pose more questions than answers concerning the role of specific bacterial virulence determinants, such as bacterial adhesins, in the pathogenesis of bacterial translocation from the GI tract. However, these preliminary findings are provocative enough to provide stimulus for further research.

5. BACTERIAL TRANSLOCATION IN HUMANS

Several studies of bacterial translocation have been performed with humans. The bacterial biotype/serotype present at the highest level in an immunosuppressed patient's feces is also the biotype/serotype most likely to cause septicemia in that patient (Tan- crede and Andremont, 1985; Wells et al., 1987). Indigenous bacteria also have been cul- tured directly from the lymph nodes of certain types of patients (Table 7). For example, indigenous GI bacteria have been cultured from the MLNs of patients with bowel cancer or bowel obstruction (Sedman et al., 1994; Vincent et al., 1988). Patients exhibiting increased intestinal permeability, such as those with Crohn's disease, ulcerative colitis, or

Table 7. Isolation of indigenous GI bacteria from the
mesenteric lymph nodes (MLN) of humans

Patient type	MLN cultures positive (%)	Reference
Bowel cancer	11	Sedman *et al.*, 1994
	65	Vincent *et al.*, 1988
Bowel obstruction	39	Sedman *et al.*, 1994
	59	Deitch *et al.*, 1989
Crohn's disease	33	Ambrose *et al.*, 1984
Ulcerative colitis	75	Peltzman *et al.*, 1991
Inflammatory bowel disease	16	Sedman *et al.*, 1994
	56	Rush *et al.*, 1988
Hemorrhagic shock	33	Moore *et al.*, 1991
	15	Moore *et al.*, 1992
Trauma	100	Brathwaite *et al.*, 1993
	81	Reed *et al.*, 1994

The indigenous GI bacteria isolated from the MLNs were identified as *E. coli*, *Klebsiella*, *Enterobacter*, *Proteus*, *Staphylococcus*, *Enterococcus*, and *Bacteroides*.

inflammatory bowel disease also produce positive MLN cultures (Ambrose et al., 1984; Peitzman et al., 1991; Sedman et al., 1994). Rush, et al. (Rush et al., 1988) demonstrated indigenous GI bacteria in the blood of patients when their systolic blood pressure decreased to <80 mm Hg and Moore et al. (Moore et al., 1992; Moore et al., 1991) cultured indigenous bacteria from the MLN of hemorrhagic shock patients in two separate studies. Brathwaite, et al. (Brathwaite et al., 1993) detected bacteria by electron microscopy in 100% of the MLNs from trauma patients. Reed, et al. (Reed et al., 1994) detected *E. coli* beta galactosidase by immunofluorescence in macrophages from 81% of the MLNs from trauma patients. A volunteer who ingested large quantities of *Candida albicans* exhibited *C. albicans* in large numbers in his urine and blood (Krause, Matheis, and Wulf, 1969). Bacterial translocation from the GI tract also is strongly suspected in the pathogenesis of human septicemia, acute respiratory death syndrome (ARDS), and multiple organ failure syndrome (MODS). Thus, evidence is accumulating that bacterial translocation from the GI tract is likely an important early step in the pathogenesis of opportunistic infections caused by the indigenous GI microflora.

6. BACTERIAL TRANSLOCATION MODEL

Our "working" model concerning the translocation of indigenous bacteria from the GI tract is presented in Fig. 2. Spontaneous" translocation of indigenous bacteria to the MLN occurs continuously at a low rate in the healthy host, but the translocating bacteria are killed in route or in situ by the host immune defenses and cultures of the MLN are usually sterile. Although not tested as yet, this low level of spontaneous translocation of indigenous bacteria to the MLN may actually be beneficial to the host by stimulating the host immune system to respond more rapidly and more effectively to more pathogenic nonindigenous microorganisms.

Oral antibiotic administration disrupts the GI ecology to promote intestinal bacterial overgrowth and translocation of indigenous bacteria to the MLN. In this first stage of translocation, the host immune defenses are able to control the numbers of

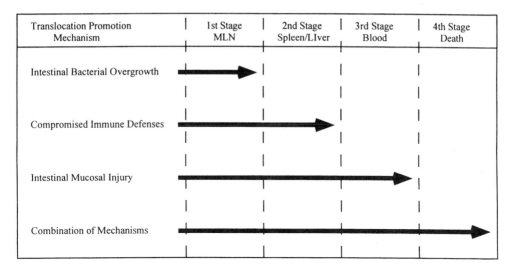

Translocation Promotion Mechanism	1st Stage MLN	2nd Stage Spleen/LIver	3rd Stage Blood	4th Stage Death
Intestinal Bacterial Overgrowth				
Compromised Immune Defenses				
Intestinal Mucosal Injury				
Combination of Mechanisms				

Figure 2. Bacterial translocation model.

translocating bacteria in the MLN and the bacteria do not spread systemically from the MLN to other organs or extraintestinal sites. The second stage of translocation occurs when the host immune system is compromised. In this stage, translocating bacteria spread from the MLN to other organs, such as the liver, spleen, or kidney. Depending upon the degree of immunodeficiency and the virulence characteristics of the translocating bacteria, the host may be able to confine the infection to these organs. If the host cannot confine the infection, then it progresses to the third stage. The third stage of translocation occurs when the translocating bacteria spread systemically to the peritoneal cavity and bloodstream. Again, the host might recover from this systemic infection depending on the degree of immunosuppression, the extent of intestinal mucosal damage, and the virulence properties of the translocating bacteria. The final fourth stage of translocation occurs when the host succumbs to bacterial infection via septic shock or multiple organ failure. This usually occurs when more than one major mechanism is operating to promote translocation, such as intestinal bacterial overgrowth plus immunosuppression or intestinal bacterial overgrowth plus shock.

7. CONCLUSION

Evidence is accumulating that bacterial translocation from the GI tract is an important initial event in the pathogenesis of opportunistic infections originating from the human GI tract. In animal models of bacterial translocation, the bacterial species most likely to translocate from the GI tract, namely *Pseudomonas aeruginosa*, *Enterococcus faecalis*, and especially the Gram-negative enteric bacilli (i.e. *Enterobacteriaceae*), are also the most common cause of septicemia in hospitalized patients. Selective antibiotic decontamination to remove the indigenous *Enterobacteriaceae* but leave intact the indigenous obligate anaerobes that exert colonization resistance against more pathogenic nonindigenous bacteria may eventually prove beneficial in certain types of patients. Oral and even systemic antibiotics, however, must be employed with caution, since intestinal bacterial overgrowth is the most efficient mechanism of initiating bacterial translocation from the GI tract to the MLN. The use of probiotics, such as *Lactobacillus acidophilus* or *Saccharomyces boulardii*, as an alternative to antibiotic therapy also requires investigation.

Maintaining a stable ecological balance in the GI tract is a major defense mechanism preventing intestinal bacterial overgrowth and subsequent bacterial translocation. Consequently, much more information is required concerning the very complex ecologic interrelationships between the host and its indigenous GI microflora if we are to understand the pathogenesis of bacterial translocation. The mechanisms whereby host immune defenses prevent bacterial translocation from the GI tract, and especially inhibit the systemic spread of translocating bacteria, also must be delineated in order to devise rational immunologic therapeutic approaches. Bacterial translocation from the GI tract has become even more relevant with the dramatic rise in the numbers of hospitalized patients with compromised immune systems and increased intestinal permeability, such as the elderly, trauma patients, and those with cancer, diabetes, transplants, invasive devices, or AIDS.

REFERENCES

Alexander, J.W., Gianotti, L., Pyles, T., Carey, M.A., and Babcock, G.F., 1990, Distribution and survival of *Escherichia coli* translocating from the intestines after thermal injury, Ann. Surg. 213:558–567.

Ambrose, M.S., Johnson, M., Burdon, D.W., and Keighley, M.R.B., 1984, Incidence of pathogenic bacteria from mesenteric lymph nodes and ileal serosa during Crohn's disease surgery, Brit J. Surg. 71:623–625.

Baker, J.W., Deitch, E.A., Berg, R., and Ma, L., 1987, Hemorrhagic shock impairs the mucosal barrier resulting in bacterial translocation from the gut and sepsis, Surg. Forum. 37:73–74.

Baker, J.W., Deitch, E.A., Ma, L., and Berg, R., 1988, Hemorrhagic shock promotes the systemic translocation of bacteria from the gut, J. Trauma. 28:896–906.

Berg, R., 1995, Bacterial translocation from the gastrointestinal tract, Trends Microbiol. 3:149–154.

Berg, R., 1996, The indigenous gastrointestinal microflora, Trends Microbiol. 4:430–435.

Berg, R., 1998, Translocation of microbes from the intestinal tract, In: Medical importance of the normal microflora, Editor: Tannock, G, Chapman & Hall, London, p. 338–370.

Berg, R., Berg, M., and Block, E., 1996, Comparison of translocation of *Escherichia coli* strains from the gastrointestinal tract, In: Germfree life and its ramifications, Editor: Hashimoto, K., et al., XII ISG Publishing Committee, Shiozawa, p. 53–58.

Berg, R., Block, E., Berg, M., and Love, J., 1996, Translocation of latex particles from the gastrointestinal tract to the mesenteric lymph nodes, In: Germfree life and its ramifications, Editor: Hashimoto, K., et al., XII ISG Publishing Committee, Shiozawa. p. 47–51.

Berg, R.D., 1980a, Inhibition of *Escherichia coli* translocation from the gastrointestinal tract by the normal cecal flora in gnotobiotic or antibiotic-decontaminated mice, Infect. Immun. 29:1073–1081.

Berg, R.D., 1980b, Mechanisms confining indigenous bacteria to the gastrointestinal tract, Amer. J. Clin. Nutr. 33:2472–2484.

Berg, R.D., 1981a, Factors influencing the translocation of bacteria from the gastrointestinal tract, In: Recent advances in germfree research, Editors: Sasaki, S., Ozawa, A., and Hashimoto, K., Tokai University Press, Tokyo, p. 411–418.

Berg, R.D., 1981b, Promotion of the translocation of enteric bacteria from the gastrointestinal tracts of mice by oral treatment with penicillin, clindamycin, or metronidazole, Infect. Immun. 33:851–861.

Berg, R.D., 1983a, Bacterial translocation from the gastrointestinal tracts of mice receiving immunosuppressive chemotherapeutic agents, Curr. Microbiol. 8:285–292.

Berg, R.D., 1983b, Translocation of indigenous bacteria from the intestinal tract, In: The intestinal microflora in health and disease, Editor: Hentges, D, Academic Press, New York, p. 333–352.

Berg, R.D., 1983c, The immune response to indigenous intestinal bacteria, In: The intestinal microflora in health and disease, Editor: Hentges, D, Academic Press, New York, p. 101–126.

Berg, R.D., 1985, Bacterial translocation from the intestines, Exp. Animals. 34:1–16.

Berg, R.D., 1992a, Bacterial translocation from the gastrointestinal tract, J. Med. 23:217–244.

Berg, R.D., 1992b, Translocation and the indigenous gut flora, In: Scientific basis of the probiotic concept, Editor: Fuller, R., Chapman & Hall, London, p. 55–85.

Berg, R.D., 1992c, Translocation of enteric bacteria in health and disease. In: Gut-derived infectious toxic shock (GITS). A major variant of septic shock, Editor: Cottier, H. and Kraft, R., S. Karger AG, Basel, Switzerland, p. 44–65.

Berg, R.D. and Garlington, A.W., 1979, Translocation of certain indigenous bacteria from the gastrointestinal tract to the mesenteric lymph nodes and other organs in a gnotobiotic mouse model, Infect. Immun. 23:403–411.

Berg, R.D. and Itoh, K., 1986, Bacterial translocation from the gastrointestinal tract-immunologic aspects, Microecol. Therapy. 16:131–145.

Berg, R.D. and Owens, W.E., 1979, Inhibition of translocation of viable *Escherichia coli* from the gastrointestinal tract of mice by bacterial antagonism, Infect. Immun. 25:820–827.

Berg, R.D., Wommack, E., and Deitch, E.A., 1988, Immunosuppression and intestinal bacterial overgrowth synergistically promote bacterial translocation, Arch. Surg. 123:1359–1364.

Brathwaite, C., Rose, S., Nagele, R., Mure, A., O'Malley, K., and Garcia-Perez, F., 1993, Bacterial translocation occurs in humans after traumatic injury: evidence using immunofluorescence, J. Trauma. 34:586–590.

Carrico, C.J., Meakins, J.L., Marshall, J.C., Fry, D., and Maier, R.V., 1986, Multiple organ failure syndrome, Arch. Surg. 121:196–208.

Deitch, E.A. and Berg, R.D., 1987, Endotoxin but not malnutrition promotes bacterial translocation of the gut flora in burned mice, J. Trauma. 27:161–166.

Deitch, E.A., Bridges, W.R., Ma, L., Berg, R., Specian, R., and Granger, N., 1989a, Role of xanthine oxidase and neutrophil generated oxy radicals in shock-induced bacterial translocation, J. Trauma. 29:1027.

Deitch, E.A., Ma, L., Ma, J.W., Grisham, M.N.G., Specian, R., and Berg, R., 1989b, Inhibition of endotoxin-induced bacterial translocation in mice, J. Clin. Invest. 84:36–42.

Deitch, E.A., Winterton, J., and Berg, R., 1987, Effect of starvation, malnutrition, and trauma on the GI tract flora and bacterial translocation, Arch. Surg. 122:1019–1025.

Deitch, E.A., Bridges, W., Baker, J., Ma, J.-W., Ma, L., Grisham, M., Granger, N., Specian, R., and Berg, R., 1988, Hemorrhagic shock-induced bacterial translocation is reduced by xanthine oxidase inhibition or inactivation, Surgery. 104:191–198.

Donnenberg, M., Newman, B., Utsalo, S., Trifillis, A., Hebel, J., and Warren, J., 1994, Internalization of *Escherichia coli* into human kidney epithelial cells: Comparison of fecal and pyelonephritis-associated strains, J. Infect. Dis. 169:831–838.

Feltis, B., Jechorek, R., Erlandsen, S., and Wells, C., 1994, Bacterial translocation and lipopolysaccharide-induced mortality in genetically macrophage-deficient op/op mice, Shock. 2:29–33.

Fuller, K.G. and Berg, R.D., 1985, Inhibition of bacterial translocation from the gastrointestinal tract by non-specific stimulation, In: Microflora control and its application to the biomedical sciences, Editor: Wostmann, B,S, Alan R. Liss, Inc., New York., p. 195–198.

Gautreaux, M., Deitch, E., and Berg, R.D., 1994a, Bacterial translocation from the gastrointestinal tract to various segments of the mesenteric lymph node complex, Infect. Immun. 62:2132–2134.

Gautreaux, M., Deitch, E., and Berg, R.D., 1994b, T-cells in the host defense against bacterial translocation from the gastrointestinal tract, Infect. Immun. 62:2874–2884.

Gautreaux, M.D., Deitch, E.A., and Berg, R.D., 1990, Immunological mechanisms preventing bacterial translocation from the gastrointestinal tract, Microecol. Ther. 20:31–34.

Gautreaux, M.D., Deitch, E.A., and Berg, R.D., 1993, T lymphocytes in host defense against bacterial translocation from the gastrointestinal tract, Infect. Immun. 62:2874–2884.

Krause, W., Matheis, H., and Wulf, K., 1969, Fungaemia and funguria after oral administration of *Candida albicans*, Lancet. 1:598–600.

Ma, L., Specian, R.D., Berg, R.D., and Deitch, E.A., 1989, Effects of protein malnutrition and endotoxin on the intestinal mucosal barrier to the translocation of indigenous flora in mice, J. Parenteral Enteral Nutr. 13:572–578.

Maejima, K., Deitch, E.A., and Berg, R.D., 1984a, Bacterial translocation from the gastrointestinal tract of rats receiving thermal injury, Infect. Immun. 43:6–10.

Maejima, K., Deitch, E.A., and Berg, R.D., 1984b, Promotion by burn stress of the translocation of bacteria from the gastrointestinal tracts of mice, Arch. Surg. 119:166–172.

Maejima, K., Shimoda, K., and Berg, R.D., 1984, Assessment of mouse strain on bacterial translocation from the gastrointestinal tract, Exp. Animals. 33:345–349.

Michetti, P., Mahan, M., Slauch, J., Mekalanos, J., and Neutra, M., 1992, Monoclonal secretory immuno-globulin A protects mice against oral challenge with the invasive pathogen *Salmonella typhimurium*, Infect. Immun. 60:1786–1792.

Moore, F., Moore, E., Poggetti, R., and Read, R., 1992, Postinjury shock and early bacteremia, Arch. Surg. 127:893–898.

Moore, F.A., Moore, E.E., Poggetti, R., McAnena, O.J., Peterson, V.M., Abernathy, C.M., and Parsons, P.E., 1991, Gut bacterial translocation via the portal vein: A clinical perspective with major torso trauma, J. Trauma. 31:629–638.

Morehouse, J., Specian, R., Stewart, J., and Berg, R.D., 1986, Promotion of the translocation of indigenous bacteria of mice from the GI tract by oral ricinoleic acid, Gastroenterology. 91:673–682.

Nolan, J., 1981, Endotoxin, reticuloendothelial function, and liver injury, Hepatology. 1:458–465.

Owens, W.E. and Berg, R.D., 1980, Bacterial translocation from the gastrointestinal tract of athymic (nu/nu) mice, Infect. Immun. 27:461–467.

Owens, W.E. and Berg, R.D., 1982, Bacterial translocation from the gastrointestinal tracts of thymectomized mice, Curr. Microbiol. 7:169-174.

Parks, D.A., Bulkley, G.B., Granger, D.N., Hamilton, S.R., and McCord, J.M., 1982, Ischemic injury in the cat small intestine: Role of superoxide radicals, Gastroenterology. 82:9–15.

Peitzman, A.B., Udekwu, A.O., Ochoa, J., and Smith, S., 1991, Bacterial translocation in trauma patients, J. Trauma. 31:1083–1087.

Penn, R.L., Maca, R.D., and Berg, R.D., 1986, Leukemia promotes the translocation of indigenous bacteria from the gastrointestinal tract to the mesenteric lymph node and other organs, Microecol. Ther. 15:85–91.

Ravin, H.A. and Fine, J., 1962, Biological implications of intestinal endotoxaemia, Fed. Proc. 21:65–68.

Reed, L., Martin, M., Manglano, R., Newson, B., Kocka, F., and Barrett, J., 1994, Bacterial translocation fol-lowing abdominal trauma in humans, Cir. Shock. 42:1–6.

Rush, B.F., Sori, A.J., Murphy, T.F., Smith, S., Flanagan, J.J., and Machiedo, G.W., 1988, Endotoxemia and bacteremia during hemorrhagic shock: the link between trauma and sepsis?, Ann. Surg. 207:549–554.

Sedman, P., Macfie, J., Sagar, P., Mitchell, C., May, J., Mancey-Jones, B., and Johnstone, D., 1994, The preva-lence of gut translocation in humans, Gastroenterology. 107:643–649.

Steffen, E.K. and Berg, R.D., 1983, Relationship between cecal population levels of indigenous bacteria and translocation to the mesenteric lymph nodes., Infect. Immun. 39:1252–1259.

Steffen, E.K., Berg, R.D., and Deitch, E.A., 1988, Comparison of the translocation rates of various indige-nous bacteria from the gastrointestinal tract to the mesenteric lymph nodes, J. Infect. Dis. 157:-1032–1037.

Tancrede, C.H. and Andremont, A.O., 1985, Bacterial translocation and gram-negative bacteremia in patients with hematological malignancies, J. Infect. Dis. 152:99–103.

Vincent, P., Colombel, J.F., Lescut, D., Fournier, L., Savage, C., Cortot, A., Quandalle, P., Vankemmel, M., and Leclerc, H., 1988, Bacterial translocation in patients with colorectal cancer, J. Infect. Dis. 158:-1395–1396.

Wells, C., Ferrieri, P., Weisdorf, D., and Rhame, F., 1987, (I do not have) The importance of surveillance stool cultures during episodes of severe neutropenia, Infect. Control. 8:317–319.

Wells, C.L., Maddus, M.A., and Simmons, R.L., 1987, The role of the macrophage in the translocation of intestinal bacteria, Arch. Surg. 122:48–53.

Winner, L., III, Mack, J., Weltzin, R., Mekalanos, J., Kraehenbuhl, J.-P., and Neutra, M., 1991, New model for analysis of mucosal immunity: Intestinal secretion of specific monoclonal immunoglobulin A from hybridoma tumors protects against *Vibrio cholerae* infection, Infect. Immun. 59:977–982.

3

INTERFERENCE WITH VIRUS AND BACTERIA REPLICATION BY THE TISSUE SPECIFIC EXPRESSION OF ANTIBODIES AND INTERFERING MOLECULES

L. Enjuanes, I. Sola, A. Izeta, J. M. Sánchez-Morgado,
J. M. González, S. Alonso, D. Escors, and C. M. Sánchez

Department of Molecular and Cell Biology
CNB, CSIC, Campus Universidad Autonoma
Cantoblanco, 28049 Madrid, Spain

SUMMARY

Historically, protection against virus infections has relied on the use of vaccines, but the induction of an immune response requires several days and in certain situations, like in newborn animals that may be infected at birth and die in a few days, there is not sufficient time to elicit a protective immune response. Immediate protection in new born could be provided either by vectors that express virus-interfering molecules in a tissue specific form, or by the production of animals expressing resistance to virus replication. The mucosal surface is the largest body surface susceptible to virus infection that can serve for virus entry. Then, it is of high interest to develop strategies to prevent infections of these areas. Virus growth can be interfered intracellularly, extracellularly or both. The antibodies neutralize virus intra- and extracellularly and their molecular biology is well known. In addition, antibodies efficiently neutralize viruses in the mucosal areas. The autonomy of antibody molecules in virus neutralization makes them functional in cells different from those that produce the antibodies and in the extracellular medium. These properties have identified antibodies as very useful molecules to be expressed by vectors or in transgenic animals to provide resistance to virus infection. A similar role could be played by antimicrobial peptides in the case of bacteria. Intracellular interference with virus growth (intracellular immunity) can be mediated by molecules of very different nature: (i) full length or single chain

Mechanisms in the Pathogenesis of Enteric Diseases 2, edited by Paul and Francis.
Kluwer Academic / Plenum Publishers, New York, 1999.

antibodies; (ii) mutant viral proteins that strongly interfere with the replication of the wild type virus (dominant-negative mutants); (iii) antisense RNA and ribozyme sequences; and (iv) the product of antiviral genes such as the Mx proteins. All these molecules inhibiting virus replication may be used to obtain transgenic animals with resistance to viral infection built in their genomes.

We have developed two strategies to target into mucosal areas either antibodies to provide immediate protection, or antigens to elicit immune responses in the enteric or respiratory surfaces in order to prevent virus infection. One strategy is based on the development of expression vectors using coronavirus derived defective RNA minigenomes, and the other relies on the development of transgenic animals providing virus neutralizing antibodies in the milk during lactation. Two types of expression vectors are being engineered based on transmissible gastroenteritis coronavirus (TGEV) defective minigenomes. The first one is a helper virus dependent expression system and the second is based on self-replicating RNAs including the information required to encode the TGEV replicase. The minigenomes expressing the heterologous gene have been improved by using a two-step amplification system based on cytomegalovirus (CMV) and viral promoters. Expression levels around $5\,\mu g$ per 10^6 cells were obtained. The engineered minigenomes will be useful to understand the mechanism of coronavirus replication and for the tissue specific expression of antigen, antibody or virus interfering molecules.

To protect from viral infections of the enteric tract, transgenic animals secreting virus neutralizing recombinant antibodies in the milk during lactation have been developed. Neutralizing antibodies with isotypes IgG1 or IgA were produced in the milk with titers of 10^6 in RIA that reduced virus infectivity by one million-fold. The recombinant antibodies recognized a conserved epitope apparently essential for virus replication. Antibody expression levels were transgene copy number independent and were related to the transgene integration site. This strategy may be of general use since it could be applied to protect newborn animals against infections of the enteric tract by viruses or bacteria for which a protective MAb has been identified. Alternatively, the same strategy could be used to target the expression of antibiotic peptides to the enteric tract in order to protect against bacterial or virus infections.

1. INTRODUCTION

Historically, protection against virus infections has relied on the use of vaccines, but the induction of an immune response requires several days and in certain situations, like in newborn animals that may be infected at birth and die in a few days, there is not sufficient time to elicit a protective immune response. Immediate protection in new born could be provided either by vectors that express virus-interfering molecules in a tissue specific form, or by the production of animals resistant to virus replication.

The possibility of expressing foreign genes in mammals by gene transfer has opened new venues in animal breeding (Brem et al., 1985; Brem and Muller, 1994; Hammer et al., 1995). An important aspect is the improvement of animal health by the obtention of transgenic animals (Castilla et al., 1998; Muller and Brem, 1996; Sola et al., 1998). Reduction of disease susceptibility of livestock will be a benefit both in terms of animal welfare and from an economical point of view, since the cost of disease has been estimated to account for 10–20% of total production cost (Muller et al., 1997).

Resistance to virus infections can be extracellular or intracellular. Intracellular interference, also named intracellular immunity, can be mediated by molecules of very different nature: (i) full length or single chain antibodies; (ii) mutant viral proteins that strongly interfere with the replication of wild type viruses (dominant-negative mutants); (iii) antisense RNA and ribozyme sequences; and (iv) products of antiviral genes such as the Mx proteins. All these molecules that inhibit virus replication may be used to obtain transgenic animals with resistance to viral infection built in their genomes. Nevertheless, in this chapter we have focused our attention on the expression of molecules such as the antibodies, microbial peptides, and interferon, that are functional either in the extracellular matrix or in cells different to the ones producing them, providing the possibility of protecting the whole tissue.

Resistance to bacteria, in addition to that mediated by well known drugs and by standard immune response, can be mediated by peptide antibiotics such as defensins, magainins, cecropins, and melittins (Boman, 1991; Wachinger et al., 1998). These small peptides were initially described in mammals, insects, and amphibians, but now it has been realized that they are more widely distributed in mammals. In principle, these antibiotics could be used in the generation of transgenic animals to increase their resistance to bacterial infection and, interestingly, to virus infection as well (Wachinger et al., 1998).

The mucosal surface is the largest body area susceptible to virus infection that can serve for virus entry. Then, it is of high interest to develop strategies to prevent infections of these areas. We have developed two strategies to target into mucosal areas molecules interfering with virus growth such as antibodies to provide immediate protection against virus infections. One strategy is based on the development of expression vectors using coronavirus derived defective RNA minigenomes, and the other one relies on the development of transgenic animals providing virus neutralizing antibodies in the milk during lactation.

1.1. Development of Expression Vectors to Target Pathogen Interfering Molecules into the Mucosal Surfaces

Two types of expression vectors are being engineered based on transmissible gastroenteritis coronavirus (TGEV) defective minigenomes (Izeta et al., 1999; Mendez et al., 1996). The first one is a helper virus dependent expression system and the second is based on self-replicating RNAs including the information required to encode the TGEV replicase. TGEV-derived vectors may have several advantages to induce mucosal immunity since: (i) TGEV infects enteric and respiratory mucosal areas (Enjuanes and Van der Zeijst, 1995) which are convenient tissues to induce secretory immunity; (ii) its tropism can be controlled by modifying the spike (S) gene making in principle possible to engineer tissue or species-specificity (Ballesteros et al., 1997); (iii) non-pathogenic strains are available to develop a safe helper virus-dependent expression system (Sánchez et al., 1992); and (iv) coronaviruses are RNA cytoplasmic viruses that replicate without a DNA intermediary making their integration into cellular chromosomes unlikely (Lai and Cavanagh, 1997). Vector systems for the expression of heterologous genes have also been developed from full-length cDNA clones of positive-strand RNA viruses such as alphaviruses including Sindbis virus, Semliki Forest virus (SFV), and Venezuelan equine encephalitis virus (VEE) (Frolov and Schlesinger, 1994; Liljeström, 1994; Pushko et al., 1997). These systems have been very useful to elicit humoral and cellular immune responses.

TGEV is a member of the *Coronaviridae* family with a plus-stranded, polyadeny-lated RNA genome of 28.5 kb (Eleouet et al., 1995). TGEV infects both enteric and respiratory tissues and causes a mortality close to one hundred percent when newborn animals are infected (Saif and Wesley, 1992). To engineer cDNAs encoding TGEV defective RNAs, three deletion mutants of 22, 10.6, and 9.7 kb (DI-A, DI-B, and DI-C, respectively) maintaining the *cis*-signals required for replication and packaging by helper viruses were isolated (Mendez et al., 1996). DI-C RNA was the most abundant and was selected to generate a cDNA encoding synthetic minigenomes that have been used for the tissue specific expression of antigens or molecules interfering with virus replication. These minigenomes expressing heterologous genes have been improved by using a two-step amplification system based on cytomegalovirus (CMV) and viral pro-moters (Izeta et al., 1998; Penzes et al., 1998). Expression levels around 2 μg per 10^6 cells were obtained and immune responses were elicited by immunizing swine with minigenomes encoding heterologous genes. These expression systems may also serve to express virus neutralizing antibodies in mucosal areas.

1.2. Interference with Virus Growth by Recombinant Antibodies

The antibodies neutralize virus intra- and extracellularly and their molecular biology is well known. In addition, antibodies efficiently neutralize viruses in the mucosal areas. The autonomy of antibody molecules in virus neutralization makes them func-tional in cells different from those producing the antibodies and in the extracellular medium. These properties have revealed the antibodies as very useful molecules to be expressed by vectors or in transgenic animals to provide resistance to virus infection.

Advances in antibody engineering have allowed the genes encoding antibodies to be manipulated so that the antigen binding domain can be intracellularly expressed (Jones and Marasco, 1997; Muller and Brem, 1994). The use of intracellular antibodies, or intrabodies, in transgenic animal research and eventual development of pathogen resistant transgenic farm animals is one of the applications. This work has concentrated mostly on the use of single chain antibody (scFv) in which the variable regions of the heavy and light chains are bound together via a linker. By adding known intracellular trafficking signals, the scFvs can be localized to specific cellular compartments such as the nucleus, the endoplasmic reticulum, the inner surface of the plasma membrane, the cytoplasm, and the mitochondria (Jones and Marasco, 1997).

Genes encoding the heavy and light chains of a hapten-specific IgM antibody were modified by site-directed mutagenesis to destroy the hydrophobic leader sequences and allow expression in the cytoplasm of non-lymphoid cells. Mutations were made in which the leader sequence of the light chain was replaced by the nuclear localization signal of the SV-40 larger T antigen. Transfectants in which the heavy chain lacking the hydrophobic leader was expressed together with a light chain carrying the nuclear localization signal were selected and a nuclear distribution of the assembled antibody was found (Biocca et al., 1990). Thus, it should be possible to target a specific antibody to the cell nucleus with the aim of interfering with viruses replicating in this compartment.

Proteins that function in the cytoplasm have also been inhibited by intrabodies. It has been found, however, that the half life of the intrabodies in the cytoplasm is shorter than in the endoplasmic reticulum, and perhaps additional modifications of the intrabody structure would allow a longer half life and therefore greater efficacy (Biocca and Cattaneo, 1995).

In the whole animal, the expression of an antibody can be temporally or spatially restricted by using a tissue-specific promoter only active at a certain time in development. Experiments to test the efficacy of antibody inhibition of HIV-1 replication have been done using scFv antibodies directed against a highly conserved domain of the HIV-1 envelope protein gp120, against the activation domain of the transcription activator protein *tat*, and against the *rev* protein, which is essential for transport of full length viral RNA from the nucleus (Marasco et al., 1993; Richardson and Marasco, 1995). Cultured cells expressing any of these antibodies have shown a marked reduction in viral titer in relationship to untransformed cells that were infected with HIV-1. The antibodies against the nuclear proteins *tat* and *rev* were effective when localized to the cytoplasm, possibly because they inhibited nuclear transport of the proteins (Mhashilkar et al., 1995).

The mucosal immune system and its predominant effector, secretory immunoglobulin A (IgA), provide the initial immunological barriers against most pathogens that invade the body at mucosal surfaces (Mestecky and McGhee, 1987). This is especially true for viruses, since resistance to infection has been strongly correlated with the presence of specific IgA antibody in mucosal secretions (Renegar and Small, 1991). At mucosal surfaces IgA antibodies are particularly stable and, since they are multivalent, might be more protective than IgG (Kilian et al., 1988). Virus neutralization by immunoglobulins is thought to result from the binding of antibody to virion attachment proteins, preventing adherence to epithelial cells. In addition, mucosal antibody interacts intracellularly with viruses preventing their replication possibly by interfering with virus assembly (Mazanec et al., 1992). IgA expressed intracellularly, or as it is transported through the epithelial cell by the polymeric immunoglobulin receptor (pIgR), may be also able to interact with intracellular pathogens such as viruses, preventing replication (Mazanec et al., 1995; Mazanec et al., 1993). It has been shown that IgA monoclonal antibodies against Sendai virus, a parainfluenza virus, colocalize with the viral hemagglutinin-neuraminidase protein within infected epithelial cells and reduce intracellular viral titers. In addition, it has been shown (Mazanec et al., 1995) that IgA interacts with influenza virus hemagglutinin (HA) protein within epithelial cells reducing viral titers in the supernatants and in cell lysates, concluding that this interference with virus replication also takes place intracellularly.

The introduction of antibody genes into cells to protect them against virus infection has been recently explored in model tissue culture systems to determine whether this strategy may potentially be applied to *in vivo* protection of mucosal surfaces by gene therapy with antibody-encoding genes, since monoclonal antibodies (MAbs) are now available for a vast range of viruses. Virus neutralizing MAbs may protect mucosal tissues against viral infections, however it is not known whether the transformation of a small percentage of the cells from a given tissue using a vector, leading to the formation of antibody secreting cells, will provide protection to the neighboring tissues.

To clarify this point, we have studied the protection of epithelial cell monolayers against TGEV infection using expression plasmids encoding virus neutralizing MAbs (Castilla et al., 1997). Immunoglobulin gene fragments encoding the variable modules of the heavy (VH) and light (VL) chains of TGEV neutralizing MAb 6A.C3 have been cloned and sequenced. The selected MAb recognizes an epitope that is located in the globular portion of the spike (S) protein (Gebauer et al., 1991). Studies by our laboratory on the mechanisms of TGEV neutralization (Suñé et al., 1990) and on its antigenic and genetic variability (Sánchez et al., 1992; Sánchez et al., 1990) have led to the identification of a mouse MAb which neutralized all the tested TGEV isolates collected in three continents throughout 40 years, and also TGEV-related coronaviruses which infect at least three animal species: porcine, canine, and feline. This MAb, 6A.C3, probably binds to an epitope essential for virus replication since no neutralization escape mutants appeared in tissue culture when this MAb was employed (Gebauer et al., 1991). A Mab with similar characteristics has been independently isolated by another group (Delmas et al., 1990).

The sequences of MAb 6A.C3 kappa and gamma 1 modules were identified as subgroup V and subgroup IIIC, respectively (Castilla et al., 1997). These chimeric immunoglobulin genes with the variable modules from the murine MAb and constant modules of human gamma 1 and kappa chains were constructed using RT-PCR. Chimeric immunoglobulins were stably or transiently expressed in murine myelomas and COS cells, respectively. The secreted recombinant antibodies had radioimmunoassay (RIA) titers higher than 10^3 and reduced the infectious virus more than 10^4-fold. Recombinant dimeric IgA showed a 50-fold enhanced neutralization of TGEV relative to a recombinant monomeric IgG_1 which contained the identical antigen binding site. Stably-transformed epithelial cloned cell lines which expressed either recombinant IgG or IgA TGEV neutralizing antibodies reduced virus production by $>10^5$-fold after infection with homologous virus, although a residual level of virus production ($<10^2$ PFU/ml) remained in less than 0.1 % of the cells. This low level persistent infection was shown not to be due to the selection of neutralization escape mutants. Although some residual virus synthesis persisted in less than 0.1% of the cells in culture, it is possible that *in vivo* defense mechanisms apart from virus neutralization, such as cytolytic T cells, could completely control virus infection. This new strategy may be particularly useful in infections where quick immune intervention is required in a defined tissue, since viral vectors could express antibody genes within two to three hours after inoculation and this expression may be targeted to specific tissues.

Three mechanisms may be responsible for the reduction in virus production: i) extracellular neutralization; ii) intracellular neutralization, and iii) modulation of virus production by antibody (Fujinami and Oldstone, 1984). Extracellular neutralization is likely to be responsible for the results of this study, because the antibody is continuously released into the medium, even during virus infection, and in the immunoglobulin gene-transformed uncloned cells about 85 to 90% of the cells did not produce the antibody yet they were still protected from TGEV infection.

Modulation of virus production by antibody binding to viral antigens on the surface of virus-infected cells is a phenomenon that operates in several virus systems (Fujinami and Oldstone, 1984). This mechanism may modulate TGEV synthesis in antibody producing ST cells. This modulation of virus synthesis probably leads to the establishment of a persistent infection, since residual virus production was often observed for at least three weeks post infection (results not shown). Antibody-induced modulation is a mechanism by which other viruses persist and escape immunologic surveillance (Fujinami and Oldstone, 1984). Experimental evidence has suggested such mechanism for measles virus, herpes simplex virus, and retrovirus.

1.3. Transgenic Animals Expressing Infectious Pathogen Specific rMAbs on B Cells

Transgenic animals to improve health and disease resistance based on specific immunity have been described (Kooyman and Pinkert, 1994; Lo et al., 1991; Storb, 1987;

Weidle et al., 1991). Pioneering studies showed the construction of transgenic mice producing functional anti-phosphorylcholine antibodies (Storb et al., 1986). Later, transgenic mice expressing chimeric anti-*Escherichia coli* immunoglobulin α heavy chain gene were developed in order to induce constitutive immunity against a pathogenic strain of *E. coli* (K99) (Kooyman and Pinkert, 1994). Because the route of *E. coli* infection was enteric, an IgA transgene was desirable. A chimeric gene construct was cloned that coded for a HC that recognized a specific *E. coli* pilus antigen. The construct comprised a κ gene promoter, murine VDJ, and bovine α-HC constant region. Expression of the immunoglobulin gene mRNA was detected before and, in some cases, only after challenge. As no differences were found when sera were analyzed for bovine IgA in control and transgenic mice, protein expression was assessed by challenge of HC founders with K99 *E. coli*. Protection was observed in the transgenic mice, however, the transgene was not transferred to the progeny.

Transgenic mice, sheep and pigs harboring genes encoding the murine α-HC and κ-LC from two different monoclonal antibodies specific for a polysaccharide such as phosphorylcholine (PC), which is potentially protective against pathogenic bacteria were generated (Lo et al., 1991). Two transgenic founders with the integration of one or both intact transgenes were produced in mice, sheep and pig. High serum levels (ranging from 0.3 to 1.3 mg/ml) of transgene rIgA were detected in transgenic mice and pigs. In the transgenic sheep no serum expression of anti-PC rMAb was found. Despite the absence of any functional mouse LC in the pigs, both animals secreted mouse transgene antibodies into their serum. The secreted rMAbs presumably included endogenous pig L chains. Allelic exclusion, i.e. the suppression of endogenous immunoglobulin rearrangement and expression, was observed in only one transgenic mouse, the endogenous immunoglobulin production of the other transgenic animals was unaffected. Unfortunately, little if any of the transgene immunoglobulin in the sera examined showed binding specificity for the antigen. Thus, a functionality in terms of the transgene rMAb could not be demonstrated.

In a second generation of transgenic animals expressing rMAbs (Weidle et al., 1991), the genes for the H (γ) and L (κ) chains of a MAb specific for 4-hydroxy-3-nitro-phenylacetate (NP) were introduced into the germ line of mice, rabbits, and pigs. During the second lactation rMAb titers higher than 0.1 mg/ml of milk were found early in lactation, and the levels declined thereafter. The transgenic rMAb bound the antigen in an ELISA test. However, in isoelectric focusing, only a small fraction of the antibody matched the mouse MAb, probably because the association of the transgenic and endogenous antibody chains (Muller et al., 1997).

1.4. Transgenic Animals Secreting Virus Neutralizing Antibodies in the Mammary Gland

To protect the enteric tract from viral infections, transgenic animals secreting virus neutralizing recombinant antibodies in the milk during lactation have been developed. Neutralizing antibodies with IgG1 or IgA isotypes were produced in the milk of transgenic mice. To this end, we used TGEV as the experimental system.

The immune response to TGEV has been characterized (Antón et al., 1995; Brim et al., 1994; VanCott et al., 1994) and full protection against this virus was provided by lactogenic immunity from immune sows (Saif and Wesley, 1992). It has also been shown that the passive oral administration of serum elicited by recombinant adenoviruses expressing the spike protein, completely protected piglets against virulent virus challenge (Torres et al., 1995).

Conventional approaches such as lactogenic immunity and artificial feeding may target the antibody to epithelial surfaces providing protection against enteric virus infections (Saif and Wesley, 1992). Alternatively, transgenic animals secreting virus neutralizing antibodies into their milk during lactation should provide immediate protection to piglets against enteric coronavirus infection (Castilla et al., 1998; Sola et al., 1998).

The mammary gland expression system is by nature very suitable for the production of proteins that function in the gastrointestinal tract and which can be orally administered (Lee et al., 1994; Lee and De Boer, 1994). Milk is now known to contain an array of bioactivities which extends the range of influence of mother over young beyond nutrition alone. Bioactivities in milk include microbial growth control, immunoregulation, and non-immune disease defense, such as lactoperoxidase, lysozyme, and lactoferrin (Schanbacher et al., 1997).

We have reported the production of the recombinant TGEV neutralizing MAb 6A.C3 of human IgG1 or porcine IgA isotypes and their secretion in the mammary gland of transgenic mice (Castilla et al., 1998; Sola et al., 1998).

To express the rIgG1 in transgenic mice, 18 founders secreting a recombinant monoclonal antibody (rMAb) neutralizing TGEV into the milk were generated (Castilla et al., 1998). The genes encoding a chimeric MAb with the variable modules of the murine TGEV specific MAb 6A.C3 and the constant modules of a human IgG_1 isotype MAb were expressed under the control of regulatory sequences derived from the whey acidic protein (WAP) which is an abundant milk protein. Antibody expression titers of 10^6 by RIA were obtained in the milk of transgenic mice which reduced TGEV infectivity with a neutralization index of 6 (10^6-fold). The antibody was synthesized at high levels throughout lactation. Integration of matrix attachment regions (MAR) sequences with the antibody genes led to a 20- to 10,000-fold increase in the antibody titer in 50% of the transgenic animals. Antibody expression levels were transgene copy number independent and were related to the site of integration. These data suggested that the MAR sequences were acting as transcription enhancer as previously suggested (Poljak et al., 1994), more than by isolating the expression cassette from negative regulatory signals from flanking genes (Bonifer et al., 1990; Jenuwein et al., 1997). The generation of transgenic animals producing virus neutralizing antibodies in milk could be a general approach to provide protection against neonatal infections of the enteric tract.

To express the rIgA, ten lines of transgenic mice secreting TGEV neutralizing rMAbs into the milk were generated (Castilla et al., 1998; Sola et al., 1998). The rMAb light and heavy chain genes were assembled by fusing the genes encoding the variable modules of the murine MAb 6A.C3, and a constant module from a porcine myeloma of IgA isotype. Seventeen out of 23 transgenic mice integrated both light and heavy chains, and at least 10 of them transmitted both genes to the progeny leading to one hundred per cent of animals secreting functional TGEV neutralizing antibody during lactation. Selected mice produced milk with TGEV specific antibody titers higher than one million as determined by RIA, neutralized virus infectivity by one million-fold, and produced up to 6 mg of antibody per ml. Antibody expression levels were transgene copy number independent and integration site dependent. Co-microinjection of genomic β-lactoglobulin gene with rMAb light and heavy chain genes led to the generation of transgenic mice carrying the three transgenes. Highest antibody titers were produced by transgenic mice that had integrated the antibody and β-lactoglobulin genes, although the number of transgenic animals generated does not allow a definitive conclusion on the enhancing effect of β-lactoglobulin co-integration. This approach may also lead to the generation of transgenic animals providing lactogenic immunity to their progeny against enteric pathogens.

The production of an active anti-CD6 rMAb in the mammary gland of transgenic mice has also been reported (Limonta et al., 1995). However, the antibody expressed by these transgenic animals did not have protective activity against infectious agents, and the antibody levels achieved were considerably lower than the TGEV neutralizing rMAbs reported above.

In principle, the expression of antibodies in transgenic animals could be regulated by an inducible promoter or it could be activated by the infectious agent itself. In that case, the cloning of the antibody genes after a viral promoter will be required. The expression of this transgene will only be induced when the infection takes place and the viral transcriptase in produced. Experiments in which the expression of an scFv antibody HIV-1 specific was controlled by the HIV-1 LTR promoter have shown that this is an effective method of inhibiting viral replication (Chen et al., 1994). This approach requires a precise characterization of the viral promoter.

1.5. Protection against Bacterial and Viral Infection by Antimicrobial Peptides

The strategy described for the protection against virus infections in mucosal areas could be extended to their protection against bacterial infection by using molecules that, such as the antibodies, inactivate the infectious agent. This is the case of antimicrobial peptides, which are key components in immunity. There are as least four types of antimicrobial peptides: defensins, magainins, cecropins, and melittins, the two first found in mammals and amphibians, respectively, and the other two found in insects. These molecules are the base of an ancient antimicrobial defense found in both animal and plant kingdoms (Boman, 1991; Lehrer et al., 1991). These peptides have been classified based on their sequence and on structural features.

Animal peptide antibiotics can be rapidly activated after injury or invasion of the host by microbial agents, combating parasitic growth immediately after infection. Antimicrobial peptides thus provide an important defense mechanism in lower animals and the first line of host defense during the time required for mobilization of specific immunity in vertebrates.

Defensins and β-defensins are found in neutrophils and in epithelial cells of mucosal tissues of mammals. They are predicted to function as the first line of host defense against microbial pathogens. Impairment of defensin activity has been implicated in chronic bacterial infections in cystic fibrosis patients (Smith et al., 1996). Interestingly, there is evidence that defensins may also be active in protection against virus infections (Wachinger et al., 1998).

Defensins act on a wide variety of bacteria but usually more efficiently on gram-positive than on gram-negative bacteria. They also work on fungi and some of them display a small degree of cytotoxicity for normal eukaryotic cells. Defensins are made as preproteins of 93–95 residues containing one defensin copy. A smaller peptide with only 12 residues and one intramolecular disulfide bond was found in bovine neutrophils (Boman, 1991).

Extracts of bovine tracheal mucosa have an abundant peptide with potent antimicrobial activity (Diamond et al., 1991). The 38-amino acid peptide, which has been named tracheal antimicrobial peptide (TAP), is produced in a proportion of 2 µg/g of wet mucosa. The size, basic charge, and presence of three intramolecular disulfide bonds is similar to, but clearly distinct from, the defensins and it has been classified as a member of the β-defensin family of antibiotic peptides found in the tracheal mucosa of the cow. The putative TAP precursor is predicted to be relative small (64 amino acids), and the mature peptide resides in the extreme carboxyterminus. The mRNA encoding this peptide is more abundant in the respiratory mucosa than in whole lung tissue. The purified peptide has antibacterial activity *in vitro* against *Escherichia coli, Staphylococcus aureus, Klebsiella pneumonia, and Pseudomonas aeruginosa.* In addition, the peptide was active against *Candida albicans*, indicating a broad spectrum of activity. This peptide appears to be, based on structure and activity, a member of a group of cysteine-rich, cationic, antimicrobial peptides found in animals, insects, and plants.

TAP gene expression in the bovine airway is inducible by lypopolysaccharide and inflammatory mediators, suggesting that it functions to protect the upper airway from infection. Limited availability of bovine TAP has precluded investigation of its potential utility in agriculture and medicine. To overcome this problem, transgenic mice expressing bTAP using an expression vector driven by control sequences from the WAP gene have been generated (Yarus et al., 1996). bTAP was purified to homogeneity from milk and showed antimicrobial activity against *E. coli*. The bTAP available from a mammary gland bioreactor will allow evaluation of bTAP for use as an antibiotic in agriculture and medicine.

The cecropins were originally identified as highly potent antibacterial peptides in immune hemolymph from the cecropia moth. All cecropins are 31–39 residues, are devoid of cysteine, and have a strongly basic N-terminal half. Although cecropins were thought to be unique to insects, a cecropin has been found in pig intestine (Lee et al., 1989), which implies that cecropins are widespread in the animal kingdom.

Cecropins A and B are highly active against several gram-positive and gram-negative bacteria, while the porcine form shows high activity only against gram-negatives. Cecropins also lyse artificial liposomes composed of phospholipids having zwitterionic or negatively charged head groups but did not lyse eukaryotic cells. The primary targets of defensins, magainins, cecropins, and melittins are the inner and outer bacterial membranes. All four groups of peptides have also been shown to form channels in artificial membranes, but it is not yet clear whether channel formation is the mechanism by which these peptides kill microorganisms.

Previously, it was reported that most cationic peptides do not induce resistance mutants *in vitro* and enhance antimicrobial activity of classical antibiotics in resistant bacteria, thus serving as anti-resistance compounds (Hancock, 1997). However, it has been recently reported (Guo et al., 1998) that increased acylation of lipid A, the major component of the outer leaflet of the outer membrane, is a cationic antimicrobial peptide resistance mechanism. In addition to antibacterial activities, amphipathic antimicrobial peptides have also been reported to act against fungi (Ahmad et al., 1995), protozoa (Bevins and Zasloff, 1990), and viruses (Wachinger et al., 1998).

Cecropins are relatively non-toxic to normal cells from multicellular organisms but, in addition to bacteria, they are toxic to protozoa and fungi, as well as infected and abnormal cells. Transgenic mice have been produced with interleukin 2 promoter/enhancer controlled expression of a synthetic cecropin-class lytic peptide that were subsequently analyzed for their resistance to *Brucella abortus* (Reed et al., 1997).

The lymphocytes of the transgenic mice could be induced to transcribe and mature cecropin mRNA after exposure to Con A. The transgenic mice showed an increased resistance to *B. abortus* as compared with non-transgenic mice.

Melittin and cecropin inhibit replication of animal viruses. Melittin is a 26 amino acid amphipathic α-helical peptide, which is a major component of bee venom (Bazzo et al., 1988; Habermann and Jentsch, 1967; Terwilliger and Eisenberg, 1982). Melittin and cecropins consist of two α-helices linked by a flexible segment and contain amphipathic structures. Whereas melittin is lytic for red blood cells at high concentrations, cecropins do not lyse erythrocytes or other eukaryotic cells (Steiner et al., 1981; Wade et al., 1992) and appear to be non-toxic for mammalian cells. Melittin has been reported to inhibit replication of murine retroviruses, tobacco mosaic virus (Marcos et al., 1995) and herpes simplex virus (Baghian et al., 1997), suggesting that melittin also displays antiviral activity. Analogous to antibacterial activity, the antiviral activity of melittin has been attributed to direct lysis of viral membranes, as demonstrated for murine retroviruses (Esser et al., 1979). However, melittin also displays antiviral activity at much lower, non-virolytic concentrations, as shown for T cells chronically infected with human immunodeficiency virus 1 (HIV-1) (Wachinger et al., 1992). Melittin and cecropins are shown to suppress production of HIV-1 by acutely infected cells. Melittin treatment of T cells reduces levels of intracellular Gag and viral mRNAs, and decrease HIV long terminal repeat (LTR) activity (Wachinger et al., 1998). HIV LTR activity is also reduced in human cells stably transfected with melittin and cecropin genes. These results indicate that antimicrobial peptides such as melittin and cecropin suppress HIV-1 replication by interfering with host cell-directed viral gene expression.

1.6. Transgenic Animals Producing γ-Interferon

(Dobrovolsky et al., 1993). The human γ-interferon (hIFN-γ) is an immuno-modulator displaying antiviral and antiproliferative properties. Large amounts of glycosylated hIFN-γ have been produced in the mammary gland of transgenic mice (Dobrovolsky et al., 1993). The concentration of hIFN-γ in the milk was 1800 IU/ml. These transgenic animals could protect their progeny from virus infections of the enteric tract during lactation.

ACKNOWLEDGMENTS

This work has been supported by grants from the Comisión Interministerial de Ciencia y Tecnología (CICYT), La Consejería de Educación y Cultura de la Comunidad de Madrid, and Fort Dodge Veterinaria from Spain, and the European Communities (Biotechnology and FAIR projects). IS, JMG, and DE received fellowships from the Department of Education and Science; AI and SA received fellowships from the Department of Education, University and Research of the Gobierno Vasco; JMS, received a fellowship from the Veterinary College of the Community of Madrid.

REFERENCES

Ahmad, I., W.R. Perkins, D.M. Lupan, M.E. Selsted, and A.S. Janoff. 1995. Liposomal entrapment of the neutrophil-derived peptide indolicidin endows it with *in vivo* anti-fungal activity. *Biochi. Biophy. Acta.* **1237**:109–114.

Antón, I.M., C. Suñé, R.H. Meloen, F. Borrás-Cuesta, and L. Enjuanes. 1995. A transmissible gastroenteritis coronavirus nucleoprotein epitope elicits T helper cells that collaborate in the *in vitro* antibody synthesis to the three major structural viral proteins. *Virology.* 212:746–751.

Baghian, A., J. Jaynes, F. Enright, and K.G. Kousolas. 1997. An amphipathic alpha-helical synthetic peptide analogue of melittin inhibits herpes simplex virus-I (HSV-1)-induced cell fusion and virus spread. *Peptides.* 18:177–183.

Ballesteros, M.L., C.M. Sanchez, and L. Enjuanes. 1997. Two amino acid changes at the N-terminus of transmissible gastroenteritis coronavirus spike protein result in the loss of enteric tropism. *Virology.* 227:378–388.

Bazzo, R., M.J. Tappin, A. Pastore, T.S. Harvey, J.A. Carver, and I.D. Campbell. 1988. The structure of melittin. A ¹H-NMR study in methanol. *Eur. J. Biochem.* 173:139–146.

Bevins, C.L. and M. Zasloff. 1990. Peptides from frog skin. *Annu. Rev. Bioch.* 59:395–414.

Biocca, S. and A. Cattaneo. 1995. Intracellular immunization: antibody targeting to subcellular compartments. *Trends Cell Biol.* 5:248–252.

Biocca, S., M.S. Neuberger, and A. Cattaneo. 1990. Expression and targeting of intracellular antibodies in mammalian cells. *EMBO J.* 9:101–108.

Boman, H.G. 1991. Antibacterial peptides: key components needed in immunity. *Cell.* 65:205–207.

Bonifer, C., M. Vidal, F. Grosveld, and A.E. Sippel. 1990. Tissue specific and protein position independent expression of the complete gene domain for chicken lysozyme in transgenic mice. *EMBO J.* 9:2843–2848.

Brem, G., B. Brenig, H.M. Goodman, R.C. Selden, F. Graf, B. Kruff, K. Springman, J. Hondele, J. Meyer, E.-L. Winnaker, and H. Krausslich. 1985. Production of transgenic mice, rabbits, and pigs by microinjection into pronuclei. *Zuchthygiene.* 20:251–252.

Brem, G. and M. Muller. 1994. Large transgenic animals. *In* Animals with novel genes. N. Maclean, editor. Cambridge University Press, Cambridge. 179–244.

Brim, T.A., J.L. VanCott, J.K. Lunney, and L.J. Saif. 1994. Lymphocyte proliferation responses of pigs inoculated with transmissible gastroenteritis virus or porcine respiratory coronavirus. *Am. J. Vet. Res.* 55:494–501.

Castilla, J., B. Pintado, I. Sola, J.M. Sánchez-Morgado, and L. Enjuanes. 1998. Engineering passive immunity in transgenic mice secreting virus-neutralizing antibodies in milk. *Nature Biotech.* 16:349–354.

Castilla, J., I. Sola, and L. Enjuanes. 1997. Interference of coronavirus infection by expression of immunoglobulin G (IgG) or IgA virus-neutralizing antibodies. *J. Virol.* 71:5251–5258.

Chen, S.Y., J. Bagley, and W.A. Marasco. 1994. Intracellular antibodies as a new class of therapeutic molecules for gene therapy. *Human Gene Therapy.* 5:595–601.

Delmas, B., D. Rasschaert, M. Godet, J. Gelfi, and H. Laude. 1990. Four major antigenic sites of the coronavirus transmissible gastroenteritis virus are located on the amino-terminal half of spike glycoprotein S. *J. Gen. Virol.* 71:1313–1323.

Diamond, G., M. Zasloff, H. Eck, M. Brasseur, W.L. Maloy, and C.L. Bevins. 1991. Tracheal antimicrobial peptide, a cysteine-rich peptide from mammalian tracheal mucosa: peptide isolation and cloning of a cDNA. *Proc. Natl. Acad. Sci. USA.* 88:3952–3956.

Dobrovolsky, V.N., O.V. Lagutin, T.V. Vinogradova, I.S. Frolova, V.P. Kuznetsov, and O.A. Larionov. 1993. Human gamma-interferon expression in the mammary gland of transgenic mice. *FEBS Letters.* 319:181–184.

Eleouet, J.F., D. Rasschaert, P. Lambert, L. Levy, P. Vende, and H. Laude. 1995. Complete sequence (20 kilobases) of the polyprotein-encoding gene 1 of transmissible gastroenteritis virus. *Virology.* 206:817–822.

Enjuanes, L. and B.A.M. Van der Zeijst. 1995. Molecular basis of transmissible gastroenteritis coronavirus epidemiology. *In* The Coronaviridae. S.G. Siddell, editor. Plenum Press, New York. 337–376.

Esser, A.F., R.M. Bartholomew, F.C. Jensen, and H.J. Muller-Eberhardt. 1979. Disassembly of viral membranes by complement independent channel formation. *Proc. Natl. Acad. Sci. USA.* 76: 5843–5847.

Frolov, I. and S. Schlesinger. 1994. Translation of Sindbis virus mRNA: effect of sequences downstream of the initiation codon. *J. Virol.* 68:8111–8117.

Fujinami, R.S. and M.B.A. Oldstone. 1984. Antibody initiates virus persistence: immune modulation and measles virus infection. *In* Concepts in viral pathogenesis. A.L. Notkins and M.B.A. Oldstone, editors. Springer-Verlag, New York. 187–193.

Gebauer, F., W.A.P. Posthumus, I. Correa, C. Suñé, C.M. Sánchez, C. Smerdou, J.A. Lenstra, R. Meloen, and L. Enjuanes. 1991. Residues involved in the formation of the antigenic sites of the S protein of transmissible gastroenteritis coronavirus. *Virology.* 183:225–238.

Guo, L., K.B. Lim, C.M. Poduje, M. Daniel, J.S. Gunn, M. Hackett, and S.I. Millers. 1998. Lipid A acylation and bacterial resistance against vertebrate antimicrobial peptides. *Cell.* **95**:189–198.

Habermann, E. and J. Jentsch. 1967. Sequence analysis of melittin from tryptic and peptic degradation products. *Hoppe-Seyler's Z. Physiol. Chem.* **348**:37–50.

Hammer, M.C., P.J. Swart, M.-P. de Béthune, R. Pauwels, E.D. Clercq, T.H. The, and D.K.F. Meijer. 1995. Antiviral effects of plasma and milk proteins: lactoferrin shows potent activity against both guman immunodficiency virus and human cytomegalovirus replicaion *in vitro. J. Infect. Dis.* **172**:380–388.

Hancock, R.E.W. 1997. Peptide antibiotics. *Lancet.* **349**:418–422.

Izeta, A., C.M. Sanchez, C. Smerdou, A. Mendez, S. Alonso, M. Balasch, J. Plana-Duran, and L. Enjuanes. 1998. The spike protein of transmissible gastroenteritis coronavirus controls the tropism of pseudorecombinant virions engineered using synthetic minigenomes. *Adv. Exp. Med. Biol.* **440**:207–214.

Izeta, A., C. Smerdou, S. Alonso, Z. Penzes, A. Mendez, J. Plana-Duran, and L. Enjuanes. 1998b. Replication and packaging of transmissible gastroenteritis coronavirus derived synthetic minigenomes. *J. Virol.* **73**: 1535–1545.

Jenuwein, T., W.C. Forrester, L.A. Fernández-Herrero, G. Laible, M. Dull, and R. Grosschedl. 1997. Extension of chromatin accessibility by nuclear matrix attachment regions. *Nature.* **385**:269–272.

Jones, S.D. and W.A. Marasco. 1997. Intracellular antibodies (intrabodies): potential applications in transgenic animal research and engineered resistance to pathogens. *In* Transgenic animals. Generation and use. L.M. Houdebine, editor. Harwood Academic Publishers, Amsterdam. 501–506.

Kilian, M., J. Mestecky, and M.W. Russell. 1988. Defence mechanisms involving Fc-dependent functions of immunoglobulin A and their subversion by immunoglobulin A proteases. *Microbio. Rev.* **52**:296–303.

Kooyman, D.L. and C.A. Pinkert. 1994. Transgenic mice expressing a chimeric anti-E. coli immunoglobulin a heavy chain gene. *Transgenic Res.* **3**:167–175.

Lai, M.M.C. and D. Cavanagh. 1997. The molecular biology of coronaviruses. *Adv. Virus Res.* **48**:1–100.

Lee, C.K., R. Weltzin, G. Soman, K.M. Georgakopoulos, D.M. Houle, and T.P. Monath. 1994. Oral administration of polymeric immunoglobulin A prevents colonization with vibrio cholerae in neonatal mice. *Infec. Imm.* **62**:887–891.

Lee, J.-Y. A. Boman, S. Chuanxin, M. Andersson, H. Jornvall, and V. Mutt. 1989. Antibacterial peptides from pig intestine: isolation of a mammalian cecropin. *Proc. Natl. Acad. Sci. USA.* **86**:9159–9162.

Lee, S.H. and H.A. De Boer. 1994. Production of biomedical proteins in the milk of transgenic dairy cows: the state of the art. *J. Cont. Release.* **29**:213–221.

Lehrer, R.I., T. Ganz, and M.E. Selsted. 1991. Defensins: endogenous antibiotic peptides of animal cells. *Cell.* **64**:229–230.

Liljeström, P. 1994. Alphavirus expression systems. *Curr. Opin. Biotech.* **5**:495–500.

Limonta, J., A. Pedraza, A. Rodríguez, F.M. Freyre, A.M. Barral, F.O. Castro, R. Lleonart, C.A. Garcia, J.V. Gavilondo, and J. de la Fuente. 1995. Production of active anti-CD6 mouse-human chimeric antibodies in the milk of transgenic mice. *Immunotechnology.* **1**:107–113.

Lo, D., V.G. Pursel, P.J. Linton, E. Sandgren, R. Behringer, C. Rexroad, R.D. Palmiter, and R.L. Brinster. 1991. Expression of mouse IgA by transgenic mice, pigs, and sheep. *Eur. J. Immunol.* **21**:1001–1006.

Marasco, W.A., W.A. Haseltine, and S. Chen. 1993. Design, intracellular expression, and activity of a human anti-human immunodeficiency virus type 1 gp120 single-chain antibody. *Proc. Natl. Acad. Sci. USA.* **90**:7889–7893.

Marcos, J.F., R.N. Beachy, R.A. Houghten, S.E. Blondelle, and E. Perez-Paya. 1995. Inhibition of plant virus infection by melittin. *Proc. Natl. Acad. Sci. USA.* **92**:12466–12469.

Mazanec, M.B., C.L. Coudret, and D.R. Fletcher. 1995. Intracellular neutralization of influenza virus by immunoglobulin A anti-hemagglutinin monoclonal antibodies. *J. Virol.* **69**:1339–1343.

Mazanec, M.B., M.E. Lamm, D. Lyn, A. Portner, and J.G. Nedrud. 1992. Comparison of IgA versus IgG monoclonal antibodies for passive immunization of the murine respiratory tract. *Virus Res.* **23**:1–12.

Mazanec, M.B., J.G. Nedrud, C.S. Kaetzel, and M.E. Lamm. 1993. A three-tiered view of the role of IgA in mucosal defense. *Immunol. Today.* **14**:430–434.

Mendez, A., C. Smerdou, A. Izeta, F. Gebauer, and L. Enjuanes. 1996. Molecular characterization of transmissible gastroenteritis coronavirus defective interfering genomes: Packaging and heterogeneity. *Virology.* **217**:495–507.

Mestecky, J. and J.R. McGhee. 1987. Immunoglobulin A (IgA): molecular and cellular interactions involved in IgA biosynthesis and immune response. *Adv. Immunol.* **40**:153–245.

Mhashilkar, A.M., J. Bagley, S.-Y. Chen, A.M. Szilvay, D.G. Helland, and W.A. Marasco. 1995. Inhibition of HIV-1 tat-mediated LTR transactivation and HIV-1 infection by anti-tat single chain intrabodies. *EMBO J.* **14**:1542–1551.

Muller, M. and G. Brem. 1994. Transgenic strategies to increase disease resistance in livestock. *Repr. Fert. Develop.* **6**:605–613.

Muller, M. and G. Brem. 1996. Intracellular, genetic or congenital immunisation—transgenic approaches to increase disease resistance of farm animals. *J. Biotechnol.* **44**:233–242.

Muller, M., U.H. Weidle, and G. Brem. 1997. Antibody encoding transgenes-their potential use in congenital and intracellular immunisation of farm animals. *In* Transgenic animals. Generation and use. L.M. Houdebine, editor. Harwood Academic Publishers, Amsterdam. 495–499.

Penzes, Z., J.M. Gonzalez, A. Izeta, M. Muntion, and L. Enjuanes. 1998. Progress towards the construction of a transmissible gastroenteritis coronavirus self-replicating RNA using a two-layer expression system. *Adv. Exp. Med. Biol.* **440**:319–327.

Poljak, L., C. Seum, T. Mattioni, and U.K. Laemmli. 1994. SARs stimulate but do not confer position independent gene expression. *Nucleic Acids Res.* **22**:4386–4394.

Pushko, P., M. Parker, G.V. Ludwing, N.L. Davis, R.E. Johnston, and J.F. Smith. 1997. Replication-helper systems from attenuated Venezuelan equine encephalitis virus: expression of heterologous genes in vitro and immunization against heterologous pathogens in vivo. *Virology.* **239**:389–401.

Reed, W.A., P.H. Elzer, F.M. Enright, J.M. Jaynes, J.D. Morrey, and K.L. White. 1997. Interleukin 2 promoter/enhancer controlled expression of a synthetic cecropin-class lytic peptide in transgenic mice and subsequent resistance to *Brucella abortus*. *Transgenic Res.* **6**:337–347.

Renegar, K.B. and P.A. Small. 1991. Immunoglobulin A mediation of murine nasal anti-influenza virus immunity. *J. Virol.* **65**:2146–2148.

Richardson, J.H. and W.A. Marasco. 1995. Intracellular antibodies: development and therapeutic potential. *TIBTECH.* **13**:306–310.

Saif, L.J. and R.D. Wesley. 1992. Transmissible gastroenteritis. *In* Diseases of Swine. A.D. Leman, B.E. Straw, W.L. Mengeling, S. D'Allaire, and D.J. Taylor, editors. Wolfe Publishing Ltd, Ames. Iowa. 362–386.

Sánchez, C.M., F. Gebauer, C. Suñé, A. Méndez, J. Dopazo, and L. Enjuanes. 1992. Genetic evolution and tropism of transmissible gastroenteritis coronaviruses. *Virology.* **190**:92–105.

Sánchez, C.M., G. Jiménez, M.D. Laviada, I. Correa, C. Suñé, M.J. Bullido, F. Gebauer, C. Smerdou, P. Callebaut, J.M. Escribano, and L. Enjuanes. 1990. Antigenic homology among coronaviruses related to transmissible gastroenteritis virus. *Virology.* **174**:410–417.

Schanbacher, F.L., R.S. Talhouk, and F.A. Murray. 1997. Biology and origin of bioactive peptides in milk. *Lives. Prod. Sci.* **50**:105–123.

Smith, J.J., S.M. Travis, E.P. Greenberg, and M.J. Welsh. 1996. Cystic fibrosis airway epithelia fail to kill bacteria because of abnormal airway surface fluid. *Cell.* **85**:229–236.

Sola, I., J. Castilla, B. Pintado, J.M. Sánchez-Morgado, B. Whitelaw, J. Clark, and L. Enjuanes. 1998. Transgenic mice secreting coronavirus neutralizing antibodies into the milk. *J. Virol.* **72**:3762–3772.

Steiner, H., D. Hultmark, A. Engstrom, H. Bennich, and H.G. Boman. 1981. Sequence and specificity of two antibacterial proteins involved in insect immunity. *Nature.* **292**:246–248.

Storb, U. 1987. Transgenic mice with immunoglobulin genes. *Ann. Rev. Immunol.* **5**:151–174.

Storb, U., C. Pinkert, B. Arp, P. Engler, K. Gollahon, J. Manz, W. Brady, and R.L. Brinster. 1986. Transgenic mice with μ and κ genes encoding antiphosphorylcholine antibodies. *J. Exp. Med.* **164**:627–641.

Suñé, C., G. Jiménez, I. Correa, M.J. Bullido, F. Gebauer, C. Smerdou, and L. Enjuanes. 1990. Mechanisms of transmissible gastroenteritis coronavirus neutralization. *Virology.* **177**:559–569.

Terwilliger, T.C. and D. Eisenberg. 1982. The structure of melittin. II. Interpretation of the stucture. *J. Biol. Chem.* **257**:6016–6022.

Torres, J.M., C.M. Sánchez, C. Suñé, C. Smerdou, L. Prevec, F. Graham, and L. Enjuanes. 1995. Induction of antibodies protecting against transmissible gastroenteritis coronavirus (TGEV) by recombinant adenovirus expressing TGEV spike protein. *Virology.* **213**:503–516.

VanCott, J.L., T.A. Brim, J.K. Lunney, and L.J. Saif. 1994. Contribution of antibody-secreting cells induced in mucosal lymphoid tissues of pigs inoculated with respiratory or enteric strains of coronavirus to immunity against enteric coronavirus challenge. *J. Immunol.* **152**:3980–3990.

Wachinger, M., A. Kleinschmidt, D. Winder, N. von Pechmann, A. Ludvigsen, M. Neumann, R. Holle, B. Salmons, V. Erfle, and R. Brack•Werner. 1998. Antimicrobial peptides melittin and cecropin inhibit replication of human immunodeficiency virus 1 by suppressing viral gene expression. *J. Gen. Virol.* **79**:731–740.

Wachinger, M., T. Saermark, and V. Erfle. 1992. Influence of amphipathic peptides on the HIV-1 production in persistently infected T-lymphoma cells. *FEBS Letters.* **309**:235–341.

Wade, D., D. Andreu, S.A. Mitchell, A.M.V. Silveira, A. Boman, H.G. Boman, and R.B. Merrifield. 1992. Antibacterial peptides designed as analogs or hybrids of cecropins and melittin. *Inter. J. Pept. Prot. Res.* **40**:429–436.

Weidle, U.H., H. Lenz, and G. Brem. 1991. Genes encoding a mouse monoclonal antibody are expressed in transgenic mice, rabbits, and pigs. *Gene.* **98**:185–191.

Yarus, S., J.M. Rosen, A.M. Cole, and G. Diamond. 1996. Production of active bovine tracheal antimicrobial peptide in milk of transgenic mice. *Proc. Natl. Acad. Sci. USA.* **93**:14118–14121.

4

COMPARATIVE PATHOGENESIS OF ENTERIC VIRAL INFECTIONS OF SWINE

Linda J. Saif

Food Animal Health Research Program
Ohio Agricultural Research and Development Center
The Ohio State University
Wooster, Ohio 44691

1. SUMMARY

At least 11 enteric viruses belonging to 6 distinct families (*Adenoviridae*, *Astroviridae*, *Caliciviridae*, *Coronaviridae*, *Parvoviridae*, and *Reoviridae*) cause diarrhea in swine mainly during the nursing and immediate post-weaning period. Most infect the small intestinal enterocytes, inducing various degrees of villous atrophy and subsequently a malabsorptive, maldigestive diarrhea. In addition rotaviruses possess an enterotoxin (NSP4) which induces a secretory diarrhea in mice. These viruses have distinct predilections for different vertical (villus/crypt) and horizontal (duodenum, jejunum, ileum, colon) replication sites in the intestine and the diarrhea intensity is often related to the extent of viral replication at these sites. In addition concurrent infections with multiple enteric viruses can produce synergistic or additive effects leading to more extensive villous atrophy throughout the intestine and more severe and prolonged diarrhea. Knowledge of enteric viral replication sites and comparative mechanisms of diarrhea induction may lead to new or improved vaccine strategies or therapeutic approaches for the prevention or treatment of these viral diarrheas.

2. INTRODUCTION

Eleven enteropathogenic viruses belonging to 6 families are associated with diarrheal infections of swine as summarized in Table 1. Most have been identified only within the past 2 decades and some, such as a porcine torovirus (Kroneman et al., 1998) and a porcine enteric parvovirus (Yasuhara et al., 1995), have only recently been further characterized following their initial detection (Scott et al., 1987; Yasuhara et al., 1989).

Mechanisms in the Pathogenesis of Enteric Diseases 2, edited by Paul and Francis.
Kluwer Academic / Plenum Publishers, New York, 1999.

Multiple serogroups (A,B,C,E) of porcine rotaviruses exist with multiple sero-types within each serogroup (A,C). Distinct serogroups and serotypes do not elicit cross-protection (Theil, 1990; Paul and Stevenson, 1992; Saif and Jiang, 1992; Saif, Rosen, and Parwani, 1994). Multiple serotypes also exist for porcine adenoviruses, but it is unclear if any cause diarrhea other than porcine adenovirus type 3 (Coussement et al., 1981; Benfield, 1990). The existence of multiple serogroups/serotypes complicates diagnosis and vaccine strategies by necessitating serogroup specific reagents and inclusion of multiple serogroups/serotypes for effective vaccines. This question of antigenic diversity has not been adequately explored for the other swine enteric viruses (caliciviruses, astroviruses, enteric parvoviruses, and porcine toroviruses).

Both enveloped and non-enveloped viruses replicate in the intestine and cause diarrhea. Interestingly, the enveloped enteric viruses also infect the upper respiratory tract to various degrees which may contribute to their pathogenesis by increasing the viral dose swallowed (Saif and Wesley, 1992). In addition both adenovirus (Coussement et al., 1981) and porcine enteric parvovirus (Yasuhara et al., 1995) infect the respiratory tract; the latter virus was also isolated from multiple organs after intranasal but not oral administration confirming its ability to also induce systemic infections.

These enteric viruses possess unique characteristics related to their intestinal tropism and replication (Saif, 1990). They are stable to low pH and proteolytic enzymes, factors important for their replication and survival in the intestine and their eventual adaptation to passage in cell culture (Saif, 1990; Theil, 1990). In fact, the porcine enteric calicivirus, the only enteric calicivirus adapted to cell culture, remains refractory to serial passage in cell culture unless the culture medium is supplemented with intestinal contents from uninfected gnotobiotic pigs (Flynn, Saif, and Moorhead et al., 1988). Most of the enteric viruses are heat labile, which may explain the prevalence of viral diarrheas during winter. Whereas coronaviruses and toroviruses are enveloped and sensitive to inactivation by common disinfectants, the other enteric viruses are non-enveloped and highly resistant to many disinfectants and environmental conditions.

The enteric viruses described in Table 1 commonly occur as enzootics in seropositive herds, most frequently in 2–3-week-old pigs and within 1–2 weeks post weaning (Saif, 1990). However, transmissible gastroenteritis virus (TGEV) and porcine epidemic diarrhea virus (PEDV) also occur as epizootics causing diarrhea in swine of all ages, but with the most severe disease and diarrhea mortality occurring in neonates (Pensaert and deBouck, 1978; Pensaert, 1992; Saif and Wesley, 1992). Because group B and C rotaviruses are less widespread than group A rotaviruses based on seroprevalence studies, they may also cause epizootic infections (Saif and Jiang, 1994). The epidemiology of TGEV infections in Europe consists mainly of enzootic infections since the appearance of the TGEV deletion mutant, PRCV; however, in North America, widespread epizootic outbreaks of TGEV continue (Saif and Wesley, 1992).

For viral diarrheas, the incubation periods are usually short, the viruses are excreted in feces in large numbers and spread to susceptible pigs via the fecal-oral route or possibly aerosols occurs rapidly. Systemic infections are generally not reported for these enteric viruses with the exception of enteric parvovirus (Yasuhara et al., 1995). Thus the localized nature of most infections is of major consideration for the design of effective vaccines and intervention strategies. One possible explanation for the localized nature of these enteric viral infections was suggested from recent in vitro studies of TGEV using polarized epithelial cells (Rossen et al., 1996). TGEV entered and exited these cells via the apical surface; in comparison, a murine coronavirus associated with systemic infections entered the same cells apically, but exited basolaterally. Whether similar effects occur in vivo in the intestine, and may account for enteric virus

Table 1. Characteristics of porcine enteropathogenic viruses

Family/Virus	Size	Nucleic acid	Discovery Year	Discovery Investigator*
Enveloped				
Coronaviridae/				
Transmissible gastroenteritis virus (TGEV)	60–220 nm	ssRNA	1946	Doyle & Hutchings
Porcine epidemic diarrhea virus (PEDV)	60–220 nm	ssRNA	1978	Pensaert & Debouck and Chasey & Cartwright
Porcine torovirus	70–240 nm	ssRNA	1987	Scott et al.
Nonenveloped				
Reoviridae/				
Rotavirus (group A)	55–70 nm	dsRNA	1975	Rodger et al.
Rotavirus (group B)	55–70 nm	dsRNA	1980	Bridger et al.
Rotavirus (group C)	55–70 nm	dsRNA	1980	Saif et al.
Rotavirus (group E)	55–70 nm	dsRNA	1986	Chasey et al.
Caliciviridae/				
Calicivirus	30–40 nm	ssRNA	1980	Bridger et al., Saif et al.
Astroviridae/				
Astrovirus	28–30 nm	ssRNA	1980	Bridger et al., Saif et al.
Adenoviridae/				
Adenovirus	70–90 nm	DNA	1981	Coussement et al.
Parvoviridae/				
Enteric Parvovirus	18–26 nm	DNA	1989	Yasuhara et al.

*See references for literature citations.

localization in villous or crypt enterocytes or systemic spread, remains speculative. Although viruses that cause localized infections of villous enterocytes do so via the luminal surface, viruses that infect primarily crypt enterocytes (parvovirus) may do so only after systemic infection followed by hematogenous (or via infected lymphoid cells) dissemination of virus to the basolateral surface of crypts.

3. COMPARATIVE PATHOGENESIS OF THE PORCINE ENTEROPATHOGENIC VIRUSES

The enteric viruses have predilections for replication in distinct vertical and longitudinal regions of the small intestine and the lesions induced are most pronounced at these sites (Table 2, Saif, 1990). Moon (1978, 1994) and Saif (1990) drew a corollary between the extent of viral replication vertically in villous enterocytes and the severity of enteric viral infections as summarized in Table 2. For example, TGEV infects and destroys absorptive cells in multiple stages of differentiation along the entire villus causing pronounced villous atrophy and often fatal diarrhea. Rotaviruses and astroviruses infect the distal tips to two-thirds of the villus, causing less severe villous atrophy and diarrhea. Group B rotaviruses infect cells on the villus tips and induce syncytia, a pathognomonic lesion distinctive of group B rotaviruses (Saif and Jiang, 1994). Adenoviruses, PEDV and caliciviruses infect enterocytes at the base and sides of the villus inducing moderate villous atrophy and diarrhea (Benfield, 1990; Bridger, 1990; Coussement et al., 1981; Flynn, Saif, and Moorhead, 1988; Pensaert, 1992). Enteric parvoviruses infect crypt enterocytes inducing severe villous atrophy, mucosal collapse, and severe hemorrhagic and often fatal diarrhea (Yasuhara, 1995).

Longitudinal segmentation of enteric viral replication sites and lesions also occurs in the intestine (Table 2, Saif, 1990). Generally, viruses that infect only limited, segmental portions of the intestine or restricted numbers of enterocytes cause mild or no villous atrophy, and diarrhea. An example is astrovirus which infects few enterocytes and causes mild or no villous atrophy and diarrhea in pigs (Saif et al., 1980; Bridger, 1990). In comparison, TGEV produces an almost continuous infection of whole villi throughout the entire small intestine which results in severe villous atrophy and often fatal diarrhea (Moon, 1994; Pensaert et al., 1970; Saif and Wesley, 1992). Other viruses produce intermediate degrees of villous atrophy and diarrhea intensity. Rotaviruses (groups A to C) generally replicate and cause villous atrophy in the distal small intestine, but usually not the colon (Paul and Stevenson, 1992; Saif and Jiang, 1994; Saif, Rosen, and Parwani, 1994; Theil, 1990). Groups A and C rotaviruses infect a higher percentage of cells than group B rotaviruses which produce scattered foci of infection in the villous tips of the distal small intestine (Saif and Jiang, 1994). Adenoviruses, PEDV and enteric parvovirus infections and lesions are restricted mainly to the jejunum and ileum, but PEDV also infects the colon (Benfield, 1990; Coussement et al., 1981; Pensaert, 1992; Yasuhara et al., 1995). In contrast to all other enteric viruses, calicivirus infections, and lesions occur mainly in the proximal small intestine (Bridger, 1990; Flynn, Saif, and Moorhead, 1988).

All the swine enteric viruses produce cytolytic infections of enterocytes leading to varying degrees of villous atrophy, crypt hyperplasia, and frequently villous fusion (Moon, 1978; 1994; Saif, 1990). Villus loss and fusion lead to reduced absorptive capacity in the small intestine and a malabsorptive, maldigestive diarrhea accompanied by dehydration and death in severe cases. Maldigestion results from loss of the digestive enzymes produced by the absorptive villous enterocytes; loss of the glucose coupled sodium transport mechanism results in malabsorption of nutrients (Argenzio, 1997; Moon, 1978; 1994). Replacement of absorptive cells by the incompletely differentiated crypt cells, which retain their secretory capacity, and the ensuing crypt hyperplasia, also lead to increased secretion in the intestine, further accentuating the diarrhea (Argenzio, 1997; Moon, 1978; 1994).

Although, it is well-established that enteric bacterial infections such as enterotoxigenic *Escherichia coli* (ETEC) induce a secretory diarrhea in pigs mediated by secretion of enterotoxins (Argenzio, 1997; Moon, 1978), recent evidence indicates that rotaviruses also possess an enterotoxin, the nonstructural protein NSP4 (Ball et al., 1996). The NSP4 and its synthetic peptides induced an age and dose-dependent diarrhea response in young rodents. Evidence indicates that NSP4 activates a signal transduction pathway that increases intracellular calcium and promotes chloride secretion (Dong et al., 1997). Although the enterotoxin potential of rotavirus NSP4 has not been confirmed in pigs, if documented, it could explain the early diarrhea seen in rotavirus-infected pigs prior to the detection of villous atrophy (Saif, Rosen, and Parwani, 1994; Theil, 1990). Furthermore, virulent and attenuated pairs of porcine rotaviruses (OSU, Gottfried) differ in their NSP4 nucleotide sequence (Zhang et al., 1998). Whereas NSP4

Table 2. The vertical and longitudinal sites of replication and villous atrophy in the intestine associated with infection by porcine enteropathogenic viruses

Virus	Diarrhea	Vertical			Longitudinal		Villous atrophy Small intestine	
		Villus	(Site)	Crypt	Small intestine	Colon	Site	Extent
I. Infect villous enterocytes								
Coronavirus–TGEV	Severe	+	Entire	–	D,J,I	–	D,J,I	Severe
Rotavirus								
Group A	Mild/severe	+	Entire	–	J,I	±	J,I	Moderate-Severe
Group B	Mild	+	(Tips)	–	D,J,I	–	D,J,I (syncytia)	Mild
Group C	Mild/severe	+		–	J,I	–	J	Mild/severe
Group E	Mild	+		–	?	–	?	?
SRSV								
Astrovirus	Mild/None	+	(Dome)	–	D,J,I	None	–	
Calicivirus	Moderate	+		–	D,J	D,J	Moderate	
II. Infect villous & crypt enterocytes								
Adenovirus	Moderate	+	(Intranuclear Inclusions)	±	J,I	+	J,I	Mild/Moderate
Coronavirus–PEDV	Moderate	+		±	D,J,I	+	J,I	Moderate
III. Infect crypt enterocytes								
Parvovirus	Severe/Hemorrhagic	?		+	J,I		J,I	Severe

from virulent OSU porcine rotavirus induced diarrhea in neonatal mice and increased intracellular calcium levels, NSP4 from attenuated OSU rotavirus or a mutated form of virulent NSP4 was avirulent in mice. The enterotoxigenicity of NSP4 has not yet been assessed in pigs.

Recovery from enteric viral infections depends on local immunity and regeneration of villi by absorptive cells from the undifferentiated crypt cell population. Villous enterocytes on the tips are continually replaced by progenitor cells originating in the crypts that differentiate and mature enzymatically as they migrate up the villus (Argenzio, 1997; Moon, 1978; 1994). The enterocyte turnover rates are slower in younger and gnotobiotic pigs, leading to less rapid repair of villous atrophy, which may contribute to the greater susceptibility of neonates to viral diarrheas (Moon, 1978; 1994). Replacement of damaged villous enterocytes by undifferentiated cells originating in crypts, that are refractory to infection by several viruses (Mebus and Newman, 1977; Pensaert et al., 1970) may partially explain the self-limiting nature of many enteric viral infections. However enteric viruses that also replicate in crypt cells may be able to replicate in the undifferentiated enterocytes which have characteristics more similar to crypt cells. Furthermore such infections may persist longer in the intestine. For example, PEDV and adenovirus both infect crypt enterocytes: PEDV appears capable of infecting regenerating cells (Pensaert, 1992); and adenovirus may persist in the intestine of infected pigs up to 45 days after exposure (Benfield, 1990; Coussement et al., 1981). In addition, the crypt hyperplasia which accompanies many enteric viral infections and increases crypt mitotic activity may predispose animals to viruses that require such rapidly dividing cells for infection.

Although these differences in viral pathogenicities can influence the severity of viral diarrheas, in the field, complex interactions among agent, host, and environment occur which further contribute to variation in the severity of enteric disease. Such factors (reviewed in Saif, 1990) include viral dose, host age, and immune status, diet, and nutrition, microbial flora, concurrent infections, hormonal influences, and environmental factors such as level of sanitation, age of weaning, level of supplemental feeding of suckling pigs, cold or heat stress, and numerous management variables. An example of a factor that influences viral pathogenicity in nursing pigs is the impact of variable levels of passive immunity on enzootic viral infections. In the field this was manifested by varied segmental distribution of villous atrophy with minimal lesions in pigs from TGEV seropositive herds with enzootic TGEV (Moxley and Olsen, 1989b). Experimentally in a pig suckling a sow previously infected with TGEV, villous atrophy was confined to the ileum and was not evident throughout most of the small intestine as seen in fully susceptible piglets (Moxley and Olsen, 1989b).

4. MULTIPLE ENTERIC VIRAL INFECTIONS

In suckling and postweaning pigs, dual or multiple enteric viral infections are common, and may be more frequent than single agent infections in post-weaning pigs (Bridger, 1990; Chu et al., 1985; Morin et al., 1983; Nagy et al., 1996; Saif et al., 1980; Theil and McCloskey, 1995). In addition dual infections with enteric viruses, and bacterial or parasitic pathogens are also frequent (Chu et al., 1985; Morin et al., 1983; Nagy et al., 1996) and in some studies such multiple infections were more common (59% of affected pigs) than single agent infections (33%) (Chu et al., 1985). Only limited data exists concerning the underlying interactive pathophysiologic mechanisms associated with multiple enteric infections in pigs. Additive or synergistic effects presumably occur in the field and have been demonstrated in some experimental studies of combined rotavirus and ETEC infections (Benfield et al., 1988; Lecce et al., 1982; Tzipori et al., 1980). For example, gnotobiotic pigs dually infected with rotavirus and ETEC had more severe clinical disease than with either pathogen alone (Benfield et al., 1988). Similarly, rotavirus infections were shown to enhance ETEC infections in postweaning pigs (Lecce et al., 1982; Tzipori et al., 1980). Although the mechanisms involved were not delineated, both virus-induced malabsorption, and enterotoxin-induced secretion would be expected to compound the diarrhea severity.

Multiple enteric viral infections are also common in individual pigs in the field. These include: coronaviruses (TGEV) and rotaviruses (Chu et al., 1985; Theil et al., 1979); caliciviruses and rotavirus (Saif et al., 1980); caliciviruses, rotaviruses, and astroviruses (Bridger, 1980; Theil and McCloskey, 1995); and coronaviruses (PEDV) and porcine reproductive, and respiratory syndrome virus (PRRSV) (Sueyoshi et al., 1996). In the latter outbreak of epidemic diarrhea in neonatal piglets, diarrhea, and dehydration were severe and piglet mortality was higher than expected with either agent alone. The PEDV antigens were detected in enterocytes of the small and large intestine and PRRSV antigens were present in macrophages in the lamina propria, Peyer's patches, and mesenteric lymph nodes of infected pigs. Although the interactive pathogenic mechanisms in these dual or multiple enteric viral infection were not elucidated, in the latter scenario PRRSV infection of intestinal macrophages in neonatal pigs may have destroyed these cells or compromised their function, thereby facilitating, and enhancing the severity of PEDV infection, leading to increased piglet mortality.

Because enteric viruses have predilections for different regions of the villus and small intestine, it is likely that dual or multiple viral infections will result in more extensive villous atrophy throughout greater regions of the intestine. Superimposing viruses that also infect crypt enterocytes (PEDV, adenovirus, parvovirus) with ones that infect villous enterocytes, results in destruction of villous and crypt enterocytes, impairing both the absorptive and regenerative capacity of the mucosa. More severe diarrhea and delayed clinical recovery is expected in such cases. Although multiple infections are common in the field, most of our understanding of disease mechanisms has been derived from studies of single agent infections. Thus there is a paucity of information regarding the pathophysiologic and interactive mechanisms contributing to diarrhea in multiple infections. This area should receive a higher research priority in the future to better address the field situation, especially as related to current high intensity swine production systems.

5. THERAPEUTIC APPROACHES TO ENHANCE MUCOSAL REPAIR AND RECOVERY FROM ENTERIC VIRAL INFECTIONS

New concepts of the pathophysiology of diarrheal diseases and potentially new therapeutic strategies are emerging based on recent knowledge of neuro-endocrine-immune communication in the intestine (Argenzio, 1997; Blikslager and Roberts, 1997). In response to enterotoxigenic bacteria and invasive pathogens, the host intestinal neuroimmune system and the mediators released (cytokines, prostaglandins, serotonin, VIP, etc) can directly and indirectly affect enterocytes and through the enteric nervous system can amplify the range and magnitude of a local stimulus. For example, recent evidence indicates that at least 60% of the cholera toxin-induced secretory response is indirectly neurally mediated in vivo (Argenzio, 1997). Thus host factors produced in response to infection by an enteric pathogen can directly contribute to the diarrheal response.

Although the pathophysiologies of viral-induced diarrheas have been less studied than bacterial or parasite-induced diarrheas, several recent concepts have emerged with important implications for clinical treatment of viral diarrheas. For both TGEV and rotavirus infections of pigs, it was shown that the neutral NaCl absorptive mechanisms were preserved, in spite of villous atrophy, but substrate-linked absorptive processes (eg coupled Na-Glucose transport) were impaired (Homaidon et al., 1991; Rhoads et al., 1991). These results indicate that the immature, undifferentiated cells retain the NaCl absorptive process, but the substrate-linked absorptive processes of the mature villous enterocytes are lost. Thus oral rehydration fluids and treatments designed to optimize the residual NaCl absorption process (addition of glutamine to such fluids or treatment with calcium blocking agents) should be useful therapeutically to treat viral diarrheas (Homaidon et al., 1991; Rhoads et al., 1991). In addition glutamine, which is the major fuel of the small intestine also promotes enterocyte proliferation (Blikslager and Roberts, 1997).

Altered intestinal ion transport is also mediated by the host inflammatory response (Argenzio, 1997). Inflammation induced by enteric viral infections is less pronounced than after many bacterial/parasite infections (Saif, Rosen, and Parwani, 1994; Sueyoshi et al., 1996; Theil, 1990) and it may also be a secondary consequence of the massive cytolytic destruction of villous enterocytes and secondary bacterial infections. The impact of cytokines released by inflammatory cells on stimulation of prostaglandins and their direct, and indirect effects on increased chloride-secretion by enterocytes (secretory diarrhea) has not been examined for enteric viral infections. Moreover inflammation can also disrupt mucosal integrity and create leaky membranes, further allowing translocation of bacteria and toxins across the intestinal epithelial barrier and initiation of systemic infections (Blikslager and Roberts, 1997). In this regard, transient increases in macromolecular permeability were observed in piglets infected with rotavirus or coronavirus (Moon, 1994) and in vitro studies showed that rotavirus infection led to enhanced toxin uptake into cells (Liprandi et al., 1997).

A number of potential therapeutic agents have been proposed as aids to enhance intestinal mucosal repair, but their impact on recovery from enteric viral infections has not been widely assessed. These include polyamines and growth factors (TGFα, EGF) to stimulate epithelial restitution and proliferation and prostaglandins to stimulate closure of tight junctions (Argenzio, 1997). In a recent study by (Zijlstra et al., 1994) supraphysiological doses of human recombinant EGF were beneficial in stimulating recovery of intestinal epithelium in rotavirus-infected pigs, but only in the proximal mid small intestine.

6. IMMUNIZATION APPROACHES TO CONTROL ENTERIC VIRAL INFECTIONS

The localized nature of most enteric viral infections is of major consideration for designing effective immunization strategies to induce intestinal immunity. However, only limited success has been achieved in the development of vaccines to prevent viral diarrheas (Saif and Jackwood, 1990; Saif and Wesley, 1992; Saif, 1996; 1998; Saif and Fernandez, 1996; Saif et al., 1997; Yuan et al., 1997). Commercial vaccines show limited efficacy in the field, including oral modified live or parenterally-administered vaccines to prevent coronavirus and rotavirus-induced diarrhea in swine (Saif and Jackwood, 1990; Saif and Wesley, 1992; Saif, 1996; 1998, Saif and Fernandez, 1996; Saif et al., 1997; Yuan et al., 1997). The existence of multiple serogroups and serotypes of porcine rotaviruses further complicates vaccine design (Paul and Stevenson, 1992; Saif and Jiang, 1994; Saif, Rosen, and Parwani, 1994; Theil, 1990).

A unique mucosal immune system, distinct from the systemic immune system has evolved to protect mucosal surfaces from pathogens (Reviewed in McGhee et al., 1992; Saif, 1996; 1998; Walker, 1994). The mucosal immune system is characterized by a ponderance of secretory (S) IgA antibodies in mucosal secretions produced by underlying plasma cells in the lamina propria. The dimeric IgA antibodies produced are selectively transported via the polymeric immunoglobulin receptor (secretory component) which is produced by crypt epithelial cells and expressed on their basolateral surface. The transported SIgA antibodies are then secreted onto mucosal surfaces. In addition, in the process of transport of dimeric IgA through epithelial cells via the polymeric Ig receptor, the IgA may function to transport viruses as immune complexes back to the intestinal lumen (Kaetzel et al., 1992) and may also inhibit intracellular viral replication or assembly (Armstrong and Dimmock, 1992; Marzanec et al., 1992; Burns et al., 1996). Although potential mechanisms for intracellular inhibition or neutralization of viral replication by SIgA are poorly understood, these findings if confirmed in vivo imply that SIgA might also promote recovery from viral infections as well as protection from reinfection. Another hallmark of the common mucosal immune system is the induction of immune responses at one mucosal site and the trafficking of effector mucosal lymphoid cells to distant mucosal sites as well as back to the site of origin (McGhee et al., 1992; Saif, 1996; 1998; Walker, 1994). For the intestine, M cells overlying Peyer's patches are specialized epithelial cells for transporting antigens from the lumen to the follicle underneath, a major inductive site for IgA responses. However compartmentalization exists within this system such that antigen stimulation at one mucosal site does not always lead to optimal protection at a distant mucosal site. This concept was confirmed by recent studies showing that use of respiratory PRCV vaccines induced poor intestinal immune responses and only partial protective immunity to enteric TGEV challenge (Saif, 1996; 1998).

Immunization strategies to induce passive and active immunity to enteric viruses in pigs have utilized porcine coronaviruses (TGEV and PRCV) and rotaviruses as models (Saif and Jackwood, 1990; Saif and Wesley, 1992; Saif, 1996; 1998, Saif and Fernandez, 1996; Saif et al., 1997; Yuan et al., 1997). Such studies revealed that the highest level of passive or active protective immunity against TGEV in pigs was achieved by oral immunization of sows or pigs with virulent TGEV and was correlated with the induction of SIgA antibodies in milk (passive immunity) or IgA antibody secreting cells (ASC) in the intestine (active immunity) (Saif and Jackwood, 1990; Saif and Wesley, 1992; Saif, 1996; 1998). The live respiratory coronavirus (PRCV) and a modified live TGEV vaccine induced only low levels of IgA antibodies to TGEV in the milk of vaccinated sows, few IgA ASC in the intestine of vaccinated pigs and only partial protection against TGEV challenge of piglets. A high dose of attenuated TGEV vaccine (10^8 PFU), much greater (3–4 logs) than used in commercial vaccines, was required to induce even low numbers of IgA ASC in the intestine (Saif, 1996; 1998) and this finding may partially explain the failure of modified live TGEV vaccines in the field (Saif and Wesley, 1992; Moxley and Olson, 1989a). Likewise for immunity to rotavirus, attenuated or inactivated rotavirus vaccines administered orally or parenterally to pigs induced few or no intestinal IgA ASC, and only partial or little protective immunity, respectively (Yuan et al., 1997). Complete protection was achieved only by virulent rotavirus and was correlated with induction of high numbers of intestinal IgA ASC (Saif and Fernandez, 1996; Saif et al., 1997; Saif, 1998).

Thus to date live oral vaccines (which presumably increase vaccine dose by intestinal replication) have been more effective than parenterally administered, or killed or subunit vaccines to induce intestinal immunity to enteric viruses, but remain less effective than the enteropathogenic viruses (which are often more stable and replicate more extensively in the intestine). Live vaccines including live recombinant organisms, because of the amplification of dose and potential targeting to intestinal M cells are likely to remain promising candidates for oral vaccines to induce mucosal immunity. However new technologies are under development to overcome at least two problems specific to oral immunization, especially using non-living vaccines: delivery of intact antigens to key mucosal lymphoid tissues (M cells of Peyer's Patches) and enhancement of immune responses within these tissues. New technologies for oral antigen delivery include use of adhesion molecules or antigens conjugated to adhesion molecules [bacterial pili, *E. coli* LT or cholera toxin (CT), etc], microspheres, liposomes, and rotavirus-like particles (McGhee et al., 1992; Saif, 1996; 1998; Saif and Fernandez, 1996; Walker, 1994). Mucosal adjuvants include avridine (a lipoidal amine), proteosomes, muramyl dipeptide, LPS, and lipid A, selected cytokines, immune stimulating complexes (ISCOMS), CT, and LT enterotoxins (McGhee et al., 1992; Saif, 1996; 1998; Saif and Fernandez, 1996; Walker, 1994). These new delivery systems and adjuvants may provide an effective means for delivery and enhanced intestinal immune responses to future recombinant vectored viral vaccines or subunit viral vaccines administered orally.

An exciting new approach with the potential to create transgenic sows which would secrete TGEV antibodies in milk and provide passive immunity against TGEV to suckling pigs has recently been proposed by Castilla, et al. (1998). This concept involves creating transgenic animals secreting a recombinant monoclonal antibody (MAb) neutralizing TGEV into the milk. To date this TGEV MAb gene has been successfully expressed in the milk of transgenic mice (Castilla et al., 1998). However, further work is needed to create transgenic lines of swine stably expressing the recombinant MAb in milk and to confirm the efficacy of this engineered milk for conferring lactogenic immunity to TGEV in suckling pigs (Saif and Wheeler, 1998).

REFERENCES

Argenzio, R.A., 1997, Neuro-immune pathobiology of infectious enteric disease. In *Mechanisms in the Pathogenesis of Enteric Diseases*, Editors: Paul, P., Francis, D., Benfield, D., Plenum Press, New York, pp. 21–30.

Armstrong, S.J. and Dimmock, N.J., 1992, Neutralization of influenza virus by low concentrations of hemagglutination-specific polymeric IgA inhibits viral fusion activity, but activation of the ribonucleoprotein is also inhibited, Virol. 66:3823–3832.

Ball, J.M., Peng, T., Zeng, C.Q.-Y., Morris, A.P., and Estes, M.K., 1996, Age-dependent diarrhea induced by a rotaviral nonstructural glycoprotein, Science 272:101–104.

Benfield, D.A., Francis, D.H., McAdaragh, J.P. Johnson, D.D., Bergeland, M.E., Rossow, K., and Moore, R., 1988, Combined rotavirus and K99 *Escherichia coli* infection in gnotobiotic pigs. Am. J. Vet. Res. 49:330–337.

Benfield, D., 1990, Enteric adenoviruses of animals. In *Viral Diarrheas of Man and Animals*. Editor: Saif, L.J. and Theil, K.W., CRC Press, Boca Raton, Florida, pp. 115–136.

Blikslager, A.T. and Roberts, M.C., 1997, Mechanisms of intestinal mucosal repair. J. Am. Vet. Med. Assoc. 211:1437–1441.

Bridger, J.C., 1980, Detection by electron microscopy of caliciviruses, astroviruses, and rotavirus-like particles in the feces of piglets with diarrhea, Vet. Rec. 107:532–533.

Bridger, J.C., 1990, Small viruses associated with gastroenteritis in animals. In *Viral Diarrheas of Man and Animals*, Editors: Saif, L.J. and Theil, K.W. CRC Press, Boca Raton, Florid, pp. 161–184.

Burns, J.W., Siadat-Pajouh, M., Krishnaney, A.A., and Greenberg, H.B., 1996, Protective effect of rotavirus VP6-specific IgA monoclonal antibodies that lack neutralizing activity, Science 272:104–107.

Castilla, J., Pintado, B., Sola, I., Sanchez-Morgado, J.M., and Enjuanes, L., 1998, Engineering passive immunity in transgenic mice secreting virus-neutralizing antibodies in milk, Nature Biotech 16:349–354.

Chasey, D., Bridger, J.C., and McCrae, M.A., 1986, A new type of atypical rotavirus in pigs, Arch. Virol. 89:235–243.

Chasey, D. and Cartwright, S.F., 1978, Virus-like particles associated with porcine epidemic diarrhea, Res. Vet. Sci. 25:255–256.

Chu, R.M., Yang, P.C., and Chang, W.F., 1985, Neonatal diarrhoea of pigs in Taiwan: aetiology, epidemiology, and treatment. In *Infectious Diarrhea in the Young*, Editors: Tzipori, S., Excerpta Medica, Amsterdam, p. 151–155.

Coussement, W., Ducatelle, R., Charlier, G., and Hoorens, J., 1981, Adenovirus enteritis in pigs, Am. J. Vet. Res. 42:1905–1911.

Dong, Y.-J., Zeng, C.Q-Y., Ball, J.M., Estes, M.K., and Morris, A.P., 1997, The rotavirus enterotoxin NSP4 mobilizes intracellular calcium in human intestinal cells by stimulating phospholipase C mediated inositol 1,4,5-triphosphate production, Proc. Natl. Acad. Sci. USA 94:3960–3965.

Doyle, L.P. and Hutchings, L.M., 1946, A transmissible gastroenteritis in pigs, J. Am. Vet. Med. Assoc. 108:257–259.

Flynn, W.T., Saif, L.J., and Moorhead, P.D., 1988, Pathogenesis of a porcine enteric calicivirus in gnotobiotic pigs, Am. J. Vet. Res. 49:819–828.

Homaidan, F.R., Torres, A., Donowitz, M., and Sharp, G.W.G., 1991, Electrolyte transport in piglets infected with transmissible gastroenteritis virus, Gastroenterology 101:895–901.

Kaetzel, C.S., Robinson, J.K., Chintalacharuvir, K.R., Vaerman, J.P., and Lamm, M.E., 1992, The polymeric immunoglobulin receptor secretory component mediates transport of immune complexes across epithelial cells, Proc. Natl. Acad. Sci. USA 88:8796–8800.

Kroneman, A., Cornelissen, A.H.M., Horzinek, M.C., deGroot, R.J., and Egberink, H.F., 1998, Identification and characterization of a porcine torovirus, J. Virol. 72:3507–3511.

Lecce, J.G., Balsbaugh, R.K., Clare, D.A., and King, M.W., 1982, Rotavirus and hemolytic enteropathogenic *Escherichia coli* in weanling diarrhea of pigs, J. Clin. Microbiol. 16:715–723.

Liprandi, F., Moros, Z., Gerder, M., Ludert, J.E., Pujol, F.H., Ruiz, M.C., Michelangeli, F., Charpilliene, A., and Cohen, J., 1997, Productive penetration of rotavirus in cultured cells induces coentry of the translator inhibitor alpha-sarcin, Virol. 237:430–438.

Marzanec, M.B., Kaetzel, C.S., Lamm, M.E., Fletcher, D., and Nerud, J.G., 1992, Intracellular neutralization of virus by IgA antibodies, Proc. Natl. Acad. Sci. USA 89:6901–6905.

McGhee, J.R., Mestecky, J., Dertzbaugh, M.T., Eldridge, J.H., Hirasawa, M., and Kiyono, H., 1992, The mucosal immune system: from fundamental concepts to vaccine development. Vaccine 10:75–88.

Mebus, C.A. and Newman, L.E., 1977, Scanning electron, light and immunofluorescent microscopy of intestine of gnotobiotic calf infected with reovirus-like agent, Am. J. Vet. Res. 38:553–558.

Moon, H.W., 1978, Mechanisms in the pathogenesis of diarrhea: a review, J. Am. Vet. Med. Assoc. 172:443–448.

Moon, H.W., 1994, Pathophysiology of viral diarrhea. In: *Viral Infections of the Gastrointestinal Tract*, 2nd edition, Editor: Kapikian, A.Z., Marcel Dekker, Inc, New York, pp. 27–52.

Morin, M., Turgeon, D., Jolette, J., Robinson, Y., Phaneuf, J.B., Sauvageau, R., Beauregard, M., Teuscher, E., Higgins, R., and Lariviere, S., 1983, Neonatal diarrhea of pigs in Quebec: infectious causes of significant outbreaks, Can. J. Comp. Med. 47:11–17.

Moxley, R.A. and Olson, L.D., 1989a, Clinical evaluation of TGE virus vaccines and vaccination procedures for inducing lactogenic immunity in sows, Am. J. Vet. Res. 50:111–118.

Moxley, R.A. and Olson, L.D., 1989b, Lesions of TGE virus infection in experimentally inoculated pigs suckling immunized sows, Am. J. Vet. Res. 50:708–716.

Nagy, B., Nagy, G.Y., Meder, M., and Moscari, E., 1996, Enterotoxigenic *E. coli*, rotavirus, porcine epidemic diarrhoea virus, adenovirus, and calici-like virus in porcine postweaning diarrhoea in Hungary, Acta Veterinaria Hungarica 44:9–19.

Paul, P.S. and Stevenson, G.W., 1992, Rotavirus and reovirus, In: *Diseases of Swine*, Editors: Leman, A.D. et al., Iowa State University Press. Ames, Iowa, pp. 331–348.

Pensaert, M., Haelterman, E.O., and Burnstein, T., 1970, Transmissible gastroenteritis of swine: virus-intestinal cell interactions. I. Immunofluorescence, histopathology, and virus production in the small intestine through the course of infection, Archiv fur die Gesamte Virusforschung 31:321–334.

Pensaert, M.B. and deBouck, P., 1978, A new coronavirus-like particle associated with diarrhea in swine, Arch. Virol. 58:243–247.

Pensaert, M.B., 1992, Porcine epidemic diarrhea, In: *Diseases of Swine*, Editors: Leman, A.D. et al., Iowa State University Press, Ames, Iowa, pp. 293–298.

Rhoads, J.M., Keku, E.O., Quinn, J., Wooseley, J., and Leece, J.G., 1991, L-glutamine stimulates jejunal sodium and chloride absorption in pig rotavirus enteritis, Gastroenterol. 100:683–669.

Rodger, S.M., Craven, J.A., and Williams, I., 1975, Demonstration of reovirus-like particles in intestinal contents of piglets with diarrhea, Aust. Vet. J., 51:536.

Rossen, J.W.A., Bekker, C.P.J., Strous, G.J.A.M., Horzinek, M.C., Dveksler, G.S., Holmes, K.V., and Rottier, P.J.M., 1996, A murine and a porcine coronavirus are released from opposite surfaces of the same epithelial cells, Virol. 224:345–351.

Saif, L.J., Bohl, E.H., Theil, K.W., Cross, R.F., and House, J.A., 1980, Rotavirus-like, calicivirus-like, and 23-nm virus-like particles associated with diarrhea in young pigs, J. Clin. Microbiol. 12:105–111.

Saif, L.J., Bohl, E.H., Theil, K.W., Kohler, E.M., and Cross, R.F., 1980, 30 nm virus-like particles resembling astrovirus in intestinal contents of a diarrheic pig, Conference of Research Workers in Animal Diseases, Abst. 149.

Saif, L.J., 1990, Comparative aspects of enteric viral infections, In: *Viral Diarrheas of Man and Animals*. Editors: Saif, L.J. and Theil, K.W., CRC Press, Boca Raton, Florida, pp. 9–31.

Saif, L.J. and Jackwood, D.J., 1990, Enteric virus vaccines: Theoretical considerations, current status, and future approaches, In: *Viral Diarrheas of Man and Animals*, Editors: Saif, L.J. and Theil, K.W., CRC Press, Boca Raton, Florida, pp. 313–329.

Saif, L.J. and Wesley, R., 1992, Transmissible gastroenteritis virus, In: *Diseases of Swine*, Editor: Leman, A.D. et al., Iowa State University Press, Ames, Iowa, pp. 293–298.

Saif, L.J. and Jiang, B.M., 1994, Nongroup A rotaviruses, In: *Rotaviruses*. Editor: Ramig, R.F., Current Topics in Microbiol and Immunology, Springer-Verlag, New York, 185:339–371.

Saif, L.J., Rosen, B., and Parwani, A., 1994, Animal Rotaviruses, In: *Virus Infections of the Gastrointestinal Tract*, 2nd edition, Editor: Kapikian, A.Z., Marcel-Dekker, Inc., New York, pp. 279–367.

Saif, L.J., 1996, Mucosal immunity: an overview and studies of enteric and respiratory coronavirus infections in a swine model of enteric disease, Vet. Immunol. Immunopathol. 54:163–169.

Saif, L.J. and Fernandez, F., 1996, Group A rotavirus veterinary vaccines, J. Infect. Dis. 171:S98–106.

Saif, L.J., Yuan, L., Ward, L., and To. T., 1997, Comparative studies of the pathogenesis, antibody immune responses, and homologous protection to porcine and human rotaviruses in gnotobiotic piglets, In: *Mechanisms in the Pathogenesis of Enteric Diseases*. Editors: Paul, P., Francis, D., and Benfield, D., Plenum Press, New York, pp. 397–403.

Saif, L.J., 1998, Enteric viral infections of pigs and strategies for induction of mucosal immunity, In: *Advances in Veterinary Science Comparative Medicine*, Editor: Shultz, R., Academic Press, (in press).

Saif, L.J. and Wheeler, M.B., 1998, WAPping gastroenteritis with transgenic antibodies, Nature Biotech 16:334–335.

Scott, A.C., Chaplin, M.J., Stack, M.J., and Lund, L.J., 1987, Porcine torovirus, Vet. Rec. 120:583.

Sueyoshi, M., Tanaka, T., Tsuda, T., Sato, K., and Ogawa, T., 1996, Concurrent infection with porcine reproductive and respiratory syndrome (PRRS) virus, and porcine epidemic diarrhea (PED) virus in pigs, Conference of Research Workers in Animal Diseases, Abst P37.

Theil, K.W., Saif, L.J., Bohl, E.H., et al., 1979, Concurrent porcine rotaviral and transmissible gastroenteritis viral infections in a 3-day-old conventional pig, Am. J. Vet. Res. 40:719–721.

Theil, K.W. and McCloskey, C.M., 1995, Detection of small round viruses in fecal specimens from recently weaned pigs by IEM using pooled weaned pig serum. Conference of Research Workers in Animal Diseases, Abst. 110.

Theil, K.W., 1990, Group A rotaviruses, In: *Viral Diarrheas of Man and Animals*, Editors: Saif, L.J. and Theil, K.W., CRC Press, Boca Raton, Florida, pp. 35–72.

Tzipori, S., Chandler, D., Makin, T., and Smith, M., 1980, *Escherichia coli* and rotavirus infections in four-week-old gnotobiotic piglets fed milk or dry food, Aust. Vet. J. 56:279–284.

Walker, R.I., 1994, New strategies for using mucosal vaccination to achieve more effective immunization, Vaccine 12:387–400.

Yuan, L., Ward, L.A., To, T.L., and Saif, L.J., 1997, Systemic and intestinal antibody-secreting cell responses to inactivated human rotavirus in a gnotobiotic pig model of diarrhea disease, J. Virol. 70:3075–3083.

Yasuhara, H., Matsui, O., Hirahara, T., Ohgitani, M., Tanaka, M., Kodama, K., Nakai, M., and Sasaki, N., 1989, Characterization of a parvovirus isolated from the diarrheic feces of a pig, Jpn. J. Vet. Sci. 51:337–344.

Yasuhara, H., Yamanaka, M., Izumida, A., Hirahara, T., Nakai, M., and Inaba, Y., 1995, Experimental infection of pigs with a parvovirus isolated from the diarrheic feces of a pig, Jpn. J. Vet. Sci. 51:337–344.

Zhang, M., Zeng, C.Q.Y., Ball, J.M., Saif, L.J., Morris, A.P., and Estes, M.K., 1998. Mutations in rotavirus nonstructural glycoprotein NSP4 in associated with altered virus virulence, J. Virol. 72:3666–3672.

Zijlstra, R.T., Odle, J., Hall, W.F., Petschow, B.W., Gelberg, H.B., and Litov, R.E., 1994, Effect of orally administered epidermal growth factor on intestinal recovery of neonatal pigs infected with rotavirus, J. Pediatr. Gastroenterol. Nutr. 19:382–389.

5

MOLECULAR EVOLUTION OF CORONA- AND TOROVIRUSES

Marian C. Horzinek

Head Virology Unit
Veterinary Faculty
Utrecht University
The Netherlands

Coronaviruses belong to the newly established *Nidovirales*—the second order (in addition to the *Mononegavirales*) in animal virus taxonomy. They comprise a group of enveloped, positive-stranded RNA viruses infecting mammals and birds. The order consists of the bigeneric family *Coronaviridae*, to which the genera *Coronavirus* and *Torovirus* have been assigned, and the monogeneric family *Arteriviridae* (Murphy et al., 1995).

Despite essential differences in genetic complexity and virion architecture between corona-, toro-, and arteriviruses, they show a striking resemblance in genome organization and replication strategy, which have been viewed as an overriding principle by the ICTV (Murphy et al., 1995) and resulted in the present classification. The name *Nidovirales* (from the Latin *nidus*, nest) refers to the 3' co-terminal nested set of subgenomic viral mRNAs that is produced during infection. Sequence similarities, though mostly restricted to the polyprotein (POL) 1b, from which the replicase-associated proteins are derived, indicate that the *Nidovirales* are phylogenetically related and may have evolved from a common ancestor. Extensive genome rearrangements through heterologous RNA recombination have resulted in a set of viruses that utilize similar replication and transcription mechanisms, but disparate strategies to package their genetic information. For a recent review, see de Vries et al. (1997).

The phylogenetic relationship between viruses in the *Nidovirales* order is not apparent from their morphology. Coronavirions are roughly spherical, 100–120 nm in diameter, and display a typical fringe of 20 nm long petal shaped spikes (peplomers). Some coronaviruses exhibit a second fringe of smaller surface projections about 5 nm in length. Torovirus particles are more pleiomorphic, spherical, oval, elongated and kidney-shaped, measuring 120 to 140 nm in their largest axis. The surface projections of toroviruses closely resemble the coronavirus peplomers. The differences in virion

Mechanisms in the Pathogenesis of Enteric Diseases 2, edited by Paul and Francis.
Kluwer Academic / Plenum Publishers, New York, 1999.

architecture become even more apparent when comparing the nucleocapsid structures. Coronaviruses possess a loosely wound, helical inner ribonucleoprotein structure and a capsid of supposedly icosahedral disposition (Risco et al., 1996), while the torovirus nucleocapsid has a compact tubular organization and exhibits kidney, disc or rod shapes in ultra-thin sections (for reviews, see Koopmans and Horzinek, 1994; Snijder and Horzinek, 1993). In view of these observations, it is not surprising that the nucleocapsid proteins (N) of the *Nidovirales* differ considerably both in sequence and in size (50, 19, and 14 kDa for corona-, toro-, and arteriviruses, respectively) and are completely unrelated.

There are also differences in the composition of the viral envelopes. The membrane of coronaviruses invariably contain (i) the 180–200 kDa spike protein (S), (ii) the 25–30 kDa triple-spanning membrane protein M, and (iii) the 9 kDa transmembrane protein E, a minor protein species, but together with M essential for virus assembly. The shorter surface projections of some coronaviruses mentioned above consist of a dimer of a 65 kDa class I membrane protein, the hemagglutin-esterase (HE), sharing 30% sequence identity with the N-terminal subunit of the hemagglutinin-esterase fusion protein (HEF) of influenza C virus. Apparently, this gene was acquired via heterologous RNA recombination, as will be discussed below.

Toroviruses also specify a 180 kDa S and a 26 kDa triple spanning M protein. Although primary sequence similarity is absent, the S and M proteins of toro- and coronaviruses are similar in size and function. There are also structural similarities: the M proteins have the same membrane topology; furthermore, heptad repeats, indicative for a coiled-coil structure first discovered in the spike proteins of coronaviruses, are also found in the torovirus peplomer. Thus, the S and M genes of these viruses may well be phylogenetically related. Toroviruses lack a homologue for the coronavirus E protein, which could indicate a key difference in their mode of assembly. The presence of a third membrane protein, the 65 kDa hemagglutinin-esterase, will be discussed in detail.

FELINE INFECTIOUS PERITONITIS

The members of the genus *Coronavirus* have been assigned to three clusters, with the prototypes mouse hepatitis virus, porcine transmissible gastroenteritis virus (to which also the feline coronaviruses belong) and avian infectious bronchitis virus, based on serological and genetic properties.

When considering molecular evolution, coronaviruses are a showcase of biologic (antigenic) and pathogenetic variability. Feline infectious peritonitis (FIP) is arguably the most enigmatic coronaviral disease, its etiology, pathobiology, and immunology having been explained largely by the Davis group of workers (Pedersen, 1976a, b; Pedersen, 1987; Pedersen et al., 1984). It is infrequent but fatal, involves immune-mediated phenomena such as antibody-dependent enhancement of infection and shows immune-complex induced pathology. The existence of a carrier-state of a harmless enteric precursor virus (conveniently termed feline enteric coronavirus; FCoV) has recently been formally proven (Herrewegh et al., 1997). The sporadic occurrence of the condition is interpreted as the result of *in-vivo* mutants that have acquired macrophage tropism—a hypothesis first formulated by Niels Pedersen.

Feline infectious peritonitis is a progressive, debilitating lethal disease of domestic and wild *Felidae*. The initial signs of naturally occurring FIP are not very characteristic. The affected cats show anorexia, chronic fever, and malaise. Occasionally, ocular and neurological disorders occur. In classical "wet" or effusive FIP these signs are accompanied by a gradual abdominal distension due to the accumulation of a viscous yellow ascitic fluid. The quantity of fluid can vary from a few milliliters to well over a liter.—There is also the "dry" or non-effusive form of FIP where little or no exudate is present. The wet and dry forms of FIP are different manifestations of the same infection. For a recent review, see Groot and Horzinek (1995).

Pathogenesis, Pathology, and Immunity

The key athogenic event leading to FIP is the infection of monocytes and macrophages. However, also the ubiquitous avirulent FCoV strains are not confined to the digestive tract and do spread beyond the intestinal epithelium and regional lymph nodes—so the difference must rather be a quantitative one. In vitro, the virulence of FCoV strains was indeed correlated with their ability to infect cultured peritoneal macrophages, the avirulent ones infected fewer macrophages and producing lower titers than virulent strains (Stoddart and Scott, 1988, 1989). Moreover, the avirulent strains were less able to sustain viral replication and to spread to other macrophages. This is no black-and-white phenomenon, rather a gradual transition, as the course of FIP is not uniform.

Humoral immunity is not protective: FCoV-seropositive cats that are experimentally challenged develop an accelerated, fulminating course of the disease, leading to the 'early death' syndrome. Clinical signs and lesions develop earlier, and the mean survival time is reduced as compared to seronegative cats. Direct evidence for the involvement of antibodies was obtained from the transfusion of purified FCoV anti-IgG into cats which developed accelerated FIP upon experimental challenge (Pedersen, 1987).

Though the vascular and perivascular lesions in FIP are thought to be immune-mediated, there is uncertainty about the actual pathogenetic mechanism. Some vascular injury may be attributed to immune-mediated lysis of infected cells: FIPV-infected white blood cells were detected in the lumen, intima, and wall of veins and in perivascular locations. Furthermore, inflammatory mediators such as cytokines, leukotrienes, and prostaglandines that are released by infected macrophages could play a role in the development of the perivascular pyogranulomas. These products could induce vascular permeability changes and provide chemotactic stimuli for neutrophils and monocytes. In response to the inflammation, the attracted cells may release additional mediators and cytotoxic substances; the monocytes would also serve as new targets for FIPV. The result would be enhanced local virus production and increased tissue damage.

Other observations point towards an immune complex (ICX) pathogenesis. Deposition of ICX and subsequent complement activation may cause an inflammatory response that extends across blood vessel walls. The resulting vascular damage would permit leakage of fluid into the intercellular space and lead to the accumulation of thoracic and abdominal exudate. The morphologic features of the vascular lesions (necrosis, polymorphonuclear cell infiltration associated with small veins and venules) indicate an Arthus type reaction. The lesions contain focal deposits of virus, IgG, and C3. Moreover, complement depletion and circulating ICX are found in cats with terminal FIP (Jacobse-Geels et al., 1980, 1982). Although FIP viruses do not infect T-cells, depletion and programmed cell death (apoptosis) has been observed in lymphoid organs of infected cats. Apoptosis was mediated by the ICX present in the serum and ascitic fluid of diseased cats (Haagmans et al., 1996).

Gross FIP lesions appear as multiple grayish-white nodules (<1 to 10 mm) in the serosal membranes, liver, lungs, spleen, omentum, intestines, and kidneys. Microscopic lesions consist of disseminated foci of necrosis and pyogranulomatous inflammation, frequently located around smaller vessels. These lesions are characterized by accumulations of fibrin and necrotic debris, and by perivascular infiltrations of macrophages, neutrophils, and lymphocytes. Histologically, disseminated perivascular pyogranulomatous inflammation and exudative fibrinous serositis in the abdominal and thoracic cavities are characteristic of the disease.

Persistent Infections and Biotypes

The fatal scenario leading to FIP may be as follows: a kitten suckled by its seropositive queen is protected by colostral antibody during the first few weeks. As the maternal antibodies wane, mucosal protection ebbs away and during an episode of maternal FCoV shedding the kitten is infected. A bout of diarrhea may be the only sign this has happened. It now develops an active immunity, but not a sterilizing one in most cases: virus and antibodies continue to co-exist in the kitten's organs, and an efficient cell-mediated immunity keeps infected macrophages and monocytes in check. In a small, socially stable cat community this animal can stay healthy.

Problems emerge when the kitten is experiencing any situation of stress, to be equated with immune suppression. Infections with FeLV or FIV are unmistakably immunosuppressive (Poland et al., 1996); Egberink et al., unpublished observations), but density (numbers of cats per surface unit), geographic change (displacement into a new environment), and other territorial factors (e.g. change in group hierarchy, dominance) are now becoming more and more important—in view of the declining prevalence of retrovirus infections. The failing immune surveillance allows the coronaviral quasispecies cloud of mutants to expand, and more macrophage-tropic mutants emerge in this stochastic process. Amongst them are some that reach high titers and outcrowd the moderate ones. This is the point when immune pathogenesis starts.

Crucial to this pathogenetic model is the evidence that coronaviruses indeed persist in individual cats—a plausible assumption based on clinical and epidemiological observations, but until recently unconfirmed. The Utrecht group has studied FCoV persistence and evolution in a closed cat breeding facility where serotype I FCoV infection was endemic (Herrewegh et al., 1995, 1997). The serotype I is represented by biotypes that are prevalent in most geographic areas, are poorly released from infected cells and usually cannot be cultivated; serotype II FCoVs are less common in the field but best-studied, and are antigenically related with canine coronaviruses.

Using the reverse transcriptase polymerase chain reaction (RT-PCR), viral RNA was detected in the feces and/or plasma of 36 out of the 42 cats tested. Of five cats, identified as FCoV shedders during an initial survey, four had detectable viral RNA in the feces when tested 111 days later. To determine whether this was due to continuous re-infection or to viral persistence, two cats were placed in strict isolation and fecal virus shedding was monitored. In one cat, shedding was found for up to seven months. The other animal was sacrificed after 124 days in order to identify the sites of virus replication. While viral genomic RNA was found in most organs tested, mRNA was detected only in the ileum, colon, and rectum. In these tissues, single FCoV-infected cells were identified by immunohistochemistry in a background of uninfected tissue.

These findings provide the first formal evidence that FCoV causes chronic enteric infections (Herrewegh et al., 1997).

To assess FCoV heterogeneity in the breeding facility and to study viral evolution during chronic infection, samples from individual cats were characterized by RT-PCR amplification of selected regions of the viral genome followed by sequence analysis. Phylogenetic comparison of nucleotides 007 to 146 of ORF7b to corresponding sequences obtained for independent European and American isolates indicated that the viruses in the breeding facility form a clade and likely have originated from a single founder infection. Comparative consensus sequence analysis of the more variable region formed by residues 079 to 478 of the S gene revealed that each cat harbored a distinct FCoV quasispecies. Moreover, FCoV appeared to be subject to immune selection during chronic infection (Herrewegh et al., 1997).

The combined data support a model in which chronically infected carriers perpetuate the endemic infection. Virtually every cat born to the breeding facility becomes infected, indicating that FCoVs are spread very efficiently. Infected cats, however, appear to resist superinfection by closely related FCoVs (Herrewegh, Ph.D.thesis Utrecht, 1997).

While the conversion of innocuous enteric coronaviruses to the lethal, FIP-inducing mutants is probably due to minute changes in one or more non-structural genes (which still need to be identified), we have recently shown that large chunks of genetic information may be shuttled between them. When studying the type II FCoV strains 79-1146 and 79-1683 (employed in most studies due to their satisfactory growth in vitro) we have found that they result from homologous RNA recombination events between FCoV type I strains and canine coronaviruses (CCV). In both cases, one template switch took place between the S and M genes, giving rise to recombinant viruses which encode a CCV-like S protein and the M, N, 7a and 7b proteins of FCoV type I (Motokawa et al., 1995; Vennema et al., 1993). Additional cross-over sites were mapped in the ORF1ab frameshifting region of strain 79-1683 and in the 5'-half of ORF 1b of strain 79-1146; this shows that the type II FCoVs have arisen from double recombination events (Herrewegh, Smeenk, Horzinek, Rottier, and de Groot 1997, unpublished results).

Serologic studies had suggested that the type II FCoVs are more closely related to CCV than to type I strains. Thus immunodominant neutralisation epitopes shared by the S proteins of CCV and FCoV type II are absent in the S of FCoV type I. The fact that the template switch occurred at different sites in strains 79-1146 and 79-1683 can only mean that they have arisen from separate recombination events. FCoV type I and CCV are the presumptive parental viruses (Motokawa et al., 1996), but the host species where the recombination took place is unknown. Cats can be experimentally infected with CCV (Barlough et al., 1984; McArdle et al., 1990, 1992; Stoddart et al., 1988), but whether CCV and FCoV readily cross species barriers in the field remains to be determined.

Two models can explain the recombination events from which the type II viruses resulted. In the most simple scenario, the recombination may have involved only two parental virus strains, with RNA replication initiating on a type I FCoV template of either negative or positive polarity (Liao and Lai, 1992), polymerase-switching to a CCV template, followed by a switch-back. Alternatively, a more complicated scheme can be envisaged in which a CCV-FCoV hybrid, arisen from a single template switch, spread into the cat population and in turn engaged in additional recombination events with (an)other type I FCoV strain(s). As explained above, FCoV type I viruses cause chronic enteric infections that may last for at least seven months (Herrewegh et al., 1997). Conceivably, persistence of FCoV would raise the odds of double infections to occur.

In general, a recombinant virus, in order to emerge and to establish itself in the field, needs not just to be viable but to have a selective advantage. Thus, the uptake of CCV sequences by the type II FCoVs may have led to increased fitness as compared to the type I FCoV. Which of the acquired genes provided the selective advantage is yet unknown. Studies on other coronaviruses have shown that the S protein plays a crucial role in eliciting protective immunity. Moreover, genetic characterization of FCoVs isolated from persistently infected cats suggested that S is subject to antigenic drift, implying that this protein is a prime target for the immune system during chronic infection. From this work, it also appeared that FCoV-infected cats develop resistance against FCoV superinfection, at least by antigenically closely related strains. Perhaps the acquisition of a CCV spike by a type I FCoV resulted in an antigenic shift, allowing the recombinant virus to escape host and/or herd immunity. However, the acquired CCV sequences may have also provided a growth advantage. In contrast to type I FCoVs, type II strains replicate efficiently in tissue culture cells and produce 50–100 fold higher titers of extracellular virus (Pedersen et al., 1984).

Both type II strains studied have retained FCoV sequences from the 5′ and 3′ end of the FCoV type I genome. One interpretation is that these FCoV sequences are required for efficient replication in the cat, and that recombinant viruses, arisen from a single template switch, are selected against. It is particularly intriguing that both strains 79-1146 and 79-1683 have retained the FCoV type I ORF1a. The POL1a polyprotein gives rise to a number of cleavage products of unknown function (reviewed in de Vries et al., 1997), some of which may be involved in specific virus-host interactions. Further genetic characterization of type II FCoVs and mapping of recombination sites will provide insight into these issues and hopefully increase our understanding of coronavirus pathobiology and evolution.

TOROVIRUSES IN UNGULATES

Thus far, two torovirus species are officially recognized: a bovine torovirus (BoTV, originally named Breda virus), evidenced in the feces of diarrheic calves (Woode, 1982), and an equine torovirus (ETV, formerly described as Berne virus), which was isolated in cell culture from rectal swabs of a horse (Weiss et al., 1983). There is serological evidence for the existence of toroviruses in other mammals (Brown et al., 1987; Weiss et al., 1984) and man (Beards et al., 1984, 1986; Brown et al., 1987, 1988; Duckmanton et al., 1997; Jamieson et al., 1998; Koopmans et al., 1993, 1997; Krishnan and Naik, 1997; Lacombe et al., 1988; Van Kruiningen et al., 1993).

During a serosurvey in Switzerland, we had already detected ETV-neutralizing antibodies in the sera of 91 out of 112 pigs tested (Weiss et al., 1984). Furthermore, several authors have reported torovirus-like particles in the feces of swine (Penrith and Gerdes, 1992; Scott et al., 1987; Woode, 1987). However, in negatively stained preparations for electron microscopy, torovirions are often pleomorphic and may appear as spherical, oval, elongated or kidney-shaped particles, carrying either a single or a double fringe of surface projections. Without additional immunological and molecular confirmation torovirions are difficult to distinguish from coronaviruses and other viral—and even non-viral—fringed particles.

A Porcine Torovirus

In a recent paper (Kroneman et al., 1998) we presented formal evidence for the existence of a porcine torovirus (PoTV). By using a reverse-transcriptase polymerase chain reaction (RT-PCR) targeted to the 3'-nontranslated region of the genome, toroviral RNA was detected in the feces of piglets. Moreover, torovirions were identified in these samples by immunoelectron microscopy. Virus shedding, as monitored by RT-PCR, started shortly after weaning and lasted for 1 or more days. Comparative sequence analysis of the N-gene indicates that PoTV is a novel torovirus closely related to, but clearly distinct from, BoTV and ETV.

The virus was detected in the feces of piglets; in fresh fecal samples, PoTV particles appeared elongated, measuring 120 nm in length and 55 nm in width. Two types of surface projections were observed, the longer of which being club-shaped, 18–20 nm in length, and most likely representing oligomers of the S protein (Horzinek et al., 1986). The shorter spikes were 6 nm long and presumably represent the HE. Surface projections of this size are also seen in BoTV, but are absent in ETV (Cornelissen et al., 1997) where the HE gene is truncated at its 5' end (Snijder et al., 1991). Preliminary observations from RT-PCR amplification and sequence analysis indicate that (like BoTV) PoTV contains an intact HE gene (A. Kroneman, Utrecht, unpublished data).

Comparative sequence analysis of the toroviral N-genes showed that BoTV and ETV are closely related, with 81% sequence identity in this region. In contrast, PoTV shared only 68% sequence identity with the N-genes of the other two viruses. The 3' non-translated regions (NTR) of PoTV, BoTV, and ETV are highly conserved, with sequence identities of about 88%. We conclude that PoTV is antigenically and genetically related to, but clearly distinct from the bovine and equine representatives of the torovirus genus and should therefore be considered as a new member species.

In a heterotypic *in vitro* neutralization assay, >80% of the adult sows in the Netherlands turned out to be positive for torovirus antibody; we had reported similar observations for Switzerland (Weiss et al., 1984). In pigs, torovirus infections are obviously as common and widespread as in cattle and horses. Piglets are infected shortly after weaning, when protection by maternal antibodies and/or lactogenic immunity has waned. Virus shedding in the feces, as monitored by RT-PCR, lasted between one to nine days, which suggests that PoTV can cause acute enteric infections.

The high percentage of seropositive animals and the time of infection shortly after weaning, when maternal immune protection has waned, is indicative for PoTV endemicity. The virus would persist on a farm because of the continuous presence of susceptible piglets and reinfection of partly immune animals. Also chronically infected carriers may exist, as has been demonstrated for other *Nidovirales* such as coronaviruses (Crouch et al., 1985; Herrewegh et al., 1995) and arteriviruses (for a review, see Plagemann and Moennig (1992). A more sensitive nested RT-PCR targeted to the conserved 3' NTR may allow the identification of long-term shedders among the adult pig population.

Recombination in Toroviruses

RNA viruses are genetically very flexible—they lack the proofreading mechanisms that operate during DNA replication. When RNA genomes are replicated, nucleotide substitutions occur at a high frequency, thereby allowing swift adaptation to selective pressure. For some viruses, homologous RNA recombination, i.e. genetic exchange between closely related RNA molecules, functions as a correction mechanism counteracting genetic drift and Muller's ratchet (Chao, 1990). At the same time, it allows the rapid horizontal spread of advantageous mutations (for a review on RNA recombination, see Lai, 1992). Heterologous RNA recombination involves non-related RNA molecules and provides a means to acquire blocks or "modules" of new genetic information either from other viruses or from the host (Goldbach and Wellink, 1988; Strauss and Strauss, 1988, 1991; Zimmern, 1987).

One remarkable example of heterologous recombination is that of the corona-virus hemagglutinin-esterase (HE) gene. In addition to the spike- (S), membrane (M), envelope (E), and nucleocapsid protein (N), some coronavirus species possess a fifth structural protein, HE (for a review, see Brian et al., 1995). This 65 kDa class I membrane protein shares 30% amino acid identity with the HE-1 subunit of the hemagglutinin-esterase fusion protein (HEF) of influenza C virus (ICV), a negative-stranded RNA virus with a segmented genome (Brian et al., 1995; Luytjes et al., 1988). It has been speculated that coronaviruses have captured the HE-module from ICV or a related virus during a mixed infection (Luytjes et al., 1988). Presumably, this event occurred after coronavirus speciation, since the HE gene is present only in the genomes of viruses related to mouse hepatitis virus (MHV), and is absent in the antigenic coro-navirus clusters represented by FIPV and infectious bronchitis virus (IBV) (Luytjes, 1995). Both in ICV and in coronaviruses, the HE displays an acetylesterase activity specific for N-acetyl-9-O-acetylneuraminic acid. The ICV HEF serves as a receptor-binding/receptor-destroying protein (Herrler et al., 1988; Vlasak et al., 1987) and it has been suggested that the coronavirus HE has similar functions (Parker et al., 1989; Vlasak et al., 1988).

We have reported HE-like sequences to occur also in the genome of ETV (Snijder et al., 1991). The equine isolate is the only torovirus that can be grown in tissue culture and is therefore the best studied. The 3'-most 15 kb of its 25–30 kb genome have been sequenced, identifying the genes for POL1b, S, M, and N (Snijder and Horzinek, 1995). In addition, a non-functional open reading frame, ORF4, was found. Translation of this ORF yielded a polypeptide sequence 30% identical to the C-terminal 142 amino acids of the HE(−1) proteins of ICV and coronavirus. These findings have led to the hypoth-esis that the HE may be part of the toroviral standard gene repertoire, and that ETV is a mutant that has lost part of its HE gene during tissue culture adaptation (Snijder et al., 1991).

During the recent genetic characterization of a BoTV strain (Breda 2), which is antigenically closely related to ETV, evidence has been provided that it carries an intact, functional gene for an HE homologue, and that the toroviral HE is a structural protein. Its origin is unknown. Although corona- and toroviruses are related, they apparently acquired their HE genes through separate heterologous RNA recom-bination events. This is best illustrated by the fact that the HE genes are located at different positions in their genomes, Snijder and Horzinek, 1995; Snijder et al., 1991; Cornelissen et al., 1997). It is also of interest that the HE sequences of ICV, corona- and toroviruses are evolutionary equidistant and that several amino acid motives, conserved in the HE(−1) of ICV and torovirus, have been lost in the coronavirus HE (Cornelissen et al., 1997). We have offered the hypothesis that ICV, coronaviruses and toroviruses each have acquired the HE-module independently from yet another source, perhaps by recombination with a host mRNA.

In general, recombinant viruses will be lost from the viral population unless the acquired genetic information results in a gain of fitness. Apparently, the HE provides a considerable selective advantage, at least during the natural infection. The role of the ICV HEF in receptor binding and entry is well-established (Herrler et al., 1988), but the function of the HE-proteins of corona- and toroviruses is not exactly known. For coronaviruses, receptor-binding and membrane fusion is mediated by the S-protein (Cavanagh, 1995). It has been suggested that the coronavirus HE may serve as an additional receptor-binding protein (Parker et al., 1989; Vlasak et al., 1988). However, recent findings suggest that MHV-infection cannot be mediated by HE alone, but requires the interaction of S with its receptor (Gagneten et al., 1995). Perhaps, HE does not play a role in viral entry but at an even earlier step of the infection. ICV, corona-, and toroviruses infect the epithelial cells of the respiratory and enteric tract. These cells are protected by a mucus layer, a gel formed by non-covalent interactions between large, highly hydrated glycoproteins, that can be up to 400 □m thick (for a review, see Mantle and Allen, 1989). This mucus layer thus presents a formidable barrier that has to be traversed before adsorption to the host cell can occur. The HE proteins may mediate viral adherence to the intestinal wall through the specific, yet reversible binding to mucopolysaccharides. In fact, the process of binding to 9-*O*-acetylated receptors, followed by cleavage and rebinding to intact receptors could, theoretically, even result in virus migration through the mucus layer and thereby not only facilitate the infection but also virus release and spread. Clearly, the role of the HE proteins during the infection of corona- and toroviruses deserves further study. More generally than just in the *Nidovirales*, they may be the result of molecular evolution by conferring a selective advantage to viruses that must penetrate through mucous layers, which shielding their epithelial targets in the respiratory, gastrointestinal, and genital tracts.

REFERENCES

Barlough, J.E., Stoddart, C.A., Sorresso, G.P., Jacobson, R.H., and Scott, F.W. (1984). Experimental inoculation of cats with canine coronavirus and subsequent challenge with feline infectious peritonitis virus. *Lab Anim Sci* **34**, 592–7.

Beards, G.M., Brown, D.W., Green, J., and Flewett, T.H. (1986). Preliminary characterisation of torovirus-like particles of humans: comparison with Berne virus of horses and Breda virus of calves. *J Med Virol* **20**, 67–78.

Beards, G.M., Hall, C., Green, J., Flewett, T.H., Lamouliatte, F., and Du Pasquier, P. (1984). An enveloped virus in stools of children and adults with gastroenteritis that resembles the Breda virus of calves. *Lancet* **1**, 1050–2.

Brian, D.A., Hogue, B.G., and Kienzle, T.E. (1995). The coronavirus hemagglutinin esterase glycoprotein. In: Siddell, S.G. (ed.) *The Coronaviridae* Plenum Press, New York, pp. 165–179.

Brown, D.W., Beards, G.M., and Flewett, T.H. (1987). Detection of Breda virus antigen and antibody in humans and animals by enzyme immunoassay. *J Clin Microbiol* **25**, 637–40.

Brown, D.W., Selvakumar, R., Daniel, D.J., and Mathan, V.I. (1988). Prevalence of neutralising antibodies to Berne virus in animals and humans in Vellore, South India. Brief report. *Arch Virol* **98**, 267–9.

Cavanagh, D. (1995). The coronavirus surface glycoprotein. In: The Coronaviridae (Siddell, S.G. Ed.) pp. 293–309. Plenum Press, New York, pp. 73–113

Chao, L. (1990). Fitness of RNA virus decreased by Muller's ratchet [see comments]. *Nature* **348**, 454–5.

Cornelissen, L.A., Wierda, C.M., van der Meer, F.J., Herrewegh, A.A., Horzinek, M.C., Egberink, H.F., and de Groot, R.J. (1997). Hemagglutinin-esterase, a novel structural protein of torovirus. *J Virol* **71**, 5277–86.

Crouch, C.F., Bielefeldt Ohmann, H., Watts, T.C., and Babiuk, L.A. (1985). Chronic shedding of bovine enteric coronavirus antigen-antibody complexes by clinically normal cows. *J Gen Virol* **66**, 1489–500.

de Vries, A.A.F., Horzinek, M.C., Rottier, P.J.M., and de Groot, R.J. (1997). The genome organisation of the Nidovirales: similarities and differences among arteri-, toro-, and coronaviruses. *Sem Virol* **8**, 33–48.

Duckmanton, L., Luan, B., Devenish, J., Tellier, R., and Petric, M. (1997). Characterization of torovirus from human fecal specimens. *Virology* **239**, 158–68.

Gagneten, S., Gout, O., Dubois-Dalcq, M., Rottier, P., Rossen, J., and Holmes, K.V. (1995). Interaction of mouse hepatitis virus (MHV) spike glycoprotein with receptor glycoprotein MHVR is required for infection with an MHV strain that expresses the hemagglutinin-esterase glycoprotein. *J Virol* **69**, 889–95.

Goldbach, R. and Wellink, J. (1988). Evolution of plus-strand RNA viruses. *Intervirology* **29**, 260–7.

Groot, R.J. de and Horzinek, M.C. (1995). Feline infectious peritonitis. In: The Coronaviridae (Siddell, S.G. Ed.) pp. 293–309. Plenum Press, New York.

Haagmans, B.L., Egberink, H.F., and Horzinek, M.C. (1996). Apoptosis and T-cell depletion during feline infectious peritonitis. *J Virol* **70**, 8977–83.

Herrewegh, A.A., de Groot, R.J., Cepica, A., Egberink, H.F., Horzinek, M.C., and Rottier, P.J. (1995). Detection of feline coronavirus RNA in feces, tissues, and body fluids of naturally infected cats by reverse transcriptase PCR. *J Clin Microbiol* **33**, 684–9.

Herrewegh, A.A., Mahler, M., Hedrich, H.J., Haagmans, B.L., Egberink, H.F., Horzinek, M.C., Rottier, P.J., and de Groot, R.J. (1997). Persistence and evolution of feline coronavirus in a closed cat- breeding colony. *Virology* **234**, 349–63.

Herrler, G., Durkop, I., Becht, H., and Klenk, H.D. (1988). The glycoprotein of influenza C virus is the hemagglutinin, esterase, and fusion factor. *J Gen Virol* **69**, 839–46.

Horzinek, M.C., Ederveen, J., Kaeffer, B., de Boer, D., and Weiss, M. (1986). The peplomers of Berne virus. *J Gen Virol* **67**, 2475–83.

Jacobse-Geels, H.E., Daha, M.R., and Horzinek, M.C. (1980). Isolation and characterization of feline C3 and evidence for the immune complex pathogenesis of feline infectious peritonitis. *J Immunol* **125**, 1606–10.

Jacobse-Geels, H.E., Daha, M.R., and Horzinek, M.C. (1982). Antibody, immune complexes, and complement activity fluctuations in kittens with experimentally induced feline infectious peritonitis. *Am J Vet Res* **43**, 666–70.

Jamieson, F.B., Wang, E.E., Bain, C., Good, J., Duckmanton, L., and Petric, M. (1998). Human torovirus: a new nosocomial gastrointestinal pathogen. *J Infect Dis* **178**, 1263–9.

Koopmans, M. and Horzinek, M.C. (1994). Toroviruses of animals and humans: a review. *Adv Virus Res* **43**, 233–73.

Koopmans, M., Petric, M., Glass, R.I., and Monroe, S.S. (1993). Enzyme-linked immunosorbent assay reactivity of torovirus-like particles in fecal specimens from humans with diarrhea. *J-Clin-Microbiol* **31**, 2738–44 issn: 0095-1137.

Koopmans, M.P., Goosen, E.S., Lima, A.A., McAuliffe, I.T., Nataro, J.P., Barrett, L.J., Glass, R.I., and Guerrant, R.L. (1997). Association of torovirus with acute and persistent diarrhea in children. *Pediatr Infect Dis J* **16**, 504–7.

Krishnan, T. and Naik, T.N. (1997). Electronmicroscopic evidence of torovirus like particles in children with diarrhoea. *Indian J Med Res* **105**, 108–10.

Kroneman, A., Cornelissen, L.A., Horzinek, M.C., de Groot, R.J., and Egberink, H.F. (1998). Identification and characterization of a porcine torovirus. *J Virol* **72**, 3507–11.

Lacombe, D., Lamouliatte, F., Billeaud, C., and Sandler, B. (1988). [Breda virus and hemorrhagic enteropathy. Reminder apropos of 1 case (letter)]. *Arch Fr Pediatr* **45**, 442.

Lai, M.M. (1992). Genetic recombination in RNA viruses. *Curr Top Microbiol Immunol* **176**, 21–32.

Liao, C.L. and Lai, M.M. (1992). RNA recombination in a coronavirus: recombination between viral genomic RNA and transfected RNA fragments. *J Virol* **66**, 6117–24.

Luytjes, W. (1995). Coronavirus gene expression: genome organization and protein synthesis. In: Siddell, S.G. (ed.) *The Coronaviridae* Plenum Press, New York, pp. 33–54.

Luytjes, W., Bredenbeek, P.J., Noten, A.F., Horzinek, M.C., and Spaan, W.J. (1988). Sequence of mouse hepatitis virus A59 mRNA 2: indications for RNA recombination between coronaviruses and influenza C virus. *Virology* **166**, 415–22.

Mantle, M. and Allen, A. (1989). Gastrointestinal mucus In: Davidson, J.S. (ed.) *Gastrointestinal secretion*. Butterworth and Co. Ltd., London, pp. 209–229.

McArdle, F., Bennett, M., Gaskell, R.M., Tennant, B., Kelly, D.F., and Gaskell, C.J. (1990). Canine coronavirus infection in cats; a possible role in feline infectious peritonitis. *Adv Exp Med Biol* **276**, 475–9.

McArdle, F., Bennett, M., Gaskell, R.M., Tennant, B., Kelly, D.F., and Gaskell, C.J. (1992). Induction and enhancement of feline infectious peritonitis by canine coronavirus. *Am J Vet Res* **53**, 1500–6.

Motokawa, K., Hohdatsu, T., Aizawa, C., Koyama, H., and Hashimoto, H. (1995). Molecular cloning and sequence determination of the peplomer protein gene of feline infectious peritonitis virus type I. *Arch Virol* **140**, 469–80.

Motokawa, K., Hohdatsu, T., Hashimoto, H., and Koyama, H. (1996). Comparison of the amino acid sequence and phylogenetic analysis of the peplomer, integral membrane and nucleocapsid proteins of feline, canine and porcine coronaviruses. *Microbiol Immunol* **40**, 425–33.

Murphy, F.A., Fauquet, C.M., Bishop, D.H.L., Ghabrial, S.A., Jarvis, A.W., Martelli, G.P., Mayo, M.A., and Summers, M.D. (1995). Virus Taxonomy. VIth Reoprt of the ICTV. Springer Verlag Wien New York.

Parker, M.D., Cox, G.J., Deregt, D., Fitzpatrick, D.R., and Babiuk, L.A. (1989). Cloning and in vitro expression of the gene for the E3 hemagglutinin glycoprotein of bovine coronavirus. *J Gen Virol* **70**, 155–64.

Pedersen, N.C. (1976a). Morphologic and physical characteristics of feline infectious peritonitis virus and its growth in autochthonous peritoneal cell cultures. *Am J Vet Res* **37**, 567–72.

Pedersen, N.C. (1976b). Serologic studies of naturally occurring feline infectious peritonitis. *Am J Vet Res* **37**, 1449–53.

Pedersen, N.C. (1987). Virologic and immunologic aspects of feline infectious peritonitis virus infection. *Adv Exp Med Biol* **218**, 529–50.

Pedersen, N.C., Boyle, J.F., and Floyd, K. (1981). Infection studies in kittens utilizing feline infectious peritonitis virus propagated in cell culture. *Am J Vet Res* **42**, 363–7.

Pedersen, N.C., Black, J.W., Boyle, J.F., Evermann, J.F., McKeirnan, A.J., and Ott, R.L. (1984). *Molecular Biology and Pathogenesis of Coronaviruses* (Rottier, P.J.M., Zeijst, B.A.M., Spaan, W.J.M., and Horzinek, M.C. Eds.) Plenum Press, New York, 365–80.

Pedersen, N.C., Evermann, J.F., McKeirnan, A.J., and Ott, R.L. (1984). Pathogenicity studies of feline coronavirus isolates 79-1146 and 79-1683. *Am J Vet Res* **45**, 2580–5.

Penrith, M.L. and Gerdes, G.H. (1992). Breda virus-like particles in pigs in South Africa [letter]. *J S Afr Vet Assoc* **63**, 102.

Plagemann, P.G.W. and Moennig, V. (1992). Lactate dehydrogenase-elevating virus, equine arteritis virus, and simian hemorrhagic fever virus: a new group of positive-strand RNA viruses. *Adv Virus Res* **4**, 99–192.

Poland, A.M., Vennema, H., Foley, J.E., and Pedersen, N.C. (1996). Two related strains of feline infectious peritonitis virus isolated from immunocompromised cats infected with a feline enteric coronavirus. *J Clin Microbiol* **34**, 3180–4.

Risco, C., Anton, I.M., Enjuanes, L., and Carrascosa, J.L. (1996). The transmissible gastroenteritis coronavirus contains a spherical core shell consisting of M and N proteins. *J Virol* **70**, 4773–7.

Scott, A.C., Chaplin, M.J., Stack, M.J., and Lund, L.J. (1987). Porcine torovirus? [letter]. *Vet Rec* **120**, 583.

Snijder, E.J. and Horzinek, M.C. (1993). Toroviruses: replication, evolution and comparison with other members of the coronavirus-like superfamily. *J-Gen-Virol* **74**, 2305–16 issn: 0022-1317.

Snijder, E.J. and Horzinek, M.C. (1995). The molecular biology of toroviruses. In: Siddell, S.G. (ed.) *The Coronaviridae* Plenum Press, New York, pp. 219–238.

Snijder, E.J., den Boon, J.A., Horzinek, M.C., and Spaan, W.J. (1991). Comparison of the genome organization of toro- and coronaviruses: evidence for two nonhomologous RNA recombination events during Berne virus evolution. *Virology* **180**, 448–52.

Stoddart, C.A., Barlough, J.E., Baldwin, C.A., and Scott, F.W. (1988). Attempted immunisation of cats against feline infectious peritonitis using canine coronavirus. *Res Vet Sci* **45**, 383–8.

Stoddart, C.A. and Scott, F.W. (1988). Isolation and identification of feline peritoneal macrophages for in vitro studies of coronavirus-macrophage interactions. *J Leukoc Biol* **44**, 319–28.

Stoddart, C.A. and Scott, F.W. (1989). Intrinsic resistance of feline peritoneal macrophages to coronavirus infection correlates with in vivo virulence. *J Virol* **63**, 436–40.

Strauss, E.G. and Strauss, J.H. (1991). RNA viruses: genome structure and evolution. *Curr Opin Genet Dev* **1**, 485–93.

Strauss, J.H. and Strauss, E.G. (1988). Evolution of RNA viruses. *Annu Rev Microbiol* **42**, 657–83.

Van Kruiningen, H.J., Colombel, J.F., Cartun, R.W., Whitlock, R.H., Koopmans, M., Kangro, H.O., Hoogkamp Korstanje, J.A., Lecomte Houcke, M., Devred, M., Paris, J.C., and et al. (1993). An in-depth study of Crohn's disease in two French families [see comments]. *Gastroenterology* **104**, 351–60.

Vennema, H., Rossen, J.W., Wesseling, J., Horzinek, M.C., and Rottier, P.J. (1993). Genomic organization and expression of the 3' end of the canine and feline enteric coronaviruses. *Adv Exp Med Biol* **342**, 11–6.

Vennema, H., Poland A., Floyd Hawkins K., and Pedersen N.C. (1995). A comparison of the genomes of FECVs and FIPVs and what they tell us about the relationships between feline coronaviruses and their evolution. *Feline Pract* **23**, 40–4.

Vlasak, R., Krystal, M., Nacht, M., and Palese, P. (1987). The influenza C virus glycoprotein (HE) exhibits receptor-binding (hemagglutinin) and receptor-destroying (esterase) activities. *Virology* **160**, 419–25.

Vlasak, R., Luytjes, W., Spaan, W., and Palese, P. (1988). Human and bovine coronaviruses recognize sialic acid-containing receptors similar to those of influenza C viruses. *Proc Natl Acad Sci U S A* **85**, 4526–9.

Weiss, M., Steck, F., and Horzinek, M.C. (1983). Purification and partial characterization of a new enveloped RNA virus (Berne virus). *J Gen Virol Reading: Society for General Microbiology Sept* **64**, 1849–58.

Weiss, M., Steck, F., Kaderli, R., and Horzinek, M.C. (1984). Antibodies to Berne virus in horses and other animals. *Vet Microbiol* **9**, 523–31.

Woode, G.N., Reed, D.E., Runnels, P.L., Herrig, M.A., and Hill, H.T. (1982). Studies with an unclassified virus isolated from diarrhoeic calves. *Veterinary Microbiology* **7**, 221–40.

Woode, G.N. (1987). Breda and Breda-like viruses: diagnosis, pathology, and epidemiology. *Ciba Found Symp* **128**, 175–91.

Zimmern, D. (1987). Evolution of RNA viruses. In: Holland, J.J., Domingo, E., and Ahlquist, P. (eds.) RNA Genetics, vol.2, pp. 211–240, CRC Press, Boca Raton FL.

6

A VIRAL ENTEROTOXIN

A New Mechanism of Virus-Induced Pathogenesis

Mary K. Estes[1]* and Andrew P. Morris[2]

[1] Division of Molecular Virology
Baylor College of Medicine
Houston, Texas 77030
[2] Department of Pharmacology
Physiology and Integrative Biology
University of Texas Health Sciences Center
Houston, Texas 77030

1. SUMMARY

Acute infectious gastroenteritis is a major cause of infant morbidity in developed countries and of infant mortality in developing areas of the world. Rotavirus is recognized as the most important etiologic agent of infantile gastroenteritis, and studies of rotavirus serve as models to understand the complex interactions between enteric viruses and the multifunctional cells of the gastrointestinal tract. Understanding such interactions is significant for microbial pathogenesis because most (>80%) infections are initiated at mucosal surfaces. Rotaviruses are pathogens that infect the mature enterocytes of the villi in the intestine and infection appears to be limited to these highly differentiated cells in immunologically competent hosts. In such hosts, infections are generally acute yet diarrheal disease can be severe and life-threatening. Disease generally is resolved within 2–5 days after infection if affected hosts receive adequate rehydration. In immunocompromised hosts, virus infections persist, virus can be detected extraintestinally and virus excretion may be detected for extended periods of time (many months).

Rotaviruses infect almost all mammalian and some avian species and much of our understanding of rotavirus pathogenesis has come from studies in animal models,

---

* Corresponding author: 713-798-3585 (phone), 713-798-3586 (fax), mestes@bcm.tmc.edu

Mechanisms in the Pathogenesis of Enteric Diseases 2, edited by Paul and Francis.
Kluwer Academic / Plenum Publishers, New York, 1999.

particularly in small animal models (mice and rabbits), but also in larger animals (cows and piglets). Studies in children are limited due to the difficulty and lack of clinical need of obtaining biopsies from infants and the inability to determine the precise time of natural infections. In all animal species where naïve animals can be infected, disease is age-dependent; for example, in mice and rabbits, diarrheal disease is the outcome of infections that occur only during the first two weeks of life (Ciarlet et al., 1998; Starkey et al., 1986; Ramig 1988; Ward et al., 1990; Burns et al., 1995), while animals remain susceptible to viral infection into adulthood. Rotavirus infections have been reported to occur repeatedly in humans from birth to old age, but the majority of infections after the first 2 years of life are asymptomatic or associated with mild gastrointestinal symptoms. The age-related resistance to rotavirus-induced diarrhea in humans is thought to be mediated primarily by acquired immunity, but it is not possible to directly test if humans also exhibit an age-dependent resistance to disease based on other factors such as intestinal development and maturation. Currently, our best understanding of the mechanisms of rotavirus pathogenesis rely on results obtained in animal models.

2. ROTAVIRUSES CAUSE DISEASE BY SEVERAL MECHANISMS

The outcome of an infection with rotavirus is clearly dependent on both host and viral factors. The host factors have been dissected by analysis of the outcome of infection in animals inoculated with well-defined viral strains. Both natural and experimental rotavirus infections are characterized by viral replication in enterocytes in the small intestine, with subsequent cell lysis and attendant villus blunting, depressed levels of mucosal disaccharidases, watery diarrhea and dehydration. A majority of studies have shown that rotaviruses can cause malabsorption secondary to destruction of enterocytes (Graham et al., 1984; Davidson et al., 1977). This mechanism is based on the observation that rotavirus infection results in histopathologic changes in the intestine. These changes are generally seen 24–36 hours after infection and the resulting blunting of the villi has been associated with reduced absorption.

Several observations suggest that malabsorption is not the entire basis of rotavirus pathogenesis. Most importantly, in several animal species, profuse diarrhea occurs *prior to* the detection of histologic changes in the intestine including prior to observations of villus blunting (Collins et al., 1989; Theil et al., 1978; McAdaragh et al., 1980; Mebus 1976; Pappenheimer and Enders, 1947; Ward et al., 1997). In addition, some animals exhibit diarrhea in the absence of clear histopathologic changes [neonatal mice infected with heterologous rotavirus strains (Burns et al., 1995)], and other adult rotavirus-infected animals (rabbits) show typical histologic changes in the intestine but do not get diarrhea (Ciarlet et al., 1998.) Finally, oral administration of epidermal growth factor to rotavirus-infected piglets can help restore intestinal mucosal dimensions and enzyme activities but such treatments do not hasten the resolution of diarrhea (Zijlstra et al., 1994). Thus, a clear association of mucosal damage and diarrhea is lacking. Explanations for this include the fact that the infection is patchy so one might observe mucosal changes in one part of the intestine but these would be insufficient to cause diarrheal disease. Vascular damage due to villus ischemia has been suggested to be involved but supporting evidence is limited. In other cases, animals with mucosal damage may release fluid into the intestinal lumen but compensatory physiologic mechanisms (colonic reabsorption of fluid) decrease fluid loss so diarrhea is not observed. Finally, other mechanisms may be involved (see below).

Viral factors involved in virulence or pathogenesis have been dissected by several approaches. First, viral genes implicated in virulence have been examined by studies of reassortants that represent genetically characterized virus strains that contain a single gene from one parental virus that is virulent and all other ten genes from a second aviru-lent parental virus. Ideally the reciprocal single gene reassortant also is analyzed in which a virus contains a single gene from an avirulent parental virus and the other 10 genes from a virulent parental virus. The analysis of reassortants has led to the association of several rotavirus genes and virulence; these putative virulence genes code for both structural and nonstructural proteins (Burke and Desselberger, 1996). Structural genes implicated in virulence include those that code for the outer capsid proteins VP4 and VP7 that are present on the surface of virions and that are likely to be involved in virus stability and virus attachment and penetration into cells. In addition, an internal protein, VP3, that functions as the capping enzyme in the process of transcription of messenger RNA has been implicated in virulence. Finally, three nonstructural proteins, NSP1 and NSP2 whose function in the replication cycle remains unclear, and NSP4, a protein known to be involved in viral morphogenesis, have been found to be virulence genes (Broome et al., 1993; Hoshino et al., 1995). The association of NSP1 with virulence has varied depending on the host species studied; it is a virulence factor for mice but not for rabbits or piglets (Broome et al., 1993; Ciarlet et al., 1998; Bridger et al., 1998).

Recent experiments have revealed that NSP4 can function as a viral enterotoxin, and this may explain the association of this gene with virulence. The discovery that NSP4 functions as an enterotoxin was unexpected because no other viral enterotoxins have been described. The remainder of this article briefly reviews the salient features about this first viral enterotoxin.

2.1. How Does the Rotavirus Enterotoxin NSP4 Cause Disease?

The rotavirus enterotoxin is a nonstructural protein called NSP4 for nonstruc-tural protein 4. This protein was initially identified as a nonstructural glycoprotein with a topology that spans the membrane of the endoplasmic reticulum (ER) and the cyto-plasmic C terminus of NSP4 functions as an intracellular receptor in viral morpho-genesis (Ericson et al., 1983; Au et al., 1989; Meyer et al., 1989; Chan et al., 1988; Taylor et al., 1993; Bergmann et al., 1989). The functioning of this protein initially was exam-ined because the rotaviruses undergo a unique morphogenesis in which newly made subviral particles bud into the endoplasmic reticulum and during this process they obtain a transient membrane envelope that is subsequently lost within the lumen of the ER as particles mature. This process also involves calcium which is required to maintain the integrity of the two outer capsid proteins as well as specific conformations necessary for the correct association of proteins as virus matures in the ER. NSP4 mobi-lizes intracellular calcium ($[Ca^{2+}]i$) release from the ER and this may also affect viral morphogenesis (Tian et al., 1994). NSP4 also possesses a membrane destabilization activity when incubated with liposomes that simulate ER membranes, and it has been hypothesized that this activity may play a role in the removal of the transient envelope from budding particles (Tian et al., 1996). Finally, NSP4 may facilitate cell death and virus release from cells (Newton et al., 1997).

The discovery that NSP4 functions as an enterotoxin was made serendipitously during studies aimed at dissecting the molecular mechanisms by which NSP4 functions

Table 1. Properties of rotavirus NSP4 or NSP4 peptide 114–135

Functions in viral morphogenesis; mediating the acquisition of a transient membrane envelope as subviral particles bud into the endoplasmic reticulum (ER)	Au et al., 1989 Meyer et al., 1989
Mobilizes $[Ca^{2+}]_i$ release from internal stores (ER)	Tian et al., 1994; Tian et al., 1995 Dong et al., 1997
Associated with virulence based on studies of reassortants	Hoshino et al., 1995
Induces an age-dependent diarrhea in mice and rats when administered by intraperitoneal or intraluminal routes but not when given intramuscularly	Ball et al., 1996 Ball et al., 1998
Does not induce histologic changes in the intestine when diarrhea is present	Ball et al., 1996 Ball et al., 1998
Induces age-dependent chloride secretion in the intestinal mucosa of young mice	Ball et al., 1996
Alters plasma membrane permeability and is cytotoxic to cells	Tian et al., 1994 Newton et al., 1997
Mutations in NSP4 from virulent/avirulent pairs of virus are associated with altered virus virulence	Kirkwood et al., 1996 Zhang et al., 1998
NSP4 induced age-dependent diarrhea and age-dependent chloride permeability changes in mice lacking the cystic fibrosis chloride transductance resistance (CFTR) channel	Morris et al., 1999
Children make antibodies and cellular immune responses to NSP4	Richardson et al., 1993 Johanssen et al., 1999
Is a novel toxin? No primary sequence similarity to other known toxins	

in morphogenesis. A synthetic peptide of NSP4 that contains amino acid residues 114–135 was conjugated to a carrier and injected into mice to produce a new antiserum. Although the mice received peptide (and no virus), they got diarrhea. Pursuit of this observation showed that both the full-length protein and the 114–135 peptide share several properties that are consistent with NSP4 being an enterotoxin.

The protein induces diarrhea in pups with a DD_{50} of 0.56 nmols while the DD_{50} of the 114–135 peptide is more than 10 fold-higher, indicating that this peptide contains only a part of the active domain of the protein. Properties that define bacterial enterotoxins include their ability to stimulate net secretion in intestinal segments in the absence of inducing histologic changes. NSP4 was shown to possess these properties, confirming that it functions as an enterotoxin. Of interest was the observation that age-dependent chloride secretion was seen in the intestinal mucosa of young mice.

These early studies and in vitro analyses of the response of human intestinal (HT29) cells to exogenously added NSP4 have led to a working model for the mechanism of action of this enterotoxin.

It is hypothesized that in young mice, rotavirus replicates in cells and the rotavirus proteins, including the nonstructural protein NSP4 are produced. It is further hypothesized that NSP4 is released from virus-infected cells by a currently unknown mechanism (either by cell lysis or by secretion), and this extracellular NSP4 can activate a signaling pathway in secretory cells. Human intestinal cells exposed to exogenously added NSP4 initiate a signaling pathway that involves activation of phospholipase C, elevation in IP_3 and mobilization of $[Ca^{2+}]i$ (Dong et al., 1997). Crypt cells isolated from mice also respond in a similar manner but mobilization of $[Ca^{2+}]i$ occurs in both young and older mice (Morris et al., 1999).

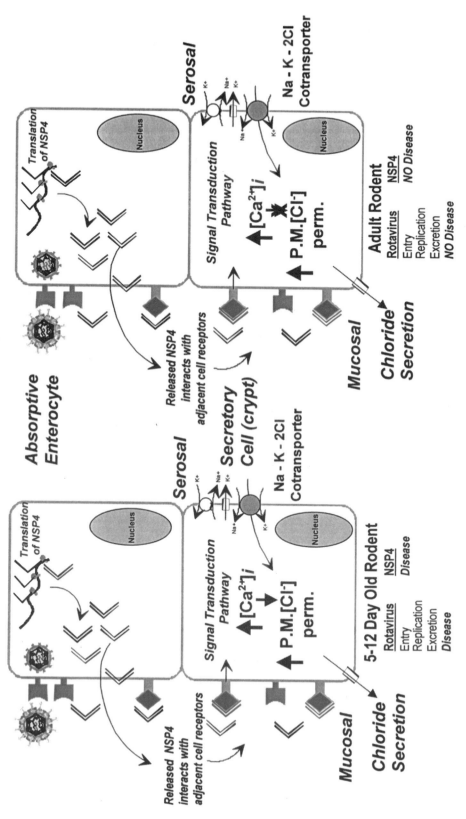

Figure 1. A proposed model of enterotoxin action. Rotavirus infected enterocytes produce virus-specific proteins including NSP4. NSP4 is released from cells by lysis or secretion and this NSP4 interacts with a receptor for NSP4 on adjacent cells. These secretory cells likely are crypt cells but might also be villus enterocytes. This triggers a signal transduction pathway that mobilizes intracellular calcium and results in increased plasma membrane chloride permeability. The plasma membrane permeability is age-dependent based on studies in CFTR knock-out mice (Morris et al., 1999).

It is hypothesized that this pathway then affects a calcium-activated chloride channel resulting in chloride secretion. Diarrhea occurs in mice lacking the cystic fibrosis transductance regulator (CFTR) channel following rotavirus infection or NSP4 treatment, indicating that a different chloride channel than CFTR mediates this effect (Angel et al., 1998; Morris et al., 1999). The chloride secretion is age-dependent in CFTR mice, indicating that age-dependent disease may result from an age-dependent induction, activation or regulation of this chloride channel (Morris et al., 1999). This pathway would be one that is activated when NSP4 is released from virus-infected cells, possibly by cell lysis, and the affected cells are hypothesized to be the secretory crypt cells. Other cell types including villus enterocytes may also be affected in a similar manner by NSP4.

An alternative pathway leading to changes in plasma membrane chloride permeability may be activated during viral infection when NSP4 is initially expressed as a transmembrane ER-specific glycoprotein within infected enterocytes. It is known that endogenous expression of NSP4 in cells can also mobilize $[Ca^{2+}]i$ from internal stores but this process occurs by a different process that is not affected by PLC inhibitors (Tian et al., 1995). Changes in the plasma membrane permeability are seen in virus-infected cells, but it remains unclear whether these effects result from expression of NSP4 or another viral protein (Michelangeli et al., 1991; Michelangeli et al., 1995).

2.2. Molecular Genetic Studies Support a Role for NSP4 in Diarrhea Induction

Confirmation of the proposed role for NSP4 in diarrhea induction by molecular genetic approaches has also been sought by studying pairs of virulent and avirulent viruses in which the avirulent virus was derived from the virulent parental virus by serial passage of virus in tissue culture. This approach was used because no reverse genetics system is available yet to allow one to construct rotaviruses containing specific genes or mutated genes by rescue of cloned genes. Comparisons of the sequences of NSP4 from two different pairs of avirulent/virulent viruses have shown that structural changes between amino acids 131 and 140 are important in pathogenesis (Zhang et al., 1998). Sequence changes in NSP4 were confirmed to have relevance to pathogenesis based on the expression and biologic testing of the virulent and avirulent NSP4 proteins and site-specific mutant forms of these proteins.

These results indicate that even a single mutation at amino acid 138 can affect the ability of NSP4 to mobilize intracellular calcium and to induce diarrhea in neonatal mice. Others have found a specific amino acid difference at position 135 in NSP4 of

Table 2. Summary of biological properties of NSP4 and NSP4 mutants

NSP4	$[Ca^{2+}]_i$ mobilization in insect cells	$[Ca^{2+}]_i$ mobilization in human intestinal epithelial cells	Diarrhea induction in neonatal mice
OSU-v NSP4	6-fold↑	10-fold↑	57%* (13/23)
OSU-a NSP4	1.4-fold↑	1.2-fold↑	16% (4/25)
OSU NSP4$_{P138S}$	No increase	No increase	0% (0/12)
OSU NSP4 $_{D131-140}$	No increase	ND	0% (0/12)

*P < 0.05 Data from Zhang et al. (1998).

symptomatic and asymptomatic human rotavirus strains (Kirkwood et al., 1996). The location of amino acid changes in NSP4 of the virulent/avirulent virus pairs downstream from the C terminus of the initial peptide tested is consistent with the finding that the 114–135 peptide does not contain the entire active domain of the protein.

These results with the virulent/avirulent NSP4 proteins raise the question of what is the basis of avirulence. Does the avirulent form of the protein fail to bind to the putative receptor on cells or does it fail to induce the signaling required to effect diarrhea induction. Experiments to test these ideas are in progress.

2.3. Can Knowledge of the Mechanisms of Action of the NSP4 Be Used to Improve Methods of Treatment and Prevention of Disease?

The discovery that rotaviruses produce an enterotoxin raises the possibility that this protein could be useful to develop new methods to prevent or treat rotavirus-induced disease. One possibility is that this protein may be used to induce protective immunity against disease. This idea is feasible based on demonstrating that passive immunity to the 114–135 peptide of NSP4 can reduce both the incidence and severity of diarrhea in neonatal mice challenged with virulent rotavirus (Ball et al., 1996). Further studies are needed to know whether this immunity was provided by lactogenic immunity or by transplacentally transferred IgG, and whether immunity to the fully active protein would induce even greater protection.

An important question is what is the relative importance of enterotoxin action in rotavirus pathogenesis in children. This question is difficult to answer in children, but future studies can be designed to determine if induction of antibody correlates with protection from disease and whether vaccination strategies that induce immunity to NSP4 improve vaccine efficacy. Sequence analysis of over 50 genes that code for NSP4 in different rotavirus strains has recently shown that there are three genetic groups (Cunliffe et al., 1997; Horie et al., 1997; Kirkwood and Palombo, 1997). An interesting question is whether antibody to one genetic type confers protective immunity to challenge with viruses that encode a different genetic type of NSP4; that is, will a single NSP4 induce both homotypic and heterotypic protection?

Limited information about antibody responses to NSP4 in children is available. One study has shown that humoral antibody responses to NSP4 are detectable in children recovering from primary rotavirus infections, but the ability to detect such responses by immunoprecipitation depends on the virus strain used as antigen; homotypic responses are detected with the greatest sensitivity (Richardson et al., 1993). Humoral and cellular immune responses to NSP4 have been detected in children and adults following rotavirus infection, and preliminary data suggest that the presence of antibody to NSP4 may be associated with protection from natural infection (Johansen et al., 1999). Whether immunity to NSP4 will provide the long sought after correlate of protection for rotavirus remains an important issue that needs to be investigated.

Understanding the mechanism of action of NSP4 may lead to new treatments for rotavirus-induced diarrhea. For example, it is possible that antibody treatment or new drugs might be developed to treat children or animals with rotavirus infection and diarrhea, specifically immunocompromised children with chronic rotavirus diarrhea. Such potential new therapies may require a more detailed understanding of the receptor for NSP4 on cells, the structure of NSP4 and whether there are distinct signaling pathways for NSP4 action when the protein is expressed endogenously versus when cells are exposed exogenously to NSP4. In the latter case, it remains to be determined how NSP4 is released from cells.

The discovery of the rotavirus enterotoxin raises interest in knowing whether other viruses encode enterotoxins. This is obviously important for understanding the mechanisms of pathogenesis for other gastroenteritis viruses such as astroviruses, caliciviruses, coronaviruses, and enteric adenoviruses. This question is also relevant for viruses such as HIV that cause a devastating enteropathy. Finally, these results emphasize the common mechanisms of pathogenesis shared among microbial pathogens.

ACKNOWLEDGMENTS

The work from our laboratories on NSP4 as an enterotoxin summarized in this review includes that of former students, postdoctoral fellows, or collaborators including Drs. Kit-Sing Au, Judy Ball, Wai-Kit Chan, Yanjie Dong, Kari Johansen, Linda J. Saif, J. Scott, L. Svensson, Peng Tian, Carl Zeng, and Mingdong Zhang. We greatly appreciate the critical work, friendship, and scientific enthusiasm of these colleagues.

REFERENCES

Angel, J., Tang, B., Feng, N., Greenberg, H.B., and Bass, D., 1998, Studies of the roles for NSP4 in the pathogenesis of homologous murine rotavirus diarrhea, J. Infect. Dis. 1177:455–458.

Au, K.S., Chan, W.K., Burns, J.W., and Estes, M.K, 1989, Receptor activity of rotavirus nonstructural glycoprotein NS28, J. Virol. 63:4553–4562.

Ball, J.M., Tian, P., Zeng, C.QY., Morris, A., and Estes, M.K., 1996, Age-dependent diarrhea is induced by a viral nonstructural glycoprotein, Science 272:101–104.

Ball, J.M., Zeng, C.QY., and Estes, M.K., 1998, Unpublished data.

Bergmann, C.C., Maass, D., Poruchynsky, M.S., Atkinson, P.H., and Bellamy, A.R., 1989, Topology of the nonstructural rotavirus receptor glycoprotein NS28 in the rough endoplasmic reticulum, EMBO J. 8:1695–1703.

Bridger, J.C., Dhaliwal, W., Adamson, M.J.V., and Howard, C.R., 1998, Determinants of rotavirus host range restriction—a heterologous bovine NSP1 gene does not affect replication kinetics in the pig, Virology 245:47–52.

Broome, R.L., Vo, P.T., Ward, R.L., Clark, H.F., and Greenberg, H.B., 1993, Murine rotavirus genes encoding outer capsid proteins VP4 and VP7 are not major determinants of host range restriction and virulence, J. Virol. 67:2448–2455.

Burke, B. and Desselberger, U., 1996, Rotavirus pathogenicity, Virology 218:299–305.

Burns, J.W., Krishnaney, A.A., Vo, P.T., Rouse, R.V., Anderson, L.J., and Greenberg, H.B., 1995, Analyses of homologous rotavirus infection in the mouse model, Virology 207:143–153.

Chan, W.K., Au, K.S., and Estes, M.K., 1988, Topography of the simian rotavirus nonstructural glycoprotein (NS28) in the endoplasmic reticulum membrane, Virology 164:435–442.

Ciarlet, M., Estes, M.K., Barone, C., Ramig, R.F., and Conner, M.E., 1998, Analysis of host range restriction determinants in the rabbit model: comparision of homologous and heterologous rotavirus infections, J. Virol. 72:2341–2351.

Ciarlet, M., Gilger, M.A., Barone, C., McArthur, M., Estes, M.K., and Conner, M.E., 1998, Rotavirus disease, but not infection and development of intestinal histopathological lesions, is age-restricted in rabbits. Virology. In Press.

Collins, J.E., Benfield, D.A., and Duimstra, J.R., 1989, Comparative virulence of two porcine group-A rotavirus isolates in gnotobiotic pigs, Am. J. Vet. Res. 50:827–835.

Cunliffe, N.A., Woods, P.A., Leite, J.P., Das, B.K., Ramachandran, M., Bhan, M.K., Hart, C.A., Glass, R.I., and Gentsch, J.R., 1997, Sequence analysis of NSP4 gene of human rotavirus allows classification into two main genetic groups, J. Med. Virol. 53:41–50.

Davidson, G.P., Gall, D.G., Petric, M., Butler, D.G., and Hamilton, J.R., 1977, Human rotavirus enteritis induced in conventional piglets. Intestinal structure and transport, J. Clin. Invest, 60:1402–1409.

Dong, Y., Zeng, C.Q.-Y., Ball, J.M., Estes, M.K., and Morris, A.P., 1997, The rotavirus enterotoxin NSP4 mobilizes intracellular calcium in human intestinal cells by stimulating phospholipase C-mediated inositol 1,4,5-trisphosphate production, Proc. Natl. Acad. Sci. USA 94:3960–3965.

Ericson, B.L., Graham, D.Y., Mason, B.B., Hanssen, H.H., and Estes, M.K., 1983, Two types of glycoprotein precursors are produced by the Simian rotavirus SA11. Virology 127:320–332.

Graham, D.Y., Sackman, J.W., and Estes, M.K., 1984, Pathogenesis of rotavirus-induced diarrhea. Preliminary studies in miniature swine piglet, Dig. Dis. Sci. 29:1028–1035.

Horie, Y., Masamune, O., and Nakagomi, O., 1997, Three major alleles of rotavirus NSP4 proteins identified by sequence analysis, J. Gen. Virol. 78:2341–2346.

Hoshino, Y., Saif, L.J., Kang, S.Y., Sereno, M.M., Chen, W.K., and Kapikian, A.Z., 1995, Identification of group A rotavirus genes associated with virulence of a porcine rotavirus and host range restriction of a human rotavirus in the gnotobiotic piglet model. Virology 209:274–280.

Johansen, K., Hinkula, J., Espinoza, F., Levi, M., Zeng, C.Q.-Y., Vesikari, T., Estes, M.K., and Svensson, L., 1999, Humoral and cell-mediated immune responses to the NSP4 enterotoxin of rotavirus, J. Med. Virol. In press.

Kirkwood, C.D., Coulson, B.S., and Bishop, R.F., 1996, G3P2 rotaviruses causing diarrheal disease in neonates differ in VP4, VP7, and NSP4 sequence from G3P2 strains causing asymptomatic neonatal infection, Arch. Virol. 141:1661–1676.

Kirkwood, C.D. and Palombo, E.A., 1997, Genetic characterization of the rotavirus nonstructural protein, NSP4, Virology 236:258–265.

McAdaragh, J.P., Bergeland, M.E., Meyer, R.C., Johnshoy, M.W., Stotz, I.J., Benfield, D.A., and Hammer, R., 1980, Pathogenesis of rotaviral enteritis in gnotobiotic pigs: a microscopic study, Am. J. Vet. Res. 41:1572–1581.

Mebus, C.A., 1976, Reovirus-like calf enteritis, Am. Dig. Dis. 21:592–599.

Meyer, J.C., Bergmann, C.C., and Bellamy, A.R., 1989, Interaction of rotavirus cores with the nonstructural glycoprotein NS28, Virology 171:98–107.

Michelangeli, F., Liprandi, F., Chemello, M.E., Ciarlet, M., and Ruiz, M.C., 1995, Selective depletion of stored calcium by thapsigargin blocks rotavirus maturation but not the cytopathic effect, J. Virol. 69:3838–3847.

Michelangeli, F., Ruiz, M.-C., Del Castillo, J.R., Ernesto Ludert, J., and Liprandi, F., 1991, Effect of rotavirus infection on intracellular calcium homeostasis in cultured cells, Virology 181:520–527.

Morris, A.P., Scott, J.K., Ball, J.M., Zeng, Q.-Y., O'Neil, W.K., and Estes, M.K., 1999, The rotaviral enterotoxin NSP4 elicits age-dependent diarrhea and calcium-mediated iodide influx into intestinal crypts of cystic fibrosis mice, Am. J. Physiol. In Press

Newton, K., Meyer, J.C., Bellamy, A.R., and Taylor, J.A., 1997, Rotavirus nonstructural glycoprotein NSP4 alters plasma membrane permeability in mammalian cells, J. Virol. 71:9458–9465.

Pappenheimer, A.M. and Enders, J.F., 1947, An epidemic disease of suckling mice. II. Inclusion in the intestinal epithelial cells, J. Exp. Med. 85:417–422.

Ramig, R.F., 1988, The effects of host age, virus dose, and virus strain on heterologous rotavirus infection of suckling mice, Microb. Pathog. 4:189–202.

Richardson, S.C., Grimwood, K., and Bishop, R.F., 1993, Analysis of homotypic and heterotypic serum immune responses to rotavirus proteins following primary rotavirus infection by using the radioimmunoprecipitation technique, J. Clin. Microbiol. 31:377–385.

Starkey, W.G., Collins, J., Wallis, T.S., Clarke, G.J., Spencer, A.J., Haddon, S.J., Osborne, M.P., Candy, D.C., and Stephen, J., 1986, Kinetics, tissue specificity and pathological changes in murine rotavirus infection of mice, J. Gen. Virol. 67:2625–2634.

Taylor, J.A., O'Brien, J.A., Lord, V.J., Meyer, J.C., and Bellamy, A.R., 1993, The RER-localized rotavirus intracellular receptor: A truncated purified soluble form is multivalent and binds virus particles, Virology 194:807–814.

Theil, K.W., Bohl, E.H., Cross, R.F., Kohler, E.M., and Agnes, A.G., 1978, Pathogenesis of porcine rotaviral infection in experimentally inoculated gnotobiotic pigs, Am. J. Vet. Res. 39:213–220.

Tian, P., Ball, J.M., Zeng, C.Q.-Y., and Estes, M.K., 1996, The rotavirus nonstructural glycoprotein NSP4 possesses membrane destabilization activity, J. Virol. 70:6973–6981.

Tian, P., Estes, M.K., Hu, Y., Ball, J.M., Zeng, C.QY., and Schilling, W.P., 1995, The rotavirus nonstructural glycoprotein NSP4 mobilizes Ca^{2+} from the endoplasmic reticulum, J. Virology 69:5763–5772.

Tian, P., Hu, Y., Schilling, W.P., Lindsay, D.A., Eiden, J., and Estes, M.K., 1994, The nonstructural glycoprotein of rotavirus affects intracellular calcium levels, J. Virol. 68:251–257.

Ward, L.A., Rosen, B.I., Yuan, L., and Saif L., 1996, Pathogenesis of an attenuated and a virulent strain of group A human rotavirus in neonatal gnotobiotic pigs, J. Gen. Virol. 77:1431–1441.

Ward, R.L., Mason, B.B., Bernstein, D.I., Sander, D.S., Smith, V.E., Zandle, G.A., and Rappaport, R.S., 1997, Attenuation of a human rotavirus vaccine candidate did not correlate with mutations in the NSP4 protein gene, J. Virol. 71:6267–6270.

Ward, R.L., McNeal, M.M., and Sheridan, J.F., 1990, Development of an adult mouse model for studies on protection against rotavirus, J. Virol. 64:5070–5075.

Zhang, M., Zeng, C.Q.-Y., Dong, Y., Ball, J.M., Saif, L.J., Morris, A.P., and Estes, M.K., 1998, Mutations in rotavirus nonstructural glycoprotein NSP4 are associated with altered virus virulence, J. Virol. 72:3666–3672.

Zijlstra, R.T., Odle, J., Hall, W.F., Petschow, B.W., Gelberg, H.B., and Litov, R.E., 1994, Effect of orally administered epidermal growth factor on intestinal recovery of neonatal pigs infected with rotavirus, J. Pediatr. Gastroenterol. Nutr. 19:382–390.

7

COMPARATIVE PATHOLOGY OF BACTERIAL ENTERIC DISEASES OF SWINE

Rodney A. Moxley and Gerald E. Duhamel

Department of Veterinary and Biomedical Sciences
Institute of Agriculture and Natural Resources
University of Nebraska-Lincoln
Lincoln, Nebraska 68583-0905

1. SUMMARY

Enteric bacterial infections are among the most common and economically significant diseases affecting swine production worldwide. Clinical signs of these infections include diarrhea, reduced growth rate, weight loss, and death of preweaned, weanling, grower-finisher, young and adult age breeding animals. The most common etiological agents include *Escherichia coli*, *Clostridium perfringens*, *Lawsonia intracellularis*, *Salmonella enterica*, and *Brachyspira* (*Serpulina*) spp. With the exception of *Brachyspira* (*Serpulina*) *hyodysenteriae*, the cause of swine dysentery, and *Lawsonia intracellularis*, the cause of proliferative enteropathy, the pathological changes seen with these agents closely resemble the diseases occurring in human beings. Histological changes in the intestines of swine with enteric bacterial infections include bacterial colonization without significant damage (e.g., certain enterotoxigenic *E. coli* and *C. perfringens* type A), attaching and effacing lesions with enteropathogenic *E. coli* and *Brachyspira pilosicoli*, the cause of colonic spirochetosis, inflammation with *S. enterica*, and necrotizing and hemorrhagic lesions with certain *C. perfringens*. Extraintestinal spread of bacteria and/or toxins occurs with some serotypes of *E. coli* and most serotypes of *S. enterica*. Enteric bacterial diseases of swine have been used as models to study the pathogenesis of similar diseases of human beings. Several of these pathogens are also important causes of food-borne disease in humans.

2. INTRODUCTION

Enteric bacteria of swine are significant causes of diarrheal disease in this species and food-borne illness in human beings (Holland, 1990; Buzby et al., 1996). Several of

Mechanisms in the Pathogenesis of Enteric Diseases 2, edited by Paul and Francis.
Kluwer Academic / Plenum Publishers, New York, 1999.

the enteric bacteria that cause natural and/or experimental disease in swine cause similar lesions or pathogenetic effects in humans, e.g., enterotoxigenic *E. coli* (ETEC; Moon et al., 1977), enterohemorrhagic *E. coli* (EHEC; Francis et al., 1986; Tzipori et al., 1986; Moxley and Francis, 1998), enteropathogenic *E. coli* (Moon et al., 1983; Tzipori et al., 1985), *Clostridium perfringens* type A (Olubunmi and Taylor, 1985), *C. perfringens* type C (Barnes and Moon, 1964; Bergeland, 1972), non-typhoid *Salmonella enterica* (Reed et al., 1986), and *Brachyspira* (*Serpulina*) *pilosicoli* (Trott et al., 1996a). Conversely, some less common enteric bacterial diseases of swine are important causes of foodborne illnesses in humans, e.g., *Campylobacter jejuni* and *Yersinia enterocolitica* (Babakhani et al., 1993; Buzby et al., 1996; Fukushima et al., 1987; Ketley et al., 1997; Thomson et al., 1998). Two important enteric bacterial pathogens of swine, namely *Lawsonia intracellularis* and *Brachyspira* (*Serpulina*) *hyodysenteriae*, do not appear to cause disease in humans. Presented herein is a brief overview of the enteric pathology and pathogenesis of important natural enteric bacterial pathogens of swine. Both infections that are useful as models of human disease and those that have no counterpart in humans are included in this review.

3. ENTERIC COLIBACILLOSIS AND EDEMA DISEASE

Enterotoxigenic *E. coli* (ETEC) commonly cause enteric disease (enteric colibacillosis) in pigs less than one day to approximately eight weeks of age. Grossly at necropsy, pigs with uncomplicated (i.e., non-septic) enteric colibacillosis may have no remarkable lesions other than those reflective of dehydration; however, mild hyperemia of the intestines is not uncommonly seen. Microscopically, coliform bacteria, aided by the expression of fimbriae on their surfaces, adhere multifocally or diffusely to the villous epithelium. This lesion is diagnostic of enteric colibacillosis. Minimal to mild neutrophilic infiltration of the epithelium and lamina propria of the small intestine is also a common lesion. The pathogenesis involves binding of fimbriae to glycoprotein or glycolipid receptors on mucus and the apical cell surfaces of villous epithelial cells, and the induction of diarrhea, largely through the effects of enterotoxins (Smyth et al., 1994; Francis et al., 1998). Fimbriae are identified antigenically; the main ones expressed by porcine ETEC strains include K88 (F4), K99 (F5), 987P (F6), F18ac (previously called F107ac and 2134P), and F41 (Smyth et al., 1994; Nagy et al., 1997). Strains that produce F5, F6, and F41 fimbriae most often cause diarrhea in pigs less than one week old, occasionally cause diarrhea in pigs one to three weeks old, and uncommonly cause diarrhea in older pigs (Alexander, 1994). Antigenic variants of F4 have been described; these include F4ab, F4ac, and F4ad (Guinee et al., 1979). F4-positive ETEC cause diarrhea in pigs less than one day old to approximately eight weeks old whereas, postweaning ETEC disease is limited to strains that produce F4 and F18ac fimbriae (Alexander, 1994; Hampson, 1994; Nagy et al., 1997). F4-positive ETEC usually adhere to epithelium in the duodenum, jejunum, and ileum, whereas F5 and F6-positive ETEC usually adhere only to the ileal epithelium. ETEC that express F18ac fimbriae (formerly called 2134P fimbriae) preferentially adhere to the ileal villous epithelium (Nagy et al., 1992).

Although fimbriae play an important role in the pathogenesis of enteric colibacillosis, the enterotoxins identify *E. coli* strains as enterotoxigenic (Gyles, 1994). Porcine ETEC strains may produce heat-stable (either STa, STb, or both) or heat-labile (LT) enterotoxins, or combinations of these (e.g., LT and STb; Gyles, 1994). STb does not significantly contribute to the diarrhea in neonatal pigs (Casey et al., 1998), hence the severe diarrhea caused by F4 ETEC strains that produce both LT and STb may largely be due to the effects of LT. LT causes increased Cl⁻ secretion from the crypt epithelial cells and impaired absorption of Na⁺ and Cl⁻ by the villous epithelial cells (Gyles, 1994). The excess electrolytes in the intestinal lumen cause an osmotic loss of water and subsequent diarrhea (Gyles, 1994).

In addition to diarrheal disease, ETEC also commonly causes a clinical syndrome in swine characterized by peracute death and hemorrhagic gastroenteritis (HGE) at necropsy (Moxley et al., 1988; Faubert and Drolet, 1995). Grossly, there is severe diffuse hyperemia and hemorrhage of the small intestine and often the large intestine. Microscopically, intestinal mucosa and submucosa are diffusely hyperemic and hemorrhagic with thrombosed blood vessels (Moxley et al., 1988; Faubert and Drolet, 1995). Based on the similarities of the lesions with experimentally-induced shock in rodent, canine, and feline models and lesions seen following the experimental induction of endotoxic shock in swine, it has been hypothesized that colibacillary HGE represents a state of endotoxic shock and/or septicemia (Moxley et al., 1988; Faubert and Drolet, 1995; Fairbrother and Ngeleka, 1994). These lesions are also markedly similar to a syndrome of neonatal children termed necrotizing enterocolitis (Cohen et al., 1991). Most colibacillary HGE cases are caused by hemolytic F4 and F18 ETEC strains, although occasional cases are caused by hemolytic edema disease strains (Moxley et al., 1988; Faubert and Drolet, 1995). Recent studies using the neonatal gnotobiotic piglet addressed the hypothesis that hemolysin is necessary for the induction of septicemia and HGE; however, deletion of the hemolysin structural gene in an ETEC strain did not reduce the incidence of septicemia/HGE in this model (Moxley et al., 1998). It was concluded that either hemolysin played no role in this condition, or that other virulence factors may have masked its effects.

Enteropathogenic *E. coli* (EPEC), also called "attaching and effacing" *E. coli*, cause diarrhea in pigs from one to eight weeks of age (Janke et al., 1989; Helie et al., 1991; Neef et al., 1994a; Zhu et al., 1994). The term "attaching and effacing" (A/E) refers to an ultrastructural lesion characterized by focal loss of microvilli on small or large intestinal epithelial cells at points where bacteria are intimately attached to the apical cell surface (Moon et al., 1983). The term EPEC, according a consensus definition reached at the Second International Symposium on EPEC in 1995, refers to *E. coli* strains that produce A/E lesions but lack Shigatoxin (Stx; Nataro and Kaper, 1998). This definition distinguishes EPEC especially from enterohemorrhagic *E. coli* (EHEC), a class of *E. coli* that causes A/E lesions and produces Stx (e.g., *E. coli* O157:H7). Based on the consensus definition, EPEC bacteria have been identified as natural pathogens of human beings (Levine, 1987; Nataro and Kaper, 1998), rabbits (Cantey and Blake, 1977), swine (Janke et al., 1989), cattle (Fischer et al., 1994) and dogs (Broes et al., 1988; Drolet et al., 1994). Most EPEC cases in swine appear to be caused by serogroup O45:K"E65" (Helie et al., 1991), although EPEC belonging to serogroup O116 also have been identified (Neef et al., 1994a).

E. coli genes that induce A/E lesion development reside on the chromosome on a 35-kb pathogenicity island called the locus of enterocyte effacement (LEE; Nataro and Kaper, 1998). The LEE of the prototype human EPEC isolate E2348/69 contains 41 predicted open reading frames arranged in at least five polycistronic operons (Nataro and Kaper, 1998). The *esc* (*E. coli* secretion) and *sep* (secretion of *E. coli* proteins) genes encode proteins that make up a type III secretion system. The *eae* (*E. coli* attaching and effacing) gene encodes the adhesin protein, intimin. The *sep* (EPEC secreted proteins) genes encode proteins that induce signal transduction events in the epithelial cell membrane which culminate in microvillous effacement. The *tir* (translocated intimin receptor) gene encodes the receptor for intimin. The Tir protein becomes inserted in the epithelial cell membrane and serves as the receptor for intimin; together, they mediate intimate attachment of the bacterium to the host cell. Tir may also nucleate actin, possibly acting as a bridge between the bacteria and the host cytoskeleton. Gnotobiotic piglets were used as a model to study the role of intimin in A/E lesion development with *E. coli* O157:H7. A/E lesions were dependent upon the production of intimin, as evidenced by the presence of A/E lesions in piglets inoculated with wild-type and complemented *eaeA* deletion mutant strains but not in those inoculated with an isogenic *eaeA* deletion mutant strain (Donnenberg et al., 1993; McKee et al., 1995).

Swine are experimentally susceptible to infection with EHEC including *E. coli* O157:H7, and are also useful as a model of Stx-induced lesions (Moxley et al., 1998). Recent surveys in the U.S. and U.K. did not detect EHEC in swine populations (Chapman et al., 1997); however, EHEC bacteria were detected in swine in Chile (Borie et al., 1997). Although EHEC bacteria have apparently not become disseminated to swine populations worldwide, other Stx-producing *E. coli* (STEC) for decades have been a widespread cause of a edema disease of swine. Edema disease is caused by F18ab-positive, Stx2e-producing, non-A/E *E. coli* strains of serogroups O138, O139, and O141 (Bertschinger and Gyles, 1994; Nagy et al., 1997). Edema disease occurs most often one to two weeks postweaning, and is characterized by neurological signs and edema in various locations, most notably the eyelids, subcutis, stomach wall, and mesocolon (Bertschinger and Gyles, 1994; MacLeod et al., 1991). Microscopically, affected pigs usually have coagulative or liquefactive infarcts (encephalomalacia) in the brain stem. Edema and brain infarcts are secondary to arteriolar necrosis. Ultrastructurally, affected arterioles have necrotic endothelium and medial myocytes, and contain platelet thrombi (Methiyapan et al., 1984). Vascular necrosis is thought to be the direct toxic effect of Stx2e. Microscopic examination of the intestine may reveal coliform bacteria adherent to small intestinal epithelium (Methiyapan et al., 1984); however, these bacteria more often are not seen, and recent in vitro studies indicate that F18ab *E. coli* bacteria bind weakly or not at all to the intestinal epithelium (Bertschinger et al., 1997). The vascular lesions in the brains of pigs with edema disease closely resemble lesions in gnotobiotic piglets inoculated orally with Stx2-producing strains of *E. coli* O157:H7 or inoculated parenterally with purified Stx1 (Francis et al., 1989; Dykstra et al., 1993). In addition, the vascular and brain lesions in both edema disease and the *E. coli* O157:H7 gnotobiotic pig model are essentially identical to the lesions seen in the brains of human patients with *E. coli* O157:H7-induced hemolytic uremic syndrome and thrombotic thrombocytopenic purpura (Tzipori et al., 1988). Additional confirmation that the brain-vascular lesions are caused by Stx have been provided by studies in which gnotobiotic piglets passively immunized against Stx2 were protected against the lesions (Chae et al., 1994).

4. CLOSTRIDIAL ENTERITIS AND ENTEROTOXEMIA

Swine and human beings are susceptible to diarrheal disease due to infection with *Clostridium perfringens*. *Clostridium perfringens* is classified (typed) on the basis of production of four major protein toxins termed α, β, ε, and ι (Songer, 1996). Types A, B,

C, D, and E have been described. Only two of these types, A and C, are known to cause enteric disease of swine, and only these two types also cause disease in humans. *Clostridium perfringens* type A enteric infection causes a mild diarrheal disease in both swine and human beings (Lindsay, 1996; Songer, 1996). In contrast, *C. perfringens* type C causes a highly lethal necrotizing enteritis in both swine and human beings. The disease in swine is called necrotizing enteritis or enterotoxemia, whereas the disease in humans is known as enteritis necroticans, pig-bel, and Darmbrand (Lawrence and Walker, 1976). The lesions of *C. perfringens* type C infection in swine and humans are markedly similar (Lawrence and Walker, 1976; Severin, et al., 1984; Taylor and Bergeland, 1992).

Clostridium perfringens type A causes a high morbidity, low mortality diarrheal disease in suckling, weanling, and grower pigs (Collins et al., 1989; Jestin et al., 1985; Johannsen et al., 1993a; Johannsen et al., 1993b; Johannsen et al., 1993c; Popoff and Jestin, 1985). Although outbreaks of diarrheal disease often have 100% morbidity, pigs remain vigorous, continue to eat or suckle, and recover spontaneously in several days. Grossly, there may be hyperemia of the small and large intestines with mild edema of the mesocolon. Microscopically, the changes vary from no lesions to epithelial slough-ing and villous atrophy with hyperemia and edema (Collins et al., 1989; Olubunmi and Taylor, 1985). Large spore-bearing Gram-positive bacilli are usually seen in large numbers in the lumen of the intestine and culture yields heavy growth of the organism.

Clostridium perfringens type A produces both α-toxin and enterotoxin (CPE) and evidence of a role for each in the porcine disease has been demonstrated (Jestin et al., 1985; Popoff and Jestin, 1985). *Clostridium perfringens* type A-induced diarrhea in human beings has been attributed largely to the effects of CPE (Lindsay, 1996). The α-toxin, a hemolytic necrotizing phospholipase, causes hydrolysis of membrane phospholipids and lysis in a wide variety of cell types including endothelial cells, ery-throcytes, platelets, leukocytes, and others (Songer, 1996). Experimental administration of α-toxin alone to one to six-hour-old piglets caused no ultrastructural changes in villi, lymphatics, or other tissues, but did cause mild edema and inflammation of the villi with minimal damage to the epithelium and blood vessels (Johannsen et al., 1993a, 1993b, 1993c). Experimentally, ligated ileal loops of pigs accumulate fluid following injection with purified CPE (Popoff and Jestin, 1985). Fecal CPE and specific serum antibodies are detected in 10- to 13-week-old pigs following natural infection (Jestin et al., 1985). Small intestinal epithelial necrosis and sloughing with villous atrophy also is seen following inoculation of four-day-old hysterectomy-derived, colostrum-deprived pigs and in eight-to-ten-week-old conventional piglets inoculated with live *C. perfringens* type A bacteria (Olubunmi and Taylor, 1985).

Clostridium perfringens type C commonly causes a disease in neonatal pigs char-acterized by necrotizing and often hemorrhagic enteritis (Taylor and Bergeland, 1992). Infection usually occurs when pigs are four days old or younger, but lesions of suba-cute to chronic enteritis may be seen in pigs up to three weeks of age. *Clostridium per-fringens* type C enteritis is diagnosed on the basis of gross and histological lesions which correspond to the length of survival of the pig. Peracute enteritis is seen in pigs 12 to 36 hours old; acute enteritis when pigs are approximately three days old; subacute enteritis when pigs are five to seven days old; and chronic enteritis when pigs are one to three weeks old (Taylor and Bergeland, 1992). Intestines in the peracute disease are usually reddish-black due to severe hemorrhage. In acute disease, the intestines are mottled reddish-tan due to a combination of hemorrhage and necrosis, often with gas pockets (emphysema) in the wall. In subacute and chronic disease, the intestinal wall appears thickened and predominantly tan in color. A diphtheritic membrane replacing the mucosa is often present. Microscopically, in all stages of the disease, there is coagulative necrosis of the mucosa, usually with emphysema and variable amounts of hemorrhage. Peracute and acute enteritis are characterized by more extensive hemorrhage; subacute and chronic enteritis by little or no hemorrhage. Also in peracute and acute enteritis, the necrotic surface is colonized by large numbers of Gram-positive bacilli with maintenance of villous architecture, although the mucosa may show coagulative necrosis. These lesions are diagnostic; however, in the subacute and chronic stages the necrotic tissue contains large numbers of mixed bacterial types, and the necrotic mucosa loses its architecture, making it more difficult to distinguish this disease from others in which mucosal necrosis is seen (e.g., *Isospora suis* and colibacillary HGE).

The characteristic lesions of *C. perfringens* type C enteritis in both swine and human beings have been attributed largely to the effects of β-toxin; however, another toxin called beta2 ($\beta2$)-toxin has recently been identified and may play a role in lesion development (Gibert et al., 1997). Type C bacteria produce at least three major toxins, α-toxin, β-toxin (also called $\beta1$), and $\beta2$-toxin encoded by the *cpa*, *cpb* (also called *cpb1*), and *cpb2* genes, respectively (Gibert et al., 1997; Songer, 1996). The α-toxin, as described above, is a hemolytic necrotizing phospholipase, whereas the $\beta1$-toxin is a highly trypsin-sensitive protein that causes increased capillary permeability, inflammation, and necrosis of intestinal mucosa. The sensitivity of $\beta1$-toxin to trypsin has been the explanation for the occurrence of the disease in pigs less than four days old in which trypsin secretion is absent, and evidence for the importance of $\beta1$-toxin has been inferred from the observations that toxoid alone prevents the disease (Taylor and Bergeland, 1992). Evidence for a role for $\beta2$-toxin in the pathogenesis of type C enteritis has come from the following studies. A novel 28-kDa protein ($\beta2$-toxin) was initially detected and purified from a *C. perfringens* type C strain isolated from a pig with necrotizing enterocolitis (Gibert et al., 1997). The purified protein was cytotoxic for Chinese hamster ovary cells and induced hemorrhagic necrosis of the intestinal mucosa in ligated intestinal loops of guinea pigs. The gene (*cpb2*) that encodes the toxin, termed $\beta2$-toxin, was cloned and detected in other *C. perfringens* type C strains from pigs with necrotizing enteritis (Gibert et al., 1997). Similar to $\beta1$-toxin, the $\beta2$-toxin is sensitive to trypsin. Type A strains also carry the *cpb2* gene, suggesting that $\beta2$-toxin may be a previously unrecognized virulence factor of at least some of these strains (Gibert et al., 1997). Further studies are needed to determine the importance and distribution of $\beta2$-toxin in various types of *C. perfringens*.

5. PROLIFERATIVE ENTEROPATHY

Proliferative enteropathy caused by the obligate intracellular bacterium *Lawsonia intracellularis*, is a distinct disease characterized by epithelial hyperplasia and the presence of curved rod-shaped bacteria free in the apical cytoplasm of enterocytes. The disease has a broad host range, and in addition to swine it affects non-human primates, hamsters, rabbits, rats, guinea pigs, ungulates such as foals, sheep, white-tailed deer, carnivores, including ferrets, arctic foxes, and dogs, and certain birds (Rowland and Lawson, 1992; McOrist et al., 1995; Joens et al., 1997; Cooper and Gebhart, 1998; Frank et al., 1998; Klein et al., in press). The recent addition of non-human primates to the wide range of species in which proliferative enteropathy has been confirmed suggest that the infection may exist unrecognized in human beings.

Proliferative enteropathy was first described in swine in 1931 under the name intestinal adenoma (Beister and Schwartze, 1931). The disease of swine has a worldwide distribution and has been referred to as porcine proliferative enteritis, porcine intestinal adenomatosis, porcine hemorrhagic enteropathy, necroproliferative enteropathy, proliferative ileitis, necrotic ileitis, necrotic enteritis, and regional ileitis. Two epidemiologically distinct clinicopathologic forms of the disease are seen in swine, a predominantly proliferative mucosal change with or without coagulative necrosis called porcine intestinal adenomatosis (PIA), and a primarily hemorrhagic form with a less prominent mucosal proliferative change, designated proliferative hemorrhagic enteropathy (PHE; Bane et al., 1998). The PIA form of the disease is seen mostly in grower and feeder aged pigs, from six to 20 weeks of age (Rowland and Lawson, 1992). It is characterized clinically by a loss of appetite with intermittent or persistent diarrhea over a period of several days or weeks. The feces are soft to watery and yellowgrey to dark brown in color. Flecks of blood are sometimes present in the stools. Although affected pigs lose weight and eventually appear stunted, mortality is infrequent. At necropsy these pigs have marked segmental thickening of the terminal small intestine which occasionally involves the cecum and upper one-third of the colon. Affected intestinal segments sometimes have adherent yellow-grey necrotic material overlying a thickened, red mucosal surface. In contrast, PHE is almost invariably seen in older finishing or breeding age animals where it has a high mortality rate. These pigs have anorexia for one to three days before they begin to pass soft, bright red to tarry black feces, and usually die within 24 to 72 hours of the onset of diarrhea. The presence of massive amounts of blood in the lumen of affected segments of intestine is the most striking change at necropsy. The thickening of the intestinal wall with PHE is not always grossly evident, but the mucosa is usually swollen, red, and may have a corrugated appearance.

Microscopically, both forms of the disease are characterized by crypt epithelial cell hyperplasia which causes the mucosa to appear thickened grossly. Hyperplastic crypt cells are also hypertrophied and contain variable numbers of short, curved bacterial rods lying free in the apical cytoplasm. The organisms are detected either by staining with silver stains such as Warthin-Starry or Dieterle's, or by immunohistochemical staining with a *L. intracellularis* monoclonal antibody, or by fluorescent rRNA in situ hybridization (Jensen et al., 1997; Boye et al., 1998). Nucleic acid-based methods involving polymerase chain reaction amplification of specific *L. intracellularis* DNA sequences have been widely used for diagnosis of the disease (Jones et al., 1993; Cooper et al., 1997; Jensen et al., 1997). A serologic test that detects *L. intracellularis* IgG serum antibody by indirect immunofluorescence has been validated for detection of animals exposed to the agent (Knittel et al., 1998). This serologic test will provide valuable information about the epidemiology and pathogenesis of proliferative enteropathy.

Because *L. intracellularis* was only recently identified as the causative agent of the disease and an infection model with organisms grown in cell culture has become available only recently, the pathogenesis of proliferative enteropathy and corresponding virulence factors of *L. intracellularis* are largely unknown (McOrist, et al., 1993; Joens et al., 1997). However, careful morphologic examination of resolving lesions of the disease in swine suggest the possibility that *L. intracellularis* disrupts normal processes of cell growth, differentiation or apoptosis in the intestinal epithelium (McOrist et al., 1996). Interruption of the intestinal homeostatic mechanism of apoptotic cell loss by *L. intracellularis* might explain the hyperplastic change characteristic of the disease (Potten, 1992; Hall et al., 1994). Conversely, the massive hemorrahage seen with PHE has been attributed to either a hypersensitivity reaction caused by massive release of intracellular organisms or a massive infection in a naive host (Love and Love, 1979). This is consistent with the observation of bacteria within membrane-bound vesicles in phagocytic cells, intracellularly in endothelial cells, and extracellularly in the connective tissue or in the lumen of lymphatics and capillaries of the lamina propria in swine (Love and Love, 1979), non-human primates (Klein et al., in press), and a foal (Duhamel and Wheeldon, 1982) with PHE.

6. SALMONELLOSIS

Salmonella enterica is important both as a pathogen of swine and as a zoonotic, food-borne pathogen of humans. Most cases of clinical salmonellosis in swine are caused by *S. enterica* serotypes Choleraesuis var. kunzendorf and Typhimurium var. Copenhagen (Ferris et al., 1997; Wilcock and Schwartz, 1992); however, swine also carry Agona, Anatum, Derby, Heidelberg, Mbandaka, Worthington, and other serotypes (Davies et al., 1997; Ferris et al., 1997). Three *S. enterica* serotypes commonly found in swine, viz., Agona, Heidelberg, and Typhimurium, are also three of the top ten serotypes isolated from human salmonellosis cases (Fedorka-Cray, 1996). Other *S. enterica* serotypes associated with food-borne disease in humans include Enteritidis, Mbandaka, Newport, and Reading (Levine et al., 1991). The number of food-borne cases in humans per year world-wide is estimated to exceed 100 billion with an estimated cost exceeding 25 billion dollars (Fedorka-Cray, 1996).

The two major forms of clinical salmonellosis in swine include septicemia and enterocolitis (Wilcock and Schwartz, 1992). Septicemia is usually caused by *S. enterica* serotype Choleraesuis var. kunzendorf. In contrast, enterocolitis is most commonly caused by serotype Typhimurium var. Copenhagen, although it is also seen in pigs infected with Typhisuis, Agona, Choleraesuis, and other serotypes. Septicemic salmonellosis occurs mainly in weaned pigs less than five months old, but may be seen occasionally in market or adult breeding swine. Gross lesions in pigs with septicemic salmonellosis include icterus, hepatomegaly, multiple pin-point foci of necrosis in the liver, and edema of the gall bladder. The spleen is often enlarged due to severe congestion. Mesenteric lymph nodes are swollen and edematous. The lung is diffusely hyperemic and edematous, and may contain foci of hemorrhage and consolidation. The fundus of the stomach is hyperemic and/or hemorrhagic. The mucosae of the ileum, cecum, and colon may be fibrinonecrotic if the pig survives the first few days of infection. Microscopically, septicemic salmonellosis is characterized by paratyphoid nodules in the liver, fibrinopurulent interstitial pneumonia, lymphadenitis, and splenitis, and fibrinoid thrombi and hyperemia of glomerular capillaries in the kidneys and mucosal vasculature of the stomach.

Enterocolitic salmonellosis most frequently occurs in pigs from weaning to about four months of age (Wilcock and Schwartz, 1992). Initially, pigs have watery, yellow diarrhea without blood or mucus. Later, blood may be seen in the feces, but usually in lesser amounts than in swine dysentery. Affected pigs are usually depressed and febrile, with anorexia and dehydration. Pigs usually only die after several days of diarrhea, and mortality is usually low. Most pigs recover but remain as carriers and may shed the organism for months. Enteric lesions can be seen in the ileum and/or any part of the large intestine. Lesions can be acute or chronic. Mild lesions are characterized by adherent debris on an inflamed mucosal surface. More severe lesions consist of deep mucosal ulcers which may be focal or coalescing. The large intestine is usually more severely affected than the ileum, with deep button ulcers in contrast to possibly just reddening and roughening of the ileal mucosa. Rectal stricture and megacolon also may be a sequela to infection with *S. enterica* serotypes Typhimurium or Agona (Wilcock and Olander, 1977).

The pathogenesis of *S. enterica* infection has been extensively studied in laboratory rodents and other species including swine. Electron microscopic studies of experimental Typhimurium infection in guinea pigs conducted over 20 years ago revealed the important role of intestinal epithelial invasion in salmonellosis (Takeuchi, 1967a; Takeuchi, 1967b). The pathogenesis of *S. enterica* infection in most species involves bacterial invasion of the intestinal epithelium and Peyer's patches, bacterial survival within macrophages, bacterial dissemination to and colonization of extraintestinal sites, and either localized lesions in these organs or development of septicemia (Ryan and Falkow, 1994). Experimental studies of early intestinal lesions in swine inoculated with various *S. enterica* serotypes revealed bacterial invasion of villous epithelial cells with spread to extraintestinal sites, small intestinal villous atrophy, and acute necropurulent enterocolitis (Arbuckle, 1975; Reed et al., 1986). Recent studies of the mechanisms of fluid accumulation in the porcine small intestine in the early stages of serotype Typhimurium infection have revealed a role for 5-hydroxytryptamine and prostaglandin E-2 (Grondahl et al., 1998). Cytokine signals were shown to be important in regulating the intestinal response of swine to *Salmonella* infection (Trebichavský et al., 1997). Other studies have shown that the persistence of serotype Cholerasuis in porcine tissues is dose dependent, with higher doses leading to immunosuppression and long-term carrier status (Gray et al., 1996).

S. enterica contains at least 60 genes that are required for virulence, the vast majority of which are located within pathogenicity islands on the chromosome (Groisman and Ochman, 1997). The best characterized pathogenicity island is *Salmonella* pathogenicity island 1 (SPI-1). SPI-1 includes genes that mediate intestinal epithelial invasion (e.g., *invA* and *orgA*), induction of neutrophil recruitment, secretion of intestinal fluid, and apoptosis of macrophages (Bäumler et al., 1998; Groisman and Ochman, 1997; Finlay and Falkow, 1997). Another pathogenicity island, SPI-2, contains at least 17 genes that encode for a two-component regulatory system designated Spi/Ssa. The SPI-2 genes also encode for proteins that mediate systemic infections (e.g., survival in macrophages). Several other genes required for virulence are found on the chromosome in "pathogenicity islets", regions smaller than SPI-1 and SPI-2. Fimbrial proteins, outer membrane proteins, and other proteins that may play a role in pathogenicity are encoded for by these genes (Groisman and Ochman, 1997).

7. SWINE DYSENTERY AND COLONIC SPIROCHETOSIS

Bacteria with the morphology of spirochetes have been described in the feces and intestines of human beings and animals for over a century, but recent advances in phenotypic and genotypic characterization have led to frequent taxonomic classification and reclassification of the pathogenic intestinal spirochetes. The agent of swine dysentery, which was originally classified as *Treponema hyodysenteriae* (Kinyon and Harris, 1979), was renamed *Serpula hyodysenteriae* (Stanton et al., 1991), and later as *Serpulina hyodysenteriae* (Stanton, 1992). However, a recent proposal was made to unify the genus *Serpulina* with that of a spirochete designated *Brachyspira aalborgi*, which had been isolated from human beings with colonic spirochetosis prior to publication of the genus *Serpulina* (Hovind-Hougen et al., 1982; Ochiai et al., 1997). Thus, in accordance with the rules of taxonomy, the etiologic agent of swine dysentery is designated *Brachyspira (Serpulina) hyodysenteriae*, and the etiologic agent of colonic spirochetosis is designated *Brachyspira (Serpulina) pilosicoli* (Trott et al., 1996a).

Swine dysentery is an economically important disease of swine that occurs mainly in grower finisher aged pigs, from 15 to 70 kg (Harris and Lysons, 1992). Suckling pigs are susceptible to the infection, but they are thought to be protected by passive transfer of maternal immunity. Diarrhea containing blood and mucus, and occasionally, fibrin, is the most consistent sign of swine dysentery. Weight loss and dehydration are also common; anorexia and increased rectal temperatures are inconsistently seen. Enteric lesions are limited to the large intestine. At the onset of diarrhea, the mucosa appears diffusely edematous and hyperemic, with abundant mucoid watery contents. Adherent flecks of mucohemorrhagic exudate and necrotic debris are seen within a few days, and rapidly progress to extensive necrosis of the mucosa which is covered with a layer of fibrinonecrotic debris. Other lesions may include swelling and edema of regional lymph nodes, and hyperemia of the gastric fundus. The spirochetes are detected in tissues either by staining with Warthin-Starry silver stain, or by immunohistochemical staining with a *Brachyspira* spp.-specific mouse monoclonal antibody (Webb et al., 1997; White et al., 1998), or by fluorescent rRNA in situ hybridization (Jensen et al., 1998). Spirochetes can be isolated from mucosal scrapings of the large intestine or feces using anaerobic culture on selective agar medium (Duhamel and Joens, 1994). The identity of the spirochetes is confirmed by amplification of *B. hyodysenteriae*-specific DNA sequences by the polymerase chain reaction (Elder et al., 1994; Leser et al., 1997). Several *B. hyodysenteriae*-specific mouse monoclonal antibodies with applications in diagnostic immunoassays also have been described for the same purpose (Achacha and Mittal, 1995; Westerman et al., 1995; Lee and Hampson, 1996).

Although the pathogenesis of swine dysentery is incompletely characterized, however, a number of important steps have been elucidated. Initial colonization of the cecum and colon by *B. hyodysenteriae* appears to involve motility-regulated mucin association followed by multiplication of the spirochetes in the mucus along the epithelial surface and in the lumen of the crypts (Kennedy et al., 1988; Milner and Sellwood, 1994; Kennedy and Yancey, 1996). Toxin-mediated epithelial cell damage is thought to be the primary pathogenetic mechanism in swine dysentery (Lysons et al., 1991; Bland et al., 1995; Witters and Duhamel, 1996). The gene encoding the toxin, which is also hemolytic, has been cloned and sequenced, and native and recombinant toxins appear to lyse cells via pore formation (Hyatt and Joens, 1997).

Porcine colonic spirochetosis (PCS), also called intestinal spirochetosis, is a non-fatal colonic disease of recently weaned, grower, and finisher pigs caused by *Brachyspira (Serpulina) pilosicoli* (Taylor et al., 1980; Duhamel et al., 1995a; Duhamel, 1998; Taylor et al., 1992; Trott et al., 1996a). Colonic infection with this spirochete or lesions consistent with colonic spirochetosis have been recognized in a wide variety of hosts in addition to swine, including human beings (Duhamel et al., 1995b; Trivett-Moore et al., 1998; Trott et al., 1997a), non-human primates (Duhamel, 1997; Duhamel et al., 1997), dogs (Duhamel et al., 1995b; Duhamel et al., 1998a), opossums (Duhamel et al., 1998b), and various species of birds (Swayne and McLaren, 1997; Webb et al.,

1997; Oxberry et al., 1998). Several epidemiological studies in the United States and Europe have indicated approximately 4.5% of healthy adult human beings with CS lesions, whereas among homosexual males, presumably infected with HIV-1, the prevalence of CS can be as high as 32.2% (Ruane et al., 1989). Overrepresentation of CS among individuals infected with HIV-1 suggests either a predisposition to an opportunistic infection or a disease association that could potentially play a role in progression of the disease. In the Eastern Highlands of Papua New Guinea B. pilosicoli infection is endemic among villagers; 93.6% of the population is affected for a calculated average duration of about 4 months (Trott et al., 1997). Brachyspira pilosicoli also has been isolated from aborigines from communities in the remote north of Western Australia, and among homosexual men in Sydney, half of them seropositive for HIV-1 (Trivett-Moore et al., 1998). Because most individuals infected with B. pilosicoli are asymptomatic, the clinical significance of the infection remains unclear. However, a healthy adult volunteer that ingested B. pilosicoli became heavily colonized and developed abdominal discomfort, nausea, and headaches that ceased with therapy 52 days after self-inoculation (Oxberry et al., 1998).

Koch's postulates to prove the role of B. pilosicoli in the causation of colonic spirochetosis of swine have been fulfilled with gnotobiotic swine (Neef et al., 1994b) and conventional swine (Duhamel, 1998; Taylor et al., 1980; Trott et al., 1996b; Thomson et al., 1997). Experimental and field investigations indicate that clinical signs of diarrhea in swine are transient and typically resolve within seven to ten days. However, clinical signs lasting for three to six weeks in a given group of pigs may be seen. Pigs as young as four weeks and as old as 20 weeks may show signs of diarrhea, and although the infection may persist, clinical signs are uncommon in pigs older than 20 weeks. Mucoid diarrhea without blood is seen at the onset of the disease, but persistent infection causes reduced performance characterized by reduced weight gain and feed-to-gain efficiency (Duhamel, 1998; MacDougald, 1997; Taylor et al., 1980; Thomson et al., 1997).

All species affected with B. pilosicoli have lesions limited to the large intestine (Taylor et al., 1980; Andrews et al., 1982; Jacques et al., 1989; Duhamel et al., 1995a; Girard et al., 1995; Trott et al., 1996; Thomson et al., 1997; Thomson et al., 1998; Duhamel, 1998). Grossly, the mesocolon may be edematous and the proximal colon is sometimes distended with gas (Taylor et al., 1980). The contents of the cecum and colon have a loose consistency and may be green to yellow in color. Fibrous tags on the serosal surface of the cecum and colon have been seen in naturally-acquired and experimentally induced infections (Christensen, 1998; Duhamel, 1998). Mucosal damage is characterized by focally coalescing superficial erosions with fibrinonecrotic exudate or adherent feed particles giving the mucosa a cobblestone appearance (Taylor et al., 1980; Duhamel, 1998; Thomson et al., 1998).

Colonization of the mucosa by spirochetes is visible on routine histopathological examination, but confirmation of B. pilosicoli can be done by either silver impregnation stain or immunohistochemical staining with a Brachyspira spp.-specific mouse monoclonal antibody (Webb et al., 1997; Duhamel, 1998; White et al., 1998). In some animals, a false brush border consisting of spirochetes intimately attached to the apical membrane of the surface colonic enterocytes by one pole and arranged in parallel arrays may be seen within the first three weeks post-infection (Taylor et al., 1980; Andrews et al., 1982; Jacques et al., 1989; Duhamel et al., 1995a; Girard et al., 1995; Trott et al., 1996b; Duhamel, 1998). At this stage, the surface epithelium may be attenuated and multifocal erosions may be present at the extrusion zone between crypt units. Clusters of spirochetes still attached to membranous debris are sloughed into the lumen of the colon appearing as rosettes of spirochetes with a clear center (Jacques et al., 1989; Duhamel et al., 1995a; Girard et al., 1995). With time, *B. pilosicoli* persist in the lumen of the colonic glands which are dilated and filled with mucus (Thomson et al., 1997; Thomson et al., 1998; Duhamel, 1998). Repair of the superficial epithelial damage is characterized by hyperplasia of the crypt epithelium with concomitant goblet cell depletion and elongation of the crypt columns and an increase in the numbers of mononuclear cells in the lamina propria (Duhamel et al., 1995a; Thomson et al., 1997; Thomson et al., 1998; Duhamel, 1998). Isolation of *B. pilosicoli* is similar to *B. hyodysenteriae*, but requires further confirmation by amplification of specific DNA sequences by polymerase chain reaction (Park et al., 1995; Fellström et al., 1997; Leser et al., 1997; Muniappa et al., 1997), or by immunoassays (Lee and Hampson, 1995).

By analogy with *B. hyodysenteriae*, the initial colonization of the colon by *B. pilosicoli* appears to be mediated by motility-regulated mucin association (Witters and Duhamel, 1998). This is followed by multiplication of the spirochetes in close proximity with the mucosal surface and inside the lumena of the crypts (Thomson et al., 1997; Duhamel, 1998). Intimate attachment of *B. pilosicoli* to the apical membrane of colonic enterocytes, causes destruction or effacement of the enterocyte microvilli (Taylor et al., 1980; Andrews et al., 1982; Jacques et al., 1989; Duhamel et al., 1995a; Girard et al., 1995; Trott et al., 1996b; Duhamel, 1998).

Comparative studies with cultured cells and infection models suggest a specific spirochete ligand and host cell membrane receptor interaction during attachment of *B. pilosicoli* (Muniappa et al., 1996; Muniappa et al., 1997; Muniappa et al., in press). Inoculation of chicks and laboratory mice with human, porcine, and canine *B. pilosicoli* have shown attachment of the spirochetes to the cecal enterocytes accompanied by focal erosions and sometimes local invasion of the gut wall (Trott et al., 1995; Muniappa et al., 1996; Muniappa et al., 1997; Sacco et al., 1997). *B. pilosicoli* can invade between enterocytes and into the lamina propria where it is seen either extracellularly or within macrophages or in capillary vessels (Muniappa et al., 1996). Ultrastructurally, the spirochetes have a propensity for colonization and damage at the extrusion zone between crypt units and local penetration into the lamina propria (Muniappa et al., 1996). Penetration of the epithelial layer may involve dissociation of intercellular junctional complexes of enterocytes by the action of a subtilisin-like serine protease present in the outer membrane of the spirochete (Muniappa and Duhamel, 1997). Members of the normal bacterial flora of the gut are present at the site of the mucosal defect and may participate in the induction of further mucosal damage. The loss of colonic function is attributable to the loss of microvillous brush border of colonized enterocytes and the local inflammatory response. This is consistent with data indicating interference with host absorption of specific amino sugars by spirochetes attached to the rectal mucosa of humans with the disease (Neutra, 1980). Translocation of *B. pilosicoli* to extraintestinal sites including the mesenteric lymph nodes and pericardial sac of experimentally inoculated pigs, and the blood stream of terminally ill human patients also has been documented (Trott et al., 1997; Hampson et al., 1998a; Hampson et al., 1998b).

REFERENCES

Achacha, M. and Mittal, K.R., 1995, Production and characterization of monoclonal antibodies against *Serpulina hyodysenteriae* and *S. innocens* and their use in serotyping, J. Clin. Microbiol. 33:2519–2521.

Alexander, T.J.L., 1994, Neonatal diarrhoea in pigs, In: *Escherichia coli* in domestic animals and humans, Editor: Gyles, C.L., CAB International, Wallingford, U.K., pp. 151–191.

Andrews, J.J. and Hoffman, L.J., 1982, A porcine colitis caused by a weakly beta hemolytic treponeme (*Treponema innocens?*), Proc. Am. Assoc. Vet. Lab. Diagn. pp. 395–402.

Arbuckle, J.B.R., 1975, Villous atrophy in pigs orally infected with *Salmonella cholerae-suis*, Res. Vet. Sci. 18:322–324.

Babakhani, F.K., Bradley, G.A., and Joens, L.A., 1993, Newborn piglet model for campylobacteriosis, Infect. Immun. 61:3466–3475.

Bane, D., Norby, B., Gardner, I., Roof, M., Knittel, J., Bush, E., and Gebhart, C., 1998, The epidemiology of porcine proliferative enteropathy, Proc. 15th Intl. Pig Vet. Soc. 3:107.

Barnes, D.M. and Moon, H.W., 1964, Enterotoxemia in pigs due to *Clostridium perfringens* type C, J. Am. Vet. Med. Assoc. 144:1391–1394.

Bäumler, A.J., Tsolis, R.M., Ficht, T.A., and Adams, L.G., 1998, Evolution of host adaptation in *Salmonella enterica*, Infect. Immun. 66:4579–4587.

Beister, H.E. and Schwartze, L.H., 1931, Intestinal adenoma in swine, Am. J. Pathol. 7:175–185.

Bergeland, M.E., 1972, Pathogenesis and immunity of *Clostridium perfringens* type C enteritis in swine, J. Am. Vet. Med. Assoc. 160:568–571.

Bertschinger, H.U. and Gyles, C.L., 1994, Oedema disease of pigs, In: *Escherichia coli* in domestic animals and humans, Editor: Gyles, C.L., CAB International, Wallingford, U.K., pp. 193–219.

Bland, A.P., Frost, A.J., and Lysons, R.J., 1995, Susceptibility of porcine ileal enterocytes to the cytotoxin of *Serpulina hyodysenteriae* and the resolution of the epithelial lesions: an electron microscopic study, Vet. Pathol. 32:24–35.

Borie, C., Monreal, Z., Guerrero, P., Sanchez, M.L., Martinez, J., Arellano, C., and Prado, V., 1997, Prevalence and characterization of enterohemorrhagic *Escherichia coli* isolated from healthy cattle and pigs slaughtered in Santiago, Chile, Archiv. Med. Vet. 29:205–212.

Boye, M., Jensen, T.K., Moller, K., Leser, T.D., and Jorsal, S.E., 1998, Specific detection of *Lawsonia intracellularis* in porcine proliferative enteropathy inferred from fluorescent rRNA in situ hybridization, Vet. Pathol. 35:153–156.

Broes, A., Drolet, R., Jacques, M., Fairbrother, J.M., and Johnson, W.M., 1988, Natural infection with an attaching and effacing *Escherichia coli* in a diarrheic puppy, Can. J. Vet. Res. 52:280–282.

Buzby, J.C., Roberts, C.T., Lin, C.T., and MacDonald, J.M., 1996, Bacterial foodborne disease: medical costs and productivity losses. U.S.D.A. Economic Research Service, AER No. 741, August, p. 70.

Cantey, J.R. and Blake, R.K., 1977, Diarrhea due to *Escherichia coli* in the rabbit: a novel mechanism, J. Infect. Dis. 135:454–462.

Casey, T.A., Herring, C.J., Schneider, R.A., Bosworth, B.T., and Whipp, S.C., 1998, Expression of heat-stable enterotoxin STb by adherent *Escherichia coli* is not sufficient to cause severe diarrhea in neonatal pigs, Infect. Immun. 66:1270–1272.

Chae, C., Moxley, R.A., Christopher-Hennings, J., Francis, D.H., and Wannemuehler, M.J., 1994, Shiga-like toxin-II-producing *Escherichia coli* O157:H7 infection in gnotobiotic piglets: protection against brain vascular lesions with SLT-II antiserum, In: Recent advances in Verocytotoxin-producing Escherichia coli infections, Editors: Karmali, M.A. and Goglio, A.G., Elsevier Science BV, Amsterdam, pp. 241–244.

Chapman, P.A., Siddons, C.A., Malo, A.T.C., and Harkin, M.A., 1997, A 1-year study of *Escherichia coli* O157 in cattle, sheep, pigs and poultry, Epidemiol. Infect. 119:245–250.

Christensen, N.H., 1998, Isolation of *Serpulina pilosicoli* from scouring finisher pigs, and control of the scouring with zinc bacitracin, Proc. 15th Int. Pig Vet. Soc. Conf. 3:418.

Cohen, I.T., Nelson, S.A., Moxley, R.A., Hirsh, M.P., Counihan, T.C., and Martin, R.F., 1991, Necrotizing enterocolitis in a neonatal piglet model, J. Pediatr. Surg. 26:598–601.

Collins, J.E., Bergeland, M.E., Bouley, D., Ducommun, A.L., Francis, D.H., and Yeske, P., 1989, Diarrhea associated with *Clostridium perfringens* type A enterotoxin in neonatal pigs, J. Vet. Diagn. Invest. 1:351–353.

Cooper, D.M., Swanson, D.L., and Gebhart, C.J., 1997, Diagnosis of proliferative enteritis in frozen and formalin-fixed, paraffin-embedded tissues from a hamster, horse, deer, and ostrich using *Lawsonia intracellularis*-specific multiplex PCR assay, Vet. Microbiol. 54:47–62.

Cooper, D.M. and Gebhart, C.J., 1998, Comparative aspects of proliferative enteritis, J. Am. Vet. Med. Assoc. 212:1446–1451.

Davies, P.R., Morrow, W.E.M., Jones, F.T., Deen, J., Fedorka-Cray, P.J., and Harris, I.T., 1997, Prevalence of salmonella in finishing swine raised in different production systems in North Carolina, USA, Epidemiol. Infect. 119:237–244.

Donnenberg, M.S., Tzipori, S., McKee, M.L., O'Brien, A.D., Alroy, J., and Kaper, J.B., 1993, The role of the *eae* gene of enterohemorrhagic *Escherichia coli* in intimate attachment in vitro and in a porcine model, J. Clin. Invest. 92:1418–1424.

Drolet, R., Fairbrother, J.M., Harel, J., and Helie, P., 1994, Attaching and effacing and enterotoxigenic *Escherichia coli* associated with enteric colibacillosis in the dog, Can. J. Vet. Res. 58:87–92.

Duhamel, G.E. and Wheeldon, E.B., 1982, Intestinal adenomatosis in a foal, Vet. Pathol. 19:447–450.

Duhamel, G.E. and Joens, L.A., 1994, Laboratory procedures for diagnosis of swine dysentery. Report to the Committee on Swine Dysentery, Am. Assoc. Lab. Diagn., Columbia, MO.

Duhamel, G.E., Muniappa, N., Gardner, I., Anderson, M.A., Blanchard, P.C., DeBey, B.M., Mathiesen, M.R., and Walker, R.L., 1995a, Porcine colonic spirochaetosis: A diarrhoeal disease associated with a newly recognized species of intestinal spirochaetes, Pig J. 35:101–110.

Duhamel, G.E., Muniappa, N., Mathiesen, M.R., Johnson, J.L., Toth, J., Elder, R.O., and Doster, A.R., 1995b, Certain canine weakly beta-hemolytic intestinal spirochetes are phenotypically and genotypically related to spirochetes associated with human and porcine intestinal spirochetosis, J. Clin. Microbiol. 33:2211–2215.

Duhamel, G.E., 1997, Intestinal spirochaetes in non-production animals. In: Intestinal spirochaetosis in domestic animals and humans, Editors: Hampson, D.J. and Stanton, T.B., CAB International, Wallingford, UK, pp. 301–320.

Duhamel, G.E., Elder, R.O., Muniappa, N., Mathiesen, M.R., Wong, V.J., and Tarara, R.P., 1997, Colonic spirochetal infections in nonhuman primates that were associated with *Brachyspira aalborgi, Serpulina pilosicoli,* and unclassified flagellated bacteria, Clin. Infect. Dis. 25(Suppl 2):S186–S188.

Duhamel, G.E., 1998, Colonic spirochetosis caused by *Serpulina pilosicoli*, Large Anim. Pract. 19:14–22.

Duhamel, G.E., Trott, D.J., Muniappa, N., Mathiesen, M.R., Tarasiuk, K., Lee, J.I., and Hampson, D.J., 1998a, Canine intestinal spirochetes consist of *Serpulina pilosicoli* and a newly identified group provisionally designated "*Serpulina canis*" sp. nov., J. Clin. Microbiol. 36:2264–2270.

Duhamel, G.E., Ganley, L., Barr, B.C., Whipple, J.P., Mathiesen, M.R., Nordhausen, R.W., Walker, R.L., Bargar, T.W., and Van Kruiningen, H.J., 1998b, Intestinal spirochetosis of North American opossums (*Didelphis virginiana*); a potential biological vector for pathogenic spirochetes, Proc. Am. Assoc. Zoo Vet. and Am. Assoc. Wildlife Vet. Joint Conf., Omaha, Neb., pp. 83–88.

Dykstra, S.A., Moxley, R.A., Janke, B.H., Nelson, E.A., and Francis, D.H., 1993, Clinical signs and lesions in gnotobiotic pigs inoculated with Shiga-like toxin I from *Escherichia coli*, Vet. Pathol. 30:410–417.

Elder, R.O., Duhamel, G.E., Schafer, R.W., Mathiesen, M.R. and Ramanathan, M., 1994, Rapid detection of *Serpulina hyodysenteriae* in diagnostic specimens by PCR, J. Clin. Microbiol. 32:1497–1502.

Fairbrother, J.M. and Ngeleka, M., 1994, Extraintestinal *Escherichia coli* infections in pigs, In: *Escherichia coli* in domestic animals and humans, Editor: Gyles, C.L., CAB International, Wallingford, U.K., pp. 221–236.

Faubert, C. and Drolet, R., 1992, Hemorrhagic gastroenteritis caused by *Escherichia coli* in piglets: clinical, pathological and microbiological findings, Can. Vet. J. 33:251–256.

Fedorka-Cray, P.J., 1996, The connection between *Salmonella*, swine, and food safety, 27th Ann. Geo. A. Young Swine Conf., University of Nebraska-Lincoln, Lincoln, Neb., pp. 25–45.

Fellström, C., Pettersson, B., Thomson, J., Gunnarsson, A., Persson, M., and Johansson, K., 1997, Identification of *Serpulina* species associated with porcine colitis by biochemical analysis and PCR, J. Clin. Microbiol. 35:462–467.

Ferris, K.E. and Miller, D.A., 1997, *Salmonella* serotypes from animals and related sources reported during July 1996-June 1997, Proc. U.S. Anim. Health Assoc.

Finlay, B.B. and Falkow, S., 1997, Common themes in microbial pathogenicity revisited, Microbiol. Mol. Biol. Rev. 61:136–169.

Fischer, J., Maddox, C., Moxley, R., Kinden, D., and Miller, M., 1994, Pathogenicity of a bovine attaching effacing *Escherichia coli* isolate lacking Shiga-like toxins, Am. J. Vet. Res. 55:991–999.

Francis, D.H., Collins, J.E., and Duimstra, J.R., 1986, Infection of gnotobiotic pigs with an *Escherichia coli* O157:H7 strain associated with an outbreak of hemorrhagic colitis, Infect. Immun. 51:953–956.

Francis, D.H., Moxley, R.A., and Andraos, C.Y., 1989, Edema disease-like brain lesions in gnotobiotic piglets infected with *Escherichia coli* serotype O157:H7, Infect. Immun. 57:1339–1342.

Francis, D.H., Grange, P.A., Zeman, D.H., Baker, D.R., Sun, R., and Erickson, A.K., 1998, Expression of mucin-type glycoprotein K88 receptors strongly correlates with piglet susceptibility to K88+ enterotoxigenic *Escherichia coli*, but adhesion of this bacterium to brush borders does not. Infect. Immun. 66:4050–4055.

Frank, N., Fishman, C.E., Gebhart, C.J., and Levy, M., 1998, *Lawsonia intracellularis* proliferative enteropathy in a weanling foal, Eq. Vet. J. 30:549–552.

Fukushima, H., Hoshina, K., Nakamura, R., and Ito, Y., 1987, Raw beef, pork, and chicken in Japan contaminated with *Salmonella* sp., *Campylobacter* sp., *Yersinia enterocolitica* and *Clostridium perfringens*—a comparative study, Zentralbl. Bakteriol. Mikrobiol. Hyg. 184:60–70.

Gibert, M., Jolivet-Renaud, C., and Popoff, M.R., 1997, Beta2 toxin, a novel toxin produced by *Clostridium perfringens*, Gene 203:65–73.

Girard, C., Lemarchand, T., and Higgins, R., 1995, Porcine colonic spirochetosis: a retrospective study of eleven cases, Can. Vet. J. 36:291–294.

Gray, J.T., Stabel, T.J., and Fedorka-Cray, P.J., 1996, Effect of dose on the immune response and persistence of *Salmonella choleraesuis* infection in swine, Am. J. Vet. Res. 57:313–319.

Groisman, E.A. and Ochman, H., 1997, How *Salmonella* became a pathogen, Trends Microbiol. 5:343–349.

Grondahl, M.L., Jensen, G.M., Nielsen, C.G., Skadhauge, E., Olsen, J.E., and Hansen, M.B., 1998, Secretory pathways in *Salmonella typhimurium*-induced fluid accumulation in the porcine small intestine, J. Med. Microbiol. 47:151–157.

Guinee, P.A.M. and Jansen, W.H., 1979, Behavior of *Escherichia coli* K antigens K88ab, K88ac, and K88ad in immunoelectrophoresis, double diffusion, and hemagglutination, Infect. Immun. 25:700–705.

Gyles, C.L., 1994, *Escherichia coli* enterotoxins, In: *Escherichia coli* in domestic animals and humans, Editor: Gyles, C.L., CAB International, Wallingford, U.K., pp. 337–364.

Hall, P.A., Coates, P.J., Ansari, B., and Hopwood, D., 1994, Regulation of cell number in the mammalian gastrointestinal tract: the importance of apoptosis, J. Cell Sci. 107:3569–3577.

Hampson, D.J., 1994, Postweaning *Escherichia coli* diarrhoea in pigs, In: *Escherichia coli* in domestic animals and humans, Editor: Gyles, C.L., CAB International, Wallingford, U.K., pp. 171–191.

Hampson, D.J., Robertson, I.D., and Oxberry, S.L., 1998a, Extraintestinal colonisation by Serpulina pilosicoli in an experimentally inoculated pig, Proc. Intl. Pig Vet. Soc. Conf., Birmingham, UK, 2:54.

Hampson, D.J., Robertson, I.D., Oxberry, S.L., and Pethick, D.W., 1998b, Evaluation of vaccination and diet for the control of Serpulina pilosicoli infection (porcine intestinal spirochaetosis), Proc. Intl. Pig Vet. Soc. Conf., Birmingham, UK 2:56.

Harris, D.L. and Lysons, R.J., 1992, Swine dysentery, In: Diseases of swine. Editors: Leman, A.D., Straw, B.E., Mengeling, W.L., D'Allaire, S., and Taylor, D.J., 7th ed., Iowa State University Press, Ames, Iowa, pp. 599–616.

Helie, P., Morin, M., Jacques, M., and Fairbrother, J.M., 1991, Experimental infection of newborn pigs with an attaching and effacing *Escherichia coli* O45:K"E65" strain, Infect. Immun. 59:814–821.

Holland, R.E., 1990, Some infectious causes of diarrhea in young farm animals, Clin. Microbiol. Rev. 3:345–375.

Hovind-Hougen, K., Birch-Andersen, A., Henrik-Nielsen, R., Orholm, M., Pederse, J.O., Teglbjærg, P.S., and Thaysen, E.H., 1982, Intestinal spirochetosis: morphological characterization and cultivation of the spirochete *Brachyspira aalborgi* gen. nov., sp. nov., J. Clin. Microbiol. 16:1127–1136.

Hyatt, D.R. and Joens, L.A., 1997, Analysis of the lytic activity of the *Serpulina hyodysenteriae* hemolysin, Infect. Immun. 65:4877–4879.

Jacques, M., Girard, C., Higgins, R., and Goyette, G., 1989, Extensive colonization of the porcine colonic epithelium by a spirochete similar to *Treponema innocens*, J. Clin. Microbiol. 27:1139–1141.

Janke, B.H., Francis, D.H., Collins, J.E., Libal, M.C., Zeman, D.H., and Johnson, D.D., 1989, Attaching and effacing *Escherichia coli* infections in calves, pigs, lambs, and dogs, J. Vet. Diagn. Invest. 1:6–11.

Jensen, T.K., Møller, K., Leser, T.D., and Jorsal, S.E., 1997, Comparison of histology, immunohistochemistry and polymerase chain reaction for detection of *Lawsonia intracellularis* in natural porcine proliferative enteropathy, Eur. J. Vet. Pathol. 3:115–123.

Jensen, T.K., Møller, K., Duhamel, G.E., Hansen, K.K., Szancer, J., and Boye, M., 1998, Fluorescent *in situ* hybridization for detection of *Serpulina hyodysenteriae* in field cases of porcine colitis associated with mixed spirochaetal infections, Proc. Intl. Pig Vet. Soc. Conf., Birmingham, UK 2:58.

Jestin, A., Popoff, M.R., and Mahe, S., 1985, Epizootiologic investigations of a diarrheic syndrome in fattening pigs, Am. J. Vet. Res. 46:2149–2151.

Joens, L.A., Nibbelink, S., and Glock, R.D., 1997, Induction of gross and microscopic lesions of porcine proliferative enteritis by *Lawsonia intracellularis*, Am. J. Vet. Res. 58:1125–1131 (correction, 58:1192).

Johannsen, U., Arnold, P., Kohler, B., and Selbitz, H.J., 1993a, Studies into experimental *Clostridium perfringens* type A enterotoxaemia of suckled piglets: experimental provocation of the disease by *Clostridium perfringens* type A intoxication and infection. Monatsh. Veterinaermed. 48:129–136.

Johannsen, U., Menger, S., Arnold, P., Kohler, B., and Selbitz, H.J., 1993b, Experimental *Clostridium perfringens* type A enterotoxaemia in unweaned piglets, Monatsh. Veterinaermed. 48:267–273.

Johannsen, U., Menger, S., Arnold, P., Kohler, B., and Selbitz, H.J., 1993c, Experimental *Clostridium perfringens* type A enterotoxaemia in unweaned piglets. II. Light- and electron-microscopic investigations on the pathology and pathogenesis of experimental *Clostridium perfringens* type A infection, Monatsh. Veterinaermed. 48:299–306.

Jones, G.F. Ward, G.E., Murtaugh, M.P., Lin, G., and Gebhart, C.J., 1993, Enhanced detection of intracellular organism of swine proliferative enteritis, ileal symbiont intracellularis, in feces by polymerase chain reaction, J. Clin. Microbiol. 31:2611–2615.

Kennedy, M.J., Rosnick, D.K., Ulrich, R.G., and Yancey, R.J., 1988, Association of *Treponema hyodysenteriae* with porcine intestinal mucosa, J. Gen. Microbiol. 134:1565–1576.

Kennedy, M.J. and Yancey, R.J., 1996, Motility and chemotaxis in *Serpulina hyodysenteriae*, Vet. Microbiol. 49:21–30.

Ketley, J.M., 1997, Pathogenesis of enteric infection by *Campylobacter*, Microbiology 143:5–21.

Kinyon, J.M. and Harris, D.L., 1979, *Treponema innocens*, a new species of intestinal bacteria, and emended description of the type strain of *Treponema hyodysenteriae* Harris et al., Int. J. Syst. Bacteriol. 29:102–109.

Klein, E.C., Gebhart, C.J., and Duhamel, G.E., Fatal outbreaks of proliferative enteropathy caused by *Lawsonia intracellularis* in young colony-raised rhesus macaques, J. Clin. Primatol., in press.

Knittel, J.P., Jordan, D.M., Schwartz, K.J., Janke, B.H., Roof, M.B., McOrist, S., and Harris, D.L., 1998, Evaluation of antmortem polymerase chain reaction and serologic methods for detection of *Lawsonia intracellularis*-exposed pigs, Am. J. Vet. Res. 59:722–726.

Lawrence, G. and Walker, P.D., 1976, Pathogenesis of enteritis necroticans in Papua New Guinea, Lancet i:125–126.

Lee, B.J. and Hampson, D.J., 1995, A monoclonal antibody reacting with the cell envelope of spirochaetes isolated from cases of intestinal spirochaetosis in pigs and humans, FEMS Microbiol. Lett. 131:179–184.

Lee, B.J. and Hampson, D.J., 1996, Production and characterisation of a monoclonal antibody to *Serpulina hyodysenteriae*, FEMS Microbiol. Lett. 136:193–197.

Leser, T.D., Møller, K., Jensen, T.K., and Jorsal, S.E., 1997, Specific detection of *Serpulina hyodysenteriae* and potentially pathogenic weakly β-haemolytic porcine intestinal spirochetes by polymerase chain reaction targeting 23S rDNA, Mol. Cell. Probes 11:363–372.

Levine, M.M., 1987, *Escherichia coli* that cause diarrhea: enterotoxigenic, enteropathogenic, enteroinvasive, enterohemorrhagic, and enteroadherent, J. Infect. Dis. 155:377–389.

Levine, W.C., Smart, A.F., Archer, D.L., Bean, N.H., and Tauxe, R.V., 1991, Foodborne disease outbreaks in nursing homes, 1975 through 1987, J. Am. Vet. Med. Assoc. 266:2105–2109.

Lindsay, J.A., 1996, *Clostridium perfringens* type A enterotoxin (CPE): more than just explosive diarrhea, Crit. Rev. Microbiol. 22:257–277.

Love, D.N. and Love, R.J., 1979, Pathology of proliferative haemorrhagic enteropathy in pigs, Vet. Pathol. 16:41–48.

Lysons, R.J., Kent, K.A., Bland, A.P., Sellwood, R., Robinson, W.F., and Frost, A.J., 1991, A cytotoxic haemolysin from *Treponema hyodysenteriae*—a probable virulence determinant in swine dysentery, J. Med. Microbiol. 34:97–102.

MacDougald, D., 1997, Clinical impact of colonic spirochetosis. Proc. Am. Assoc. Swine Pract., Quebec City, Canada, p. 497.

MacLeod, D.L., Gyles, C.L., and Wilcock, B.P., 1991, Reproduction of edema disease of swine with purified Shiga-like toxin-II variant, Vet. Pathol. 28:66–73.

McKee, M.L., Melton-Celsa, A.R., Moxley, R.A., Francis, D.H., and O'Brien, A.D., 1995, Enterohemorrhagic *Escherichia coli* O157:H7 requires intimin to colonize the gnotobiotic pig intestine and to adhere to HEp-2 cells, Infect. Immun. 63:3739–3744.

McOrist, S., Jasni, S., Mackie, R.A., MacIntyre, N., Neef, N., and Lawson, G.H.K., 1993, Reproduction of porcine proliferative enteropathy with pure cultures of Ileal Symbiont Intracellularis, Infect. Immun. 61:4286–4292.

McOrist, S., Gebhart, C.J., Boid, R., and Barns, S.M., 1995, Characterization of *Lawsonia intracellularis* gen. nov., sp. nov., the obligately intracellular bacterium of porcine proliferative enteropathy, Int. J. Syst. Bacteriol. 45:820–825.

McOrist, S., Roberts, L., Jasni, S., Rowland, A.C., Lawson, G.H.K., Gebhart, C.J., and Bosworth, B., 1996, Developed and resolving lesions in porcine proliferative enteropathy: possible pathogenetic mechanisms, J. Comp. Pathol. 115:35–45.

Methiyapun, P., Pohlenz, J.F.L., and Bertschinger, H.U., 1984, Ultrastructure of the intestinal mucosa in pigs experimentally inoculated with an edema disease-producing strain of *Escherichia coli* (O139:K12:H1), Vet. Pathol. 21:516–520.

Milner, J.A. and Sellwood, R., 1994, Chemotactic response to mucin by *Serpulina hyodysenteriae* and other porcine spirochetes: Potential role in intestinal colonization, Infect. Immun. 62:4095–4099.

Moon, H.W., Nagy, B., and Isaacson, R.E., 1977, Intestinal colonization and adhesion by enterotoxigenic *Escherichia coli*: ultrastructural observations on adherence to ileal epithelium of the pig, J. Infect. Dis. 136S:124–129.

Moon, H.W., Whipp, S.C., Argenzio, R.A., Levine, M.M., and Giannella, R.A., 1983, Attaching and effacing activities of rabbit and human enteropathogenic *Escherichia coli* in pig and rabbit intestines, Infect. Immun. 41:1340–1351.

Moxley, R.A., Erickson, E.D., and Briesch, S., 1988, Shock associated with enteric colibacillosis in suckling and weaned swine, Proc 29th Ann Geo A Young Conf, University of Nebraska, Lincoln, Neb., pp. 33–38.

Moxley, R.A. and Francis, D.H., 1998, Overview of animal models, In: *Escherichia coli* O157:H7 and other Shiga toxin-producing *E. coli* infections, Editors: Kaper, J.B. and O'Brien, A.D., ASM Press, Washington, D.C., pp. 249–260.

Muniappa, N., Duhamel, G.E., Mathiesen, M.R., and Barger, T.W., 1996, Light microscopic and ultrastructural changes in the ceca of chicks inoculated with human and canine *Serpulina pilosicoli*, Vet. Pathol. 33:542–550.

Muniappa, N. and Duhamel, G.E., 1997, Outer membrane-associated serine protease of intestinal spirochetes, FEMS Microbiol. Lett. 154:159–164.

Muniappa, N., Mathiesen, M.R., and Duhamel, G.E., 1997, Laboratory identification and enteropathogenicity testing of *Serpulina pilosicoli* associated with porcine colonic spirochetosis, J. Vet. Diagn. Invest. 9:165–171.

Muniappa, N., Ramanathan, M.R, Tarara, R.P., Westerman, R.B., Mathiesen, M.R., and Duhamel, G.E., Attachment of human and rhesus *Serpulina pilosicoli* to cultured cells and comparison with a chick infection model, J. Spiro. Tick-borne Dis., in press.

Nagy, B., Casey, T.A., Whipp, S.C., and Moon, H.W., 1992, Susceptibility of porcine intestine to pilus-mediated adhesion by some isolates of piliated enterotoxigenic *Escherichia coli* increases with age, Infect. Immun. 60:1285–1294.

Nagy, B., Whipp, S.C., Imberechts, H., Bertschinger, H.U., Dean-Nystrom, E.A., Casey, T.A., and Salajka, E., 1997, Biological relationship between F18ab and F18ac fimbriae of enterotoxigenic and verotoxigenic *Escherichia coli* from weaned pigs with oedema disease or diarrhoea, Microb. Pathog. 22:1–11.

Nataro, J.P. and Kaper, J.B., 1998, Diarrheagenic *Escherichia coli*, Clin. Microbiol. Rev. 11:142–201.

Neef, N.A., McOrist, S., Lysons, R.J., Bland, A.P., and Miller, B.G., 1994a, Development of large intestinal attaching and effacing lesions in pigs in association with the feeding of a particular diet, Infect. Immun. 62:4325–4332.

Neef, N.A., Lysons, R.J., Trott, D.J., Hampson, D.J., Jones, P.W., and Morgan, J.H., 1994b, Pathogenicity of porcine intestinal spirochetes in gnotobiotic pigs, *Infect. Immun.* 62:2395–2403.

Neutra, M.R., 1980, Prokaryotic-eukaryotic cell junctions: Attachment of spirochetes and flagellated bacteria to primate large intestinal cells, J. Ultrastruct. Res. 70:186–203.

Ochiai, S., Adachi, Y., and Mori, K., 1997, Unification of the genera *Serpulina* and *Brachyspira*, and proposals of *Brachyspira hyodysenteriae* comb. nov., *Brachyspira innocens* comb. nov. and *Brachyspira pilosicoli* comb. nov., Microbiol. Immunol. 41:445–452.

Olubunmi, P.A. and Taylor, D.J., 1985, *Clostridium perfringens* type A in enteric diseases of pig, Trop. Vet. 3:28–33.

Oxberry, S.L., Trott, D.J., and Hampson, D.J., 1998, *Serpulina pilosicoli*, waterbirds and water: potential sources of infection for humans and other animals, Epidemiol. Infect. 121:219–225.

Park, N.Y., Chung, C.Y., McLaren, A.J., Atyeo, R.F., and Hampson, D.J., 1995, Polymerase chain reaction for identification of human and porcine spirochaetes recovered from cases of intestinal spirochaetosis, FEMS Microbiol. Lett. 125:225–230.

Popoff, M.R. and Jestin, A., 1985, Enteropathogenicity of purified *Clostridium perfringens* enterotoxin in the pig, Am. J. Vet. Res. 46:2147–2148.

Potten, C.S., 1992, The significance of spontaneous and induced apoptosis in the gastrointestinal tract of mice, Cancer Metastasis Rev. 11:179–195.

Reed, W.M., Olander, H.J., and Thacker, H.L., 1986, Studies on the pathogenesis of *Salmonella typhimurium* and *Salmonella choleraesuis* var *kunzendorf* infection in weanling pigs, Am. J. Vet. Res. 47:75–83.

Rowland, A.C. and Lawson, G.H.K., 1992, Porcine proliferative enteropathies, In: Diseases of swine. Editors: Leman, A.D., Straw, B.E., Mengeling, W.L., D'Allaire, S., and Taylor, D.J., 7th ed., Iowa State University Press, Ames, Iowa, pp. 560–569.

Ruane, P.J., Nakata, M.M., Reinhardt, J.F., and George, W.L., 1989, Spirochete-like organisms in the human gastrointestinal tract, Rev. Infect. Dis. 11:184–196.

Ryan, K.J. and Falkow, S., 1994, *Enterobacteriaceae*, In: Sherris Medical Microbiology: an introduction to infectious diseases. Editor: Ryan, K.J., 3rd ed., Appleton and Lange, Norwalk, Conn., pp. 321–324.

Sacco, R.E., Trampel, D.W., and Wannemuehler, M.J., 1997, Experimental infection of C3H mice with avian, porcine, or human isolates of *Serpulina pilosicoli*, Infect. Immun. 65:5349–5353.

Severin, W.P.J., de la Fuente, A.A., and Stringer, M.F., 1984, *Clostridium perfringens* type C causing necrotizing enteritis, J. Clin. Pathol. 942–944.

Smyth, C.J., Marron, M., and Smith, S.G.J., 1994, Fimbriae of *Escherichia coli*, In: *Escherichia coli* in domestic animals and humans, Editor: Gyles, C.L., CAB International, Wallingford, U.K., pp. 399–435.

Songer, J.G., 1996, Clostridial enteric diseases of domestic animals, Clin. Microbiol. Rev. 9:216–234.

Stanton, T.B., Jensen, N.S., Casey, T.A., Tordoff, L.A., Dewhirst, F.E., and Paster, B.J., 1991, Reclassification of *Treponema hyodysenteriae* and *Treponema innocens* in a new genus, *Serpula* gen. nov., as *Serpula hyodysenteriae* comb. nov. and *Serpula innocens* comb. nov., Int. J. Syst. Bacteriol. 41:50–58.

Stanton, T.B., 1992, Proposal to change the genus designation *Serpula* to *Serpulina* gen. nov. containing the species *Serpulina hyodysenteriae* comb. nov. and *Serpulina innocens* comb. nov., Int. J. Syst. Bacteriol. 42:189–190.

Swayne, D.E. and McLaren, A.J., 1997, Avian intestinal spirochaetes and avian intestinal spirochaetosis, In: Intestinal spirochaetosis in domestic animals and humans, Editors: Hampson, D.J. and Stanton, T.B., CAB International, Wallingford, UK, pp. 267–300.

Takeuchi, A., 1967a, Electron microscope studies of experimental *Salmonella* infection. I. Penetration into the intestinal epithelium by *Salmonella typhimurium*, Am. J. Pathol. 50:109–136.

Takeuchi, A., 1967b, Electron-microscope studies of experimental *Salmonella* infection in the preconditioned guinea pig. II. Response of the intestinal mucosa to the invasion by *Salmonella typhimurium*, Am. J. Pathol. 50:137–161.

Taylor, D.J., Simmons, J.R., and Laird, H.M., 1980, Production of diarrhea and dysentery in pigs by feeding pure cultures of a spirochete differing from *Treponema hyodysenteriae*, Vet. Rec. 106:326–332.

Taylor, D.J., 1992, Spirochetal diarrhea, In: Diseases of swine. Editors: Leman, A.D., Straw, B.E., Mengeling, W.L., D'Allaire, S., and Taylor, D.J., 7th ed., Iowa State University Press, Ames, Iowa, pp. 584–587.

Taylor, D.L. and Bergeland, M.E., 1992, Clostridial Infections, In: Diseases of swine. Editors: Leman, A.D., Straw, B.E., Mengeling, W.L., D'Allaire, S., and Taylor, D.J., 7th ed., Iowa State University Press, Ames, Iowa, pp. 454–459.

Taylor, D.J., Sanford, S.E., Jones, J.E.T., and Yager, J.A., 1992, Miscellaneous bacterial infections, In: Diseases of swine. Editor: Leman, A.D., Straw, B.E., Mengeling, W.L., D'Allaire, S., and Taylor, D.J., 7th ed., Iowa State University Press, Ames, Iowa, pp. 627–649.

Thomson, J.R., Smith, W.J., Murray, B.P., and McOrist, S., 1997, Pathogenicity of three strains of *Serpulina pilosicoli* in pigs with a naturally acquired intestinal flora, Infect. Immun. 65:3693–3700.

Thomson, J.R., Smith, W.J., and Murray, B.P., 1998, Investigations into field cases of porcine colitis with particular reference to infection with *Serpulina pilosicoli*, Vet. Rec. 142:235–239.

Trebichavský, I., Dlabač, V., Řeháková, Z., Zahradníčková, and Šplíchal, I., 1997, Cellular changes and cytokine expression in the ilea of gnotobiotic piglets resulting from peroral *Salmonella typhimurium* challenge, Infect. Immun. 65:5244–5249.

Trivett-Moore, N.L., Gilbert, G.L., Law, C.L.H., Trott, D.J., and Hampson, D.J., 1998, Isolation of *Serpulina pilosicoli* from rectal biopsy specimens showing evidence of intestinal spirochetosis, J. Clin. Microbiol. 36:261–265.

Trott, D.J., McLaren, A.J., and Hampson, D.J., 1995, Pathogenicity of human and porcine intestinal spirochetes in one-day-old specific-pathogen-free chicks: an animal model of intestinal spirochetosis. Infect Immun. 63:3705–3710.

Trott, D.J., Stanton, T.B., Jensen, N.S., Duhamel, G.E., Johnson, J.L., and Hampson, D.J., 1996a, *Serpulina pilosicoli* sp. nov., the agent of porcine intestinal spirochetosis, Int. J. Syst. Bacteriol. 46:206–215.

Trott, D.J., Huxtable, C.R., and Hampson, D.J., 1996b, Experimental infection of newly weaned pigs with human and porcine strains of *Serpulina pilosicoli*, Infect. Immun. 64:4648–4654.

Trott, D.J., Combs, B.G., Mikosza, A.S.J., Oxberry, S.L., Robertson, I.D., Passey, M., Taime, J., Sehuko, R., Alpers, M.P., and Hampson, D.J., 1997a, The prevalence of *Serpulina pilosicoli* in humans and domestic animals in the Eastern Highlands of Papua New Guinea, Epidemiol. Infect. 119:369–379.

Trott, D.J., Jensen, N.S., Saint Girons, I., Oxberry, S.L., Stanton, T.B., Lindquist, D., and Hampson, D.J., 1997b, Identification and characterization of *Serpulina pilosicoli* isolates recovered from the blood of critically ill patients, J. Clin. Microbiol. 35:482–485.

Tzipori, S., Robins-Browne, R.M., Gonis, G., Hayes, J., Withers, M., and McCartney, E., 1985, Enteropathogenic *Escherichia coli* enteritis: evaluation of the gnotobiotic piglet as a model of human infection, Gut 26:570–578.

Tzipori, S., Wachsmuth, I.K., Chapman, C., Birner, R., Brittingham, J., Jackson, C., and Hogg, J., 1986, The pathogenesis of hemorrhagic colitis caused by *Escherichia coli* O157:H7 in gnotobiotic piglets, J. Infect. Dis. 154:712–716.

Tzipori, S., Chow, C.W., and Powell, H.R., 1988, Cerebral infection with *Escherichia coli* O157:H7 in humans and gnotobiotic piglets, J. Clin. Pathol. 41:1099–1103.

Webb, D.M., Duhamel, G.E., Mathiesen, M.R., Muniappa, N., and White, A.K., 1997, Cecal spirochetosis associated with *Serpulina pilosicoli* in captive juvenile ring-necked pheasants, Avian Diseases 41:997–1002.

Westerman, R.B., Phillips, R.M., and Joens, L.A., 1995, Production and characterization of monoclonal antibodies specific for lipooligosaccharide of *Serpulina hyodysenteriae*, J. Clin. Microbiol. 33:2145–2149.

White, A., Hansen-Lardy, L., Brodersen, B., Kelling, C.L., Hesse, R., and Duhamel, G.E., 1998, Enhanced immunohistochemical detection of infectious agents in formalin-fixed, paraffin-embedded tissues following heat-mediated antigen retrieval, J. Vet. Diagn. Invest. 10:214–217.

Wilcock, B.P. and Olander, H.J., 1977, The pathogenesis of porcine rectal stricture. II. Experimental salmonellosis and ischemic proctitis, Vet. Pathol. 14:43–55.

Wilcock B.P. and Schwartz, K.J., 1992, Salmonellosis, In: Diseases of swine, Editors: Leman, A.D., Straw, B.E., Mengeling, W.L., D'Allaire, S., and Taylor, D.J., 7th ed., Iowa State University Press, Ames, Iowa, pp. 570–583.

Witters, N.A. and Duhamel, G.E., 1996, Cell membrane permeability- and mitochondrial dysfunction-inducing activities in cell free supernatants from *Serpulina hyodysenteriae* serotypes 1 and 2, Comp. Immunol. Microbiol. Infect. Dis. 19:233–244.

Witters, N.A. and Duhamel, G.E., 1998, Differential modulation of *Serpulina pilosicoli* motility-regulated mucin chemotaxis by supplementing growth medium with fecal extract or purified mucin, Proc. Conf. Res. Wrks. Anim. Dis. abst. #55.

Zhu, C., Harel, J., Jacques, M., Desautels, C., Donnenberg, M.S., Beaudry, M., and Fairbrother, J.M., 1994, Virulence properties and attaching-effacing activity of *Escherichia coli* O45 from swine post-weaning diarrhea, Infect. Immun. 62:4153–4159.

8

MECHANISMS AND IMPACT OF ENTERIC INFECTIONS

Richard L. Guerrant,[1] Aldo A. M. Lima,[2] Manuel Barboza,[2]
Sharon Young,[1] Terezinha Silva,[2] Leah Barrett,[1] Yongde Bao,[3]
Jay Fox,[3] and Sean Moore[1]

[1] Division of Geographic and International Medicine
University of Virginia
Charlottesville, Virginia
[2] Clinical Research Unit
Federal University of Ceará
Fortaleza, CE, Brazil
[3] Department of Microbiology
University of Virginia
Charlottesville, Virginia

1. SUMMARY

The increased recognition of both old and new enteric pathogens and their potential impact requires an improved understanding of pathogenesis and effective interventions. While the overwhelming mortality (>3 million children per year) due to diarrheal diseases is well-recognized, the potential long-term impacts of enteric infections and early childhood diarrhea morbidity are just beginning to be appreciated. Furthermore, several enteric infections are now being recognized as causes of growth shortfalls with or without diarrhea; i.e., malnutrition may be one of the greatest yet of the "emerging infectious diseases."

The increased appreciation of this extended impact calls for further quantification and improved understanding of the deranged physiology. In particular, persistent diarrheal illnesses exhibit common themes of blunted villi, disruption of intestinal barrier function and varying degrees of sub-mucosal inflammation for which lactulose/mannitol permeability and fecal lactoferrin provide respective quantification. Finally, such improved understanding will allow targeted interventions among those most vulnerable, which will enable further documentation of cost effectiveness and the potential for improved human development which is critical to reducing the

Mechanisms in the Pathogenesis of Enteric Diseases 2, edited by Paul and Francis.
Kluwer Academic / Plenum Publishers, New York, 1999.

widening disparity and population overgrowth which increasingly threaten our global security.

2. INTRODUCTION

In providing an overview of the impact of enteric infections, we shall first introduce emerging enteric infections, and then suggest that the potential impact of long-term morbidity may well exceed even the staggering mortality from diarrheal diseases. We shall then suggest that malnutrition may well be one of the greatest of the emerging enteric infections.

Turning to pathogenesis, after a brief review of host defenses, a focus on microbial virulence traits will include discussion of four example enterotoxins that have served as unique probes for cell signaling processes. These included continued new understandings of the mechanisms of action of cholera toxin, the paradigm of mammalian particulate guanylate cyclase activation, *E. coli* STa, the newly recognized cause of persistent diarrhea, enteroaggregative *E. coli*, with its ability to trigger host-cell cytokine responses, and finally, the leading cause of nosocomial diarrhea throughout the world, *Clostridium difficile* and its remarkable toxins, A and B, which trigger cytokine responses and inactivate the host signaling peptide, RHO.

We shall then conclude with examples of how this improved understanding of pathophysiology can be applied in both simple diagnostics as well as novel approaches to therapy of enteric infections throughout the world.

3. EMERGING ENTERIC INFECTIONS

As demonstrated by the impressive outbreaks in recent years of *Cyclospora* and imported Guatemalan raspberries as well as *Cryptosporidium* in water-borne outbreaks and enterohemorrhagic *E. coli* in industrialized areas, health threats that once seemed far away now threaten to come rolling up to our threshold today. Both the direct impact of the globalization of our food supply and the indirect impact of often increasing disparity and poverty with its associated population overgrowth raise the needs like never before to address enteric infections that threaten the health of the poor in the tropics.

As shown in Table 1, numerous enteric infections have been recognized only in the last two or three decades, many of which are the focus of important papers in this meeting and review. These include the increasingly versatile numbers and types of enteropathogenic *E. coli*, including those that make the cholera-like toxin, LT, those producing the heat-stable toxin STa or STb, the classical enteropathogenic *E. coli* (EPEC) which orchestrate a remarkable attaching and effacing pathogenesis, the newly recognized *Shiga*-like toxin producing enterohemorrhagic *E. coli* (EHEC), including O157 and others), *Shigella*-like invasive *E. coli*, and the enteroaggregative *E. coli* increasingly associated with persistent diarrhea in developing as well as developed areas. Other emerging enteric bacterial infections include the explosion of the seventh El Tor cholera pandemic throughout Latin America since 1991 and the emergence of *Vibrio cholerae* O139 in South Asia since 1992. Finally, with *Helicobacter pylori*, the new recognition of likely major infectious etiologies of

Table 1. Emerging enteric infections (recognized since 1970)

Bacterial:
Cholera—Latin America 1991
V. cholerae O139, S. Asia since 1992
E. coli O157 (and other EHEC), US 1982–1998; Japan 1996
Enteroaggregative E. coli (persistent diarrhea in tropics; AIDS diarrhea in US)
Multidrug resistant Salmonella sp. (incl. Quinolone-resistant S. typhi in Vietnam)

Parasitic:
Cryptosporidiosis—esp. US 1993
Cyclospora—Nepal, Carribbean, Peru, US/raspberries 1996–98
Microsporidia—worldwide, especially with AIDS
Metrochis—Canada 1996
Ancyclostoma caninum (Eos. Enteritis)—Australia 1990's

Viral:
Torovirus, Astrovirus, Rotavirus, Calicivirus (Norwalk-like, et al.)

peptic ulcer disease, gastric carcinoma, and gastrointestinal lymphoma have now been recognized.

Emerging parasitic infections include three newly recognized enteric protozoa in humans, Cryptosporidiosis, Cyclosporidosis, and Microsporidiosis. While long known to the veterinary world, except for occasional anecdotal reports, it was the AIDS epidemic that brought these to prominent attention in humans. Now that we recognize *Cryptosporidium* and *Cyclospora*, it is increasingly appreciated that these are huge threats to normal as well as immunocompromised hosts.

Finally, numerous viral enteric pathogens have been recognized within the last three decades, including rotaviruses, caliciviruses, astroviruses, enteric adenoviruses, toroviruses, and others that are the focus of several papers in this conference.

4. EMERGING RECOGNITION OF THE MORBIDITY AS WELL AS MORTALITY IMPACT OF DIARRHEAL DISEASES AND ENTERIC INFECTIONS

As noted in Table 2, diarrheal diseases constitute one of the leading causes of mortality worldwide. Widely appreciated are the estimated 3.1 million deaths per year, which translate to over 8400 children who die each day from diarrheal diseases.

Not as well understood is the morbidity impact of often six to eight or more dehydrating, malnourishing diarrheal illnesses among children in their most critical first

Table 2. Leading causes of global mortality and morbidity*

	Mortality	Mortality (% DALYS)
1. Infectious Diseases	16.5 (32%)	36.4%
2. Cancer	6.1 (11.8%)	5.9%
3. Heart Diseases	5.0 (9.7%)	3.1%
4. Cerebrovascular Disease	4.0 (7.8%)	3.2%
5. Chronic Lung Disease	3.0 (5.8%)	3.5%

*Adapted from R.L. Guerrant Am. J. Trop. Med. Hyg., 59 (1), 1998, pp. 3–16.

couple of years of life. Indeed, the increasingly popular disability-adjusted life year (DALY) calculation which emphasizes not only years of life lost but also years lost to disability with a new emphasis on disabling illnesses like chronic diseases, counts only the few days of overt illness with estimated 10% disability for just the few days of overt illness with diarrheal diseases. However, poorly quantified and not even counted is the likely substantial long-term developmental impact of these devastating childhood diarrheal diseases. Even pilot studies, analogous to those conducted with the treatment of intestinal helminth infections, have begun to reveal substantial long-term growth as well as physical fitness and cognitive function defects that appear to relate directly to early childhood diarrheal burdens, effects that are observed four to six years later at six to nine years of age (Guerrant et al., 1998a). While intuitively not surprising, the quantification of these potential long-term developmental impacts will be of tremendous importance in assessing the impact and cost effectiveness of key interventions for diarrheal diseases. In Brazil, for example, an approximate 4% decrement in physical fitness at six to nine years of age is associated with diarrhea in the first two years of life. In a study in Zimbabwe, a 4% improvement in physical fitness after treatment for schistosomiasis was associated with a fully 16.6% improvement in work productivity (Ndamba et al., 1993).

5. MALNUTRITION AS AN EMERGING INFECTIOUS DISEASE

Long recognized are the frequency of enteric infections that often are even more common in asymtomatic individuals than in those with overt diarrheal illnesses. However, only recently have specific asymptomatic infections with *Cryptosporidium* and now with enteroaggregative *E. coli* and, at least in some populations, *Giardia lamblia*, been associated with nutritional shortfalls, even in the absence of overt diarrheal illnesses. Since these "asymptomatic" infections may be even more common than currently recognized, it is entirely possible that malnutrition may be one of the most important of all of the emerging infectious disease, as shown in Fig. 1.

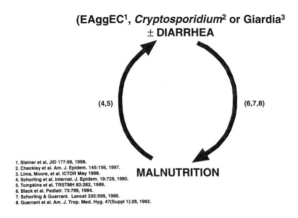

**(EAggEC[1], *Cryptosporidium*[2] or Giardia[3]
± DIARRHEA**

(4,5)   (6,7,8)

1. Steiner et al, JID 177:88, 1998.
2. Checkley et al. Am. J. Epidem. 145:156, 1997.
3. Lima, Moore, et al. ICTDR May 1998.
4. Schorling et al. Internat. J. Epidem. 19:728, 1990.
5. Tompkins et al. TRSTMH 83:282, 1989.
6. Black et al. Pediatr. 73:799, 1984.
7. Schorling & Guerrant. Lancet 335:599, 1990.
8. Guerrant et al. Am. J. Trop. Med. Hyg. 47(Suppl 1):28, 1992.

MALNUTRITION

Figure 1. Enteric Infections.

6. PERSISTENT DIARRHEA DISRUPTS INTESTINAL BARRIER FUNCTION

Among the themes of this conference is the remarkable thread of altered histopathology seen with several infections that cause persistent diarrhea and possibly malnutrition. This includes villus blunting, crypt hypertrophy, often with or without an inflammatory infiltrate in the lamina propria. Indeed, such as deranged histopathology is seen with *Cryptosporidium*, *Cyclospora* or *Microsporidium* infections (Guerrant and Thielman, 1998). Furthermore, we have documented substantial disruptions of intestinal barrier function as measured by lactulose:mannitol permeability ratios in patients with AIDS with or without diarrhea (worse with diarrhea) as well as in children with persistent diarrhea in Northeast Brazil (Bao et al., 1996; Lima et al., 1997) (Fig. 2a and b). As the potential role of cytokines in triggering secretion as well as of glutamine in reconstructing the damaged barrier function has been raised by studies by Argenzio and by Lima and Guerrant, the potential for a novel, effective therapy may emerge (Argenzio et al., 1994; Lima et al., 1992; Lima et al., 1998a; Guerrant et al., 1998b).

Indeed, we find disrupted intestinal barrier function in children with persistent diarrhea due to *Cryptosporidium* or other causes and are investigating the potential of glutamine and micronutrients in repairing this damaged barrier function.

7. ENTERIC HOST DEFENSES VS. MICROBIAL VIRULENCE TRAITS

As shown in Fig. 3, the key host mechanisms in the gastrointestinal tract include normal hygiene (i.e., the chance of acquiring most enteric infections is dependent upon the number of organisms ingested, even though some, such as *Shigella* or parasite cysts may require only a very few organisms). A second host defense is normal gastric acidity, followed by intestinal mucus, cellular and humoral immunity, normal motility and our important normal enteric microbial flora.

Conversely, the traits that enable the microorganism to be an enteric pathogen include adherence, enterotoxin or cytotoxin production, invasion or penetration of the intestinal mucosa. Indeed, the entire repertoire of traits enabling an enteric pathogen to cause disease can be illustrated by the versatile *E. coli*. Whether by the production of cholera-like LT, STa or b, *Shiga*-like toxin (EHEC), attachment then effacement (EPEC) or the triggering of cytokine responses (enteroaggregative *E. coli*), these versatile traits are often encoded on transmissible genetic elements on plasmids or bacteriophage. As shown in Table 3, four of these enteric microbial toxins have served as unique probes for basic cell signaling.

8. CHOLERA TOXIN AND *E. COLI* LT

Often felt to be the best understood of enteric pathogens, *Vibrio cholerae* causes devastating epidemic dehydrating diarrhea via the action of its remarkable enterotoxin. Indeed, choleratoxin has provided one of the most helpful probes in understanding the G protein regulation of adenylate cyclase, the mechanism by which the isotonic

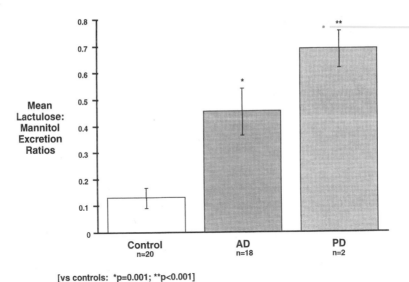

Figure 2a. Disruption of Intestinal Barrier Function in Children with Acute and Persistent Diarrhea in Fortaleza, Brazil.

diarrhea occurs. However, some have suggested that prostaglandins may be even more important than cyclic AMP in causing secretory diarrhea (Peterson et al., 1990, 1991, 1992) and we have found that the activating factor appears to be involved distal to cyclic AMP but perhaps proximal to a protein synthesis dependent increase in prostaglandin production to elicit either fluid secretion or CHO cell elongation Guerrant et al., 1994; Thielman et al., 1997).

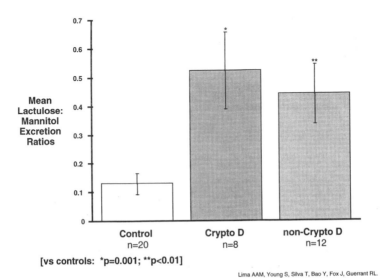

Figure 2b. Disruption of Intestinal Barrier Function in Children with Cryptosporidial and non-Cryptosporidial Diarrhea in Fortaleza, Brazil.

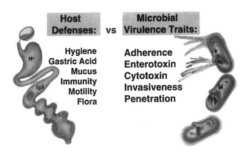

Figure 3. The 2 casts of actors in enteric infections.

9. *E. COLI* STA, THE PARADIGM OF PARTICULATE GUANYLATE CYCLASE ACTIVATORS

Although a violation of the ying-yang hypothesis that cyclic GMP would be expected to have an opposite effect from that of cyclic AMP, the activation of particulate guanylate cyclase by *E. coli* STa and the discovery that cyclic GMP in fact elicits a secretory response led to the appreciation of cyclic GMP as a mediator of fluid secretion as well (Hughes et al., 1978; Field et al., 1978; Guerrant et al., 1980).

Furthermore, *E. coli* STa is the first of a family of activators of particulate guanylate cyclase that now include several microbial heat stable toxins and the key mammarian mediators, guanylin, uroguanylin and perhaps others (Bobak et al., 1992; Fonteles et al., 1998).

10. ENTEROAGGREGATIVE *E. COLI*: POTENTIAL EFFECTS VIA UP-REGULATION OF HOST CYTOKINE RELEASE

One of the leading emerging enteric infections associated with persistent diarrhea in many tropical areas, including India, Mexico, Brazil (Nataro et al., 1998), as well as in patients with AIDS in the U.S. (Wanke et al., 1998) is enteroaggregative *E. coli* (EAgg EC). While EAgg EC have several potential virulence traits, including a heat stable toxin and potential cytotoxins, we have found that EAgg EC are associated with intestinal inflammation as determined by fecal lactoferrin and with not only persistent diarrhea but growth shortfalls even in the absence of diarrhea (Steiner et al., 1998). Indeed, Steiner and colleagues have shown that EAgg EC trigger epithelial cell interleukin 8 release via an apparent heat stable extracellular protein released by EAgg EC. Thus, EAgg EC may well represent the type of pathogenesis (perhaps shared by

Table 3. Enteric microbial toxins: unique probes for signaling & secretion

Choleratoxin	causes	cholera	via	cAMP
E. coli STa		turista		cGMP
Eagg E. coli		Persistent diarrhea		IL-8
C. difficile Toxin A		Nosocomial diarrhea		rho

C. difficile toxin A and by whole viable *Helicobacter pylori* organisms) that effect host cell derangement via triggering the host cell to release potent pro-inflammatory cytokines.

11. *CLOSTRIDIUM C. DIFFICILE* TOXIN A, AN INACTIVATOR OF HOST CELL RHO

Among the largest microbial toxins known, toxins A and B of *C. difficile* appear to have at least part of their remarkable effects via the monoglucosylation of host cell RHO, thus inactivating this critical intracellular signaling pathway. While the amino 1/3 of both toxins A and B inactivate RHO, only toxin A with amino acid repeating units at the carboxy 1/3 appear to trigger potent host cell cytokine release. Whether differences in the enterotoxicity and cytotoxicity of these two toxins in different cell systems is partially or entirely dependent on different binding portions of the molecules is under current study. In any case, it is now clear that *C. difficile* toxins provide yet another example of the unique pharmacologic interruption of host cell signaling pathways by a novel mechanism. Understanding these microbial toxin effects will not only shed light on basic cell signaling processes but also on understanding and hopefully interrupting microbial pathogenesis to control the major problem of *C. difficile* colitis without the harmful effects (via increasingly widespread resistance) of potent antibiotics.

12. CLUES TO CONTROL: IMPROVED DIAGNOSTICS AND TREATMENTS DERIVED FROM UNDERSTANDING PATHOGENESIS

As suggested earlier in this report, an improved understanding of pathogenesis may well lead to simpler, improved means of diagnosis or treatment. As an example of the former, an improved understanding of inflammatory diarrhea and the neutrophil marker lactoferrin has led us to develop a simple diagnostic test for fecal lactoferrin to identify inflammatory diarrheas. Although ideopathic inflammatory bowel disease may also be positive, the predominant microbial diarrheas that are inflammatory happen to be those for which fecal culture and possible antimicrobial therapy are available. These include *Salmonella*, *Shigella* and *Campylobacter* infections or, in the hospital, *C. difficile* antibiotic associated colitis. Indeed, the use of fecal lactoferrin can vastly improve the cost effectiveness of stool culture (Choi et al., 1996; Miller et al., 1994; Guerrant et al., 1994).

Regarding novel approaches to therapy, as suggested above, glutamine, as the major enterocyte energy source, may well provide a key "provisionally essential" amino acid to repair the damaged intestinal barrier function due to a wide range of disruptive microbial infections. In addition, we have found that glutamine is also at least as effective if not more effective that glucose in driving sodium co-transport and thus can provide a highly effective oral rehydration as well as nutrition therapy (ORNT). Indeed, in preliminary studies, we now find that glutamine does appear to speed repair of disrupted mucosal barrier function as determined by lactulose:mannitol permeability ratios (Lima et al., 1998b). Finally, in order to improve its stability, we developed highly stable derivatives that also drive intestinal sodium co-transport and may be even more effective in repairing damaged intestinal barrier function (U.S. patent # 5,561,111).

13. CONCLUSIONS

With the increased recognition of new pathogens and new appreciation of the potential long-term impact of persistent and acute diarrheal illnesses, a new understanding of pathogenesis becomes more important than ever before. Microbial interactions with the host, perhaps synergistic with host impairments such as immunologic or micronutrient deficiencies may disrupt intestinal barrier and absorptive function and thus may constitute a major cause of malnutrition as well as overt diarrhea.

Not only do microbial toxins like choleratoxin, STa, enteroaggregative *E. coli*, and *C. difficile* toxins A and B offer powerful probes to understanding basic cell signaling, but, with growing limits on antimicrobial therapy, an understanding of these pathways may open critical novel pharmacologic and physiologic means to better control the devastating impact of enteric infections in our hospitals and around the world.

ACKNOWLEDGMENT

Much of this work was supported through NIH ICIDR Grant U0 1AI26512-10 from the National Institutes of Allergy and Infectious Diseases, NIH, Bethesda, Maryland.

REFERENCES

Argenzio R.A., Rhoads J.M., Armstrong M., and Gomez G. Glutamine stimulates prostaglandin-sensitive Na(+)-H+ exchange in experimental porcine cryptosporidiosis [see comments]. Gastroenterol 1994;106:1418–1428.

Bao Y.D., Silva T.J., Guerrant R.L., Lima A.M., and Fox J.W. Direct analysis of mannitol, lactulose and glucose in urine samples by high-performance anion-exchange chromatography with pulse amperometric detection—clinical evaluation of intestinal permeability in human immunodeficiency virus infection. Journal of Chromatography 1996;685:105–112.

Bobak D.A. and Guerrant R.L. New developments in enteric bacterial toxins. [Review]. Advances in Pharmacology Adv Pharmacol 1992;23:85–108.

Choi S.W., Park C.H., Silva T.M.J., Zaenker EI, and Guerrant RL. To culture or not to culture: Fecal lactoferrin screening for inflammatory bacterial diarrhea. J Clin Microbiol 1996;34:928–932.

Fonteles M.C., Greenberg R.N., Monteiro H.S., Currie M.G., and Forte L.R. Natriuretic and kaliuretic activities of guanylin and uroguanylin in the isolated perfused rat kidney. American Journal of Physiology. 1998;275:t–7.

Field M., Graf Jr. L.H., and Mata L.J. Heat stable enterotoxin of *E. coli*. *In vitro* effects on guanylate cyclase activity, cyclic GMP concentration, and ion transport in small intestine. Proc Natl Acad Sci USA 1978;75:2800–2804.

Guerrant R.L., Hughes J.M., Chang B., Robertson D.C., and Murad F. Activation of intestinal guanylate cyclase by heat-stable enterotoxin of *E. coli*: Studies of tissue specificity, potential receptors and intermediates. J Infect Dis 1980;142:220–228.

Guerrant R.L., Fang G.D., Thielman N.M., and Fonteles M.C. Role of platelet activating factor (PAF) in the intestinal epithelial secretory and Chinese hamster ovary (CHO) cell cytoskeletal responses to cholera toxin. Proc Natl Acad Sci USA 1994;91:9655–9658.

Guerrant R.L., Martins C.A.P., and Silva T. Fecal lactoferrin as a marker of fecal leukocytes. J Clin Microbiol 1994;32:2629–2630.

Guerrant R.L. and Thielman N.M. Emerging enteric protozoa: *Cryptosporidium, Cyclospora,* and Microsporidia. In: Scheld W.M., Armstrong D., and Hughes J.M., eds. Emerging Infections. Washington, DC: ASM Press, 1998:233–245.

Guerrant D.I., Moore S.R., Lima A.A.M., Patrick P., Schorling J.B., and Guerrant R.L. Early childhood diarrhea, correlates with impaired physical fitness but not activity levels, five years later in a poor urban community in Northeast Brazil. Submitted. Lancet 1998a.

Guerrant R.L. and Lima A.A.M. Glutamine-based ORNT drives sodium transport *in vitro,* reverses cholera-induced secretion in rabbit loops and sppds repair of disrupted intestinal barrier function in children with diarrhea or malnutrition. Presented at the 34th U.S. Japan Cholera Conference, Shonan Village, Japan, Nov. 30, 1998 1998b. (Abstract).

Hughes J.M., Murad F., Chang B., and Guerrant R.L. Role of cyclic GMP in the action of heat-stable enterotoxins of *Escherichia coli.* Nature 1978;271:755–756.

Lima A.A.M., Barboza Jr. M.S., Silva T.M.J., McAuliffe I., and Guerrant R.L. Enteroaggregative *E. coli* associated with persistent diarrhea: Pathophysiology and treatment with glutamine-based oral rehydration and nutrition therapy (ORNT). 6th Annual Meeting of the NIAID International Centers for Tropical Research (ICTDIR), May 5–7, Bethesda, MD 1997.

Lima A.A.M., Soares A.M., Freire Jr. J.E., and Guerrant R.L. Cotransport of sodium with glutamine, alanine and glucose in the isolated rabbit ileal mucosa. Braz J Med Biol Res 1992;25:637–640.

Lima A.A., Barboza M.S., and Melo A.S., et al. Long-term impact and control of physiologic derangements from early childhood diarrhea in a cohort followed from birth in Northeast Brazil. ASTMH in San Juan, PR October 1998a (Abstract).

Lima A.A.M., Barboza Jr. M.S., and Melo A.S., et al. Magnitude, impact and control of persistent diarrhea and malnutrition in a prospective cohort study of children in Northeast Brazil. 7th Annual Meeting of the NIAID International Centers for Tropical Research (ICTDIR), May 2, Bethesda, MD 1998b (Abstract).

Miller J.R., Barrett L.J., Kotloff K., and Guerrant R.L. A rapid test for infectious and inflammatory enteritis. Arch Intern Med 1994;154:2660–2664.

Nataro J.P., Steiner T., and Guerrant R.L. Enteroaggregative *Escherichia coli.* Emerging. Infectious Diseases 1998;4:251–261.

Ndamba J., Makaza N., Munjoma M., Gomo E., and Kaondera K.C. The physical fitness and work performance of agricultural workers infected with Schistosoma mansoni in Zimbabwe. Annals. of Tropical. Medicine & Parasitology 1993;87:553–561.

Peterson J.W. and Ochoa G. Role of prostaglandins and cAMP in the secretory effects of cholera toxin. Science 1989;245:857–859.

Peterson J.W., Jackson C.A., and Reitmeyer J.C. Synthesis of prostaglandins in cholera toxin-treated Chinese hamster ovary cells. Microbial Pathogenesis 1990;9:345–353.

Peterson J.W., Reitmeyer J.C., Jackson C.A., and Ansare G.A.S. Protein synthesis is required for cholera toxin-induced stimulation or arachidonic acid metabolism. Biochimica et Biophysica Acta 1991;-1092:79–84.

Steiner T.S., Lima A.M., Nataro J.P., and Guerrant R.L. Enteroaggregative *Escherichia coli* produce intestinal inflammation and growth impairment and cause interleukin-8 release from intestinal epithelial cells. Journal of Infectious Diseases 1998;177:88–96.

Thielman N.M., Marcinkiewicz M., Sarosiek J., Fang G.D., and Guerrant R.L. The role of platelet activating factor in Chinese hamster ovary cell responses to cholera toxin. J Clin Invest 1997;99:1999–2004.

Wanke C.A., Gerrior J., Blais V., Mayer H., and Acheson D. Successful treatment of diarrheal disease associated with enteroaggregative *E. coli* in adults infected with human immunodeficiency virus. Journal of Infectious Diseases 1998; (in press).

9

INSULIN MODULATES INTESTINAL RESPONSE OF SUCKLING MICE TO THE *ESCHERICHIA COLI* HEAT-STABLE ENTEROTOXIN

Ahmad M. Al-Majali,[1] Elikplimi K. Asem,[2] Carlton Lamar,[2]
J. Paul Robinson,[2] James Freeman,[1] and A. Mahdi Saeed[1]

Departments of Veterinary Pathobiology[1] and
Basic Medical Sciences[2]
School of Veterinary Medicine
Purdue University
West Lafayette, Indiana 47907

1. SUMMARY

Effect of insulin on the response of suckling mice to the enterotoxigenic *Escherichia coli* heat-stable enterotoxin (STa) was studied. Four groups (8–10 in each group) of two day old Swiss Webster suckling mice were used. Five, 10, 25, and 50 µg of insulin were given orally to half the mice in each group respectively. The rest of the mice in each group were given normal saline as intra-litter controls. After 7 days, the suckling mouse assay for STa was performed on three mice from each insulin-treated and control groups. Enterocyte suspensions were prepared from mice in all groups. Intestinal tissue samples were taken for electron microscopy. Interaction of STa with its putative receptor on the enterocytes was evaluated using indirect immunofluorescence and flow cytometry. The suckling mouse assay revealed a significant increase in the gut weight to body weight ratio in all mice in the insulin treated groups compared to control mice ($p < 0.05$). Flow cytometry and indirect immunofluorescence analyses suggested that insulin had an up-regulatory effect on the STa receptor level. Similarly, insulin was found to increase intestinal brush border membrane differentiation as indicated by the increase in the inward movement of milk particles through the intestinal mucosa. Insulin seems to modify the structure-function of the brush border membrane including the response of suckling mice to STa. This study may provide further insights into the mechanism of STa/receptor interaction in diarrhea in newborn animals and human infants.

Mechanisms in the Pathogenesis of Enteric Diseases 2, edited by Paul and Francis.
Kluwer Academic / Plenum Publishers, New York, 1999.

2. INTRODUCTION

Enterotoxigenic strains of *Escherichia. coli* (ETEC) produce peptide toxins which alter intestinal water balance and lead to acute diarrheal illnesses in humans and animals. A large (85–90 kDa), heat-labile toxin (LT) produced by many ETEC has been well described and shares many structural and functional homologies with cholera toxin, including the ability to ADP-ribosylate and irreversibly activate intestinal adenylate cyclase (Sears and Kaper, 1996). The other classes of *E. coli* toxins are low molecular weight, heat-stable toxins (ST). There are two types of ST, STa and STb. STb has mostly been observed in ETEC infecting pigs and calves, but has not been well characterized (Dreyfus et al., 1985; Epstein et al., 1986). STa, on the other hand, has been purified to homogeneity (Staples et al., 1980; Saeed and Greenberg, 1985). STa producing-*E. coli* is a major cause of diarrhea in newborn animals and human infants. STa is composed of 18 amino acids and has a molecular weight of 2 kDa. Slight variations in toxin size were observed in ETEC from some host species, but heterogeneity in the size of STa is not reflected in a difference in their mechanism of action, or potencies (Rao et al., 1981; Saeed and Greenberg, 1985). STa has been observed to dramatically alter guanosine 3′,5′-cyclic monophosphate (cGMP) metabolism via the activation of intestinal guanylate cyclase followed by a blockade of inward ion transport and subsequent secretion of water into the intestinal lumen (Guandalini et al., 1982; Rao et al., 1981; Wada et al., 1994). Guanylate cyclase has been identified as the receptor for STa by cloning and expression analysis of the STa receptor gene from rat, human, and pig intestinal DNA libraries (de Sauvage et al., 1991; Schulz et al., 1990; Wada et al., 1994). It was reported that guanylate cyclase C, which is part of the extracellular domain of the membranous guanylate cyclase, is an *N*-linked glycoprotein receptor that accounts for multiple heat-stable enterotoxin-binding proteins in the intestine (Vaandrager et al., 1993).

Growth factors such as insulin and epidermal growth factor (EGF) are commonly found in milk of lactating women and other mammals (Steeb et al., 1995). A major site for the synthesis of these circulating growth factors is the liver, but insulin-like growth factor-I (IGF-I) is also produced locally in other tissues (Simmons et al., 1995; Steeb et al., 1995). The biological effect of growth factors is mediated by their binding to specific receptors on the plasma membrane. The number of these receptors on the membranes can be regulated by the concentration of growth factors in the environment (Ziegler et al., 1995). One major site for the action of growth factors is the intestinal brush border membrane. Many studies have attempted to explain normal developmental patterns for different intestinal disaccharidase, alkaline phosphatase and peptidase. Some reports suggest the involvement of some growth factors in regulating intestinal brush border membrane disaccharidase (Menard et al., 1981; Steeb et al., 1995). The differentiation of the absorptive surface of the intestinal epithelial cells is characterized by increases in sucrase and lactase activities (Menard et al., 1981; Schmidt et al., 1988).

This study was initiated to explore the effect of insulin on the intestinal response to STa. The effect of insulin on the intestinal brush border membrane differentiation was studied using electron microscopy and brush border enzymes assays. Flow cytometry and indirect immunofluorescence were utilized to study the modulating effect of insulin on the STa/receptor interaction.

3. MATERIAL AND METHODS

3.1. STa Purification

STa was isolated and purified to homogeneity by growing ETEC strains in a chemically defined medium, desalting, and concentrating by batch adsorption chromatography on Amberlite XAD-2 resin, reversed phase silica, and preparative reverse-phase high performance liquid chromatography (RV-HPLC). This rapid purification scheme resulted in high yields of pure STa, which exhibited biochemical homology to STa purified by different procedures. No contamination was detected in the HPLC-purified STa. This procedure has been described in detail and homogeneity of the purified STa was established as described (Saeed and Greenberg, 1985).

3.2. Insulin Feeding of Suckling Mice

Four litters (8–10 mice in each group) of two day old Swiss Webster suckling mice were used. Half the mice in each litter received 5, 10, 25, and 50 µg of insulin (isophane insulin suspension, USP, Eli Lilly & Company, Indianapolis, IN) respectively. The rest of suckling mice in each litter received normal saline and were kept as intra-litter controls. All mice were given insulin or saline orally each day for 7 days using a 0.5-ml syringe and 50-µm diameter polyethylene tube. We assumed that all mice had a similar chance to suckle their mothers during the seven-day experiment.

3.3. Suckling Mouse Assay

Mice were separated from their mothers immediately before use and randomly divided into groups of three. These mice were starved for two hours before inoculation. Each mouse was inoculated orally with a diarrheagenic dose of HPLC-purified STa (0.1 ml PBS containing 1 µg STa) with one drop of 2% Evans blue. After 3 hours, mice were killed by cervical dislocation, the abdomen was opened, and the entire intestine (excluding the stomach) was removed with forceps. The intestines from each group were pooled and weighed. The ratio of the intestinal weight to the remaining carcass weight was calculated. Animals with no dye in the intestine or with dye within the peritoneal cavity were excluded from the calculations. The minimum amount of STa that induced a gut to remaining body weight ratio of 0.087 or higher was considered one mouse unit (mu) (Giannella, 1976).

3.4. Electron Microscopy

One half centimeter of small intestine from each mouse of the different groups was fixed in 3% glutaraldehyde, and then postfixed in 1% osmium tetraoxide. Tissues were dehydrated, infiltrated in different concentrations of epon and incubated under high vacuum. Thin sections were prepared and stained with uranyl acetate and lead acetate and viewed in a JEOL, JEM-100, CX electron microscope.

3.5. Isolation of Suckling Mouse Enterocytes

Enterocyte suspensions were prepared as described previously (Al-Majali et al., 1998). The population of cells harvested was monitored by periodic wet mount examination through the whole procedure to assess the quantity and quality of the isolated enterocytes. Cell counts were determined and cell viability was assessed by exclusion of 0.2% trypan blue by cells. Dry smears were fixed in 100% methanol for both immunofluorescence and Giemsa staining. The remaining cells were used for flow cytometric analysis.

3.6. Immunofluorescence Assay

Intestinal epithelial cells isolated from suckling mouse intestines were washed 3 times in 10 mM PBS (pH 7.2) to remove any traces of the DTT solution. Smears of enterocytes were made on glass slides, air-dried, and then fixed in absolute methanol for 10 min. Slides were incubated with STa, rabbit anti-STa antibody and anti-rabbit-IgG-FITC conjugated antibody as was described by Saeed et al. (1987). As negative controls, similar samples were incubated with STa and the anti-rabbit-IgG-FITC-conjugated antibody without the anti-STa antibody.

3.7. Flow Cytometry Analysis

Enterocytes were prepared for flow cytometry following the procedure reported by Al-Majali et al. (1998). Flow cytometric analysis was preformed using an Epics ELITE flow cytometer (Coulter Electronics, Hileah, FL.). Flow cytometer was set to read 5000 cells from each enterocyte preparation. Fluorochrome excitation was done using 15 mW of 488 nm argon laser light. FITC-conjugated beads were run and the mean fluorescent intensity was set at a fixed value.

3.8. Statistics

Statistical analysis of the data was preformed by using the two-tailed student t-test for unpaired samples. Differences were analyzed for significance at $p < 0.05$.

4. RESULTS

4.1. Effect of Insulin on the Response of Suckling Mouse to the Heat-Stable Enterotoxin

Results of the suckling mouse assay indicated that the gut weight to remaining body weight ratios in all of the insulin-fed suckling mouse groups were directly related to the amount of insulin that was given (Fig. 1).

4.2. Effect of Insulin on Intestinal Development and Differentiation

Cell number and viability were relatively higher in insulin-fed suckling mice groups than mice of the control groups (Fig. 2). The increases in cell number and viability were directly related to the amount of insulin that was fed in each group (Fig. 2). Electron microscopy revealed a significant increase in the number of lipid endocytes (fat particles) in the intestinal mucosa of insulin-fed suckling mice (Fig. 3). This increase in lipid endocytes was proportional to the amount of insulin that was fed in each group

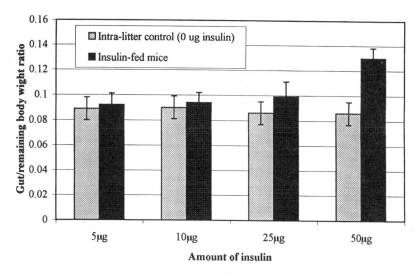

Figure 1. Ratio of gut weight to remaining body weight of control mice and suckling mice that were fed different doses of insulin (5, 10, 25, 50 µg) and challenged with 1 µg of STa. Each litter of suckling mice included mice that were fed the stated dose of insulin (■) for 7 days and mice (intra-litter control) that were fed saline without insulin (▢). Each point represents the mean of three readings ± SEM.

of suckling mice. The lipid endocytes were mostly concentrated in the apical part of the epithelial cell mucosa. This increase in lipid particles was due to an increase in the uptake of milk particles at the intestinal absorptive surface. Electron microscopic studies did not reveal any significant changes in the morphology of the intestinal mucosa nor the ultrastructural characteristics of the absorptive surface in samples obtained from mice fed different doses of insulin.

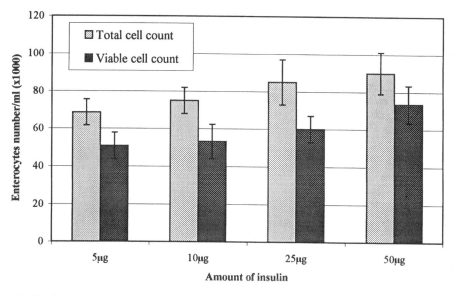

Figure 2. Number and viability of enterocytes obtained from control mice and mice fed 5, 10, 25, and 50 µg of insulin. Each point represents the mean of three readings ± SEM.

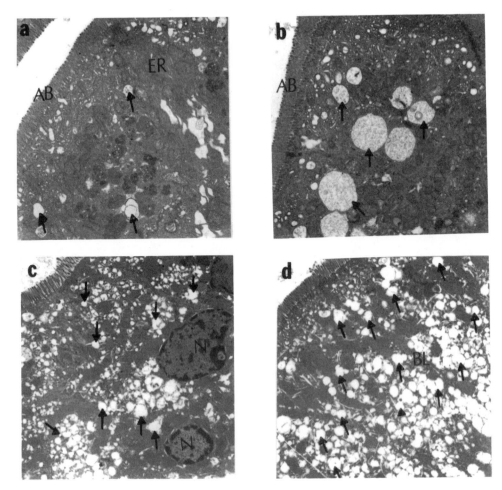

Figure 3. Transmission electron micrographs of small intestine epithelium (5000X) of suckling mice that were fed different amounts of insulin. a; epithelium of control group; b, c, d; epithelium of mice fed 5, 10, 25 µg of insulin respectively. **Arrows**; Fat droplets (lipid endocytes), **AB**; Absorptive surface, **N**; Nucleus, **BL**; Basolateral membrane, **ER**; Endoplasmic reticulum.

4.3. Effect of Insulin on STa Interaction with Its Receptor

4.3.1. Indirect Immunofluorescence Assay. Indirect immunofluorescence study of STa-susceptible mice revealed the localization of intensely stained areas mostly at the brush border membrane region of the enterocytes. It was found that in feeding suckling mice fed insulin for 7 days, there was increased intensity of fluorescence staining on the brush border membrane of enterocytes (Fig. 4). This increase in fluorescence intensity was directly proportional to the amount of insulin that was given to each group of the suckling mice (Table 1).

4.3.2. Flow Cytometry. Flow cytometric histograms revealed a significant increase in fluorescence intensity among enterocytes from insulin-treated mice when compared with that of control mice. The staining results of freshly isolated enterocytes

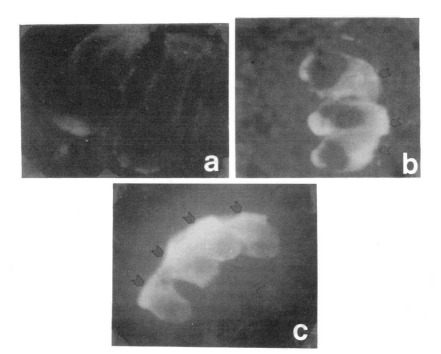

Figure 4. Fluorescence micrographs (1000X) of enterocytes obtained from the different insulin-fed groups. A: Negative control, no anti-STa antibody was added; B and C: Enterocytes obtained from mice that were fed 10 and 50 μg of insulin, respectively. All cells were incubated with STa, rabbit anti-STa antibody, and anti-rabbit-IgG-FITC conjugated antibody. Arrowheads indicate the location of the brush border membrane of the enterocytes.

Table 1. Intensities of fluorescence on enterocytes observed with indirect immunofluoresence and flow cytometric analysis of samples obtained from mice that were fed increased doses of insulin. Enterocytes were reacted with STa, rabbit anti-STa antibody, and anti-rabbit-IgG-FITC-conjugated antibody

Doses of insulin (μg)[a]	Fluorescence intensity	
	Using indirect immunofluorescence assay	Using flow cytometry (%) of fluorescence intensity[b]
0[c]	+	25.4
5	++	31.1
10	+++	33
25	++++	64.7
50	++++	82.3

[a]Mice groups that were fed different doses of insulin for 7 days.
[b]Statistical analysis indicated significant difference ($P < 0.05$) between the values of fluorescent intensities for control and treated groups.
[c]Enterocytes from the intra-litter control mice that were fed saline without insulin.

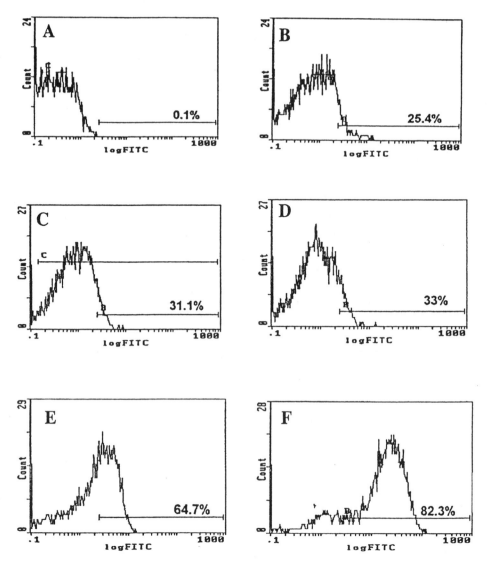

Figure 5. Representative flow cytometric histograms for enterocytes obtained from the intestine of suckling mice. A: negative control, no STa added; B: Control, no insulin was given; C, D, E, and F: Treated mice fed 5, 10, 25, and 50 ug of insulin, respectively, for 7 days. All cells were incubated with STa, rabbit anti-STa antibody, and anti-rabbit-IgG-FITC conjugated antibody.

from insulin-treated and control mice are shown in Table 1 and Fig. 5. The increase in fluorescence intensity of the surface of enterocytes was directly proportional to the amount of insulin that was fed to each group of suckling mice ($p < 0.005$) (Table 1). No fluorescence was noticed on the enterocytes of the control groups where no STa was added. A similar observations were made upon repeating the experiment.

5. DISCUSSION

Diarrheal disease caused by *Escherichia coli* that produce heat-stable enterotoxin (STa) is common in newborn animals and human infants. The reason for higher prevalence and greater severity of the disease in younger subjects is not well elucidated. In order to formulate efficacious control and prevention methods, a clear understanding of the disease mechanism is necessary. Insulin and IGF-I have been identified throughout the small and large intestine in animals and man (Rouyer-Fessard et al., 1990). IGF-I and insulin are present in breast milk (0–80 microunit/liter for insulin and 1.3–7 ηg/ml for IGF-I), and free IGF-I has been found in human saliva (Costigan et al., 1988; Grosvenor et al., 1992; Koldvsky and Strbak, 1995). In this study, we hypothesized that insulin, as a growth factor, may exert a modulating effect on the intestinal epithelium of newborn animals and may modify their response to diarrheagenic toxins. We, therefore, investigated the effect of insulin on the interaction of suckling mice enterocytes to the *E. coli* STa using electron microscopy, brush border enzyme analysis, indirect immunofluorescence and flow cytometric analysis.

The suckling mouse assay is considered specific for differentiating between STa and other enterotoxins produced by enterotoxigenic *E. coli* cultures (Wada et al., 1994). Insulin-fed mice had a gut weight to remaining body weight ratio higher than the control group, when both groups were inoculated with similar diarrheagenic doses of STa. These findings suggest that insulin had a modulating effect on intestinal epithelium response to *E. coli* STa. The small intestine in mice acquires its capability to respond to insulin during the suckling period (Menard et al., 1981; Menard and Dagenais, 1993). The fact that insulin is able to increase epithelial cell proliferation in both small and large intestines supports, at least in the mouse model, the view that the developmental pattern of epithelial cell proliferation and differentiation is under some modulatory influence of insulin. Results of electron microscopic studies suggest that insulin has increased the absorptive surface as indicated by the increase in the inward movement of milk particles (Fig. 3). It was reported that IGF, epidermal growth factor (EGF), transforming growth factor α (TGF) and β have important modulatory roles in small intestinal crypt cell proliferation, particularly after intestinal injury (Arsenault and Menard, 1984; Menard and Dagenais, 1993; Potten et al., 1995). A premature rise in the circulating insulin level induces significant increase in epithelial cell labeling indices. This suggests an important role of insulin in modulating intestinal cell proliferation and modulation. Insulin was reported to increase brush border membrane enzyme activity, namely that was trehalase, glucoamylase, sucrase and lactase (Menard et al., 1981). Increasing the amount of insulin in the intestinal lumen causes an increase in its own receptors in that area (Heaton and Gelehrter, 1981; Menard and Dagenais, 1993). The fact that insulin up-regulates production of its own receptor (Heaton and Gelehrter, 1981) may explain the dose-dependent effect of the insulin on the STa-receptor binding. This study suggest that insulin may modulate the STa receptor number on the brush border membrane. This up-regulation of STa binding can be either through the increase of the STa receptor density or increase in the affinity of these receptors to the STa toxin. The flow cytometric analysis demonstrated that enterocytes from both insulin-fed groups and control group contained STa receptors. However, the fluorescence intensity suggesting receptor activity was higher on the enterocytes of the insulin-fed groups compared to the control (Fig. 5). No fluorescence was observed on the enterocytes of the negative control group where no STa was added. Our flow cytometry results suggest that due to the elevation of intestinal cell proliferation and differentiation in response to insulin, there was an increase in the STa binding. The biological function of insulin within the small intestine is not completely known. It was reported that the presence of insulin and IGF-I receptors on the brush border membrane suggest an autocrine/paracrine role for these growth factors (Simmons et al., 1995; Steeb et al., 1995).

In summary, the results of this study suggest that insulin has a modulatory effect on the response of suckling mouse intestine to STa. The changes in the structural function of the intestinal brush border membrane due to the effect of insulin may modify the STa/receptor interaction. Knowledge of this modification may provide insights into how to intervene with the STa/receptor interaction.

REFERENCES

Al-Majali, A., Asem, E., Lamar, C., Robinson, J.P., Freeman, M.J., and Saeed, A.M., 1998, Effect of dietary insulin on the response of suckling mice enterocytes to *Escherichia coli* heat-stable enterotoxin, Vet. Res. 29 [In Press].

Arsenault, P. and Menard, D., 1984, Insulin influences the maturation and poliferation of suckling mouse intestinal epithelial mucosa inserum-free organ culture, Biol. Neonate 49:229–236.

Costigan, D.C., Guyda, H.J., and Posner, B.I., 1988, Free insulin-like growth factor-I (IGF-I) andIGF-II in human saliva, J. Clin. Endocrinol. Metab. 66:1014–1018.

de Suavage, F.J., Camerato, T.R., and Goeddel, D.V., 1991, Primary structure and functional expression of the human receptor for *Escherichia coli* heat-stable enterotoxin. J. Biol. Chem. 266:17912–17918.

Dreyfus, L.A., Frantz, J.C.F., and Robertson, D.C., 1983, Chemical properties of heat-stable enterotoxins Produced by enetrotoxigenic *Escherichia coli* of different host origins, Infect. Immun. 42:539–548.

Epstein, S.A., Giannella, R.A., and Brandwein, H.J., 1986, Activation of guanylate cyclase by *E. coli* heat-stable enterotoxin (STa), FEBS Lett. 203:44–48.

Giannella, R.A., 1976, Suckling mouse model for detection of heat-stable *Escherichia coli* enterotoxin: characteristics of the model, Infect. Immun. 4:95–99.

Grosvenor, C.E., Picciano, M.F., and Baumurucker, C.R., 1992, Hormones and growth factors in milk, Endocr. Rev. 14:710–728.

Guandalini, S., Rao, M.C., Smith, P.L., and Field, M., 1982, cGMP modulation of ilealion transport: invitro effects of *Escherichia coli* heat-stable entrotoxin, Am. J. Physiol. 243:G36–G41.

Heaton, J.H. and Gelehrter, T.D., 1981, Desensitization of hepatoma cells to insulin action, evidence for a post-research mechanism, J. Biol. Chem. 256:12257–12262.

Koldovsky, O. and Strbak, V., 1995, Hormones and growth factors in human milk, In: Handbook of milk composition, Editor: Jensen, R.G., Academic Press, San Diego, pp. 428–432.

Menard, D. and Dagenais, P., 1993, Stimulatory effects of insulin on DNA synthesis in suckling mouse colon, Biol. Neonate 63:310–315.

Menard, D., Malo, C., and Calvert, R., 1981, Insulin accelerates the development of intestinal brush border hydrolytic activities of suckling mice, Dev. Biol. 85:150–155.

Potten, C.S., Owen, G., Hewitt, D., Chadwick, C.A., Hendry, H., Lord, B.I., and Woolford, L.B., 1995, Stimulation and inhibition of proliferation in the small intestinal crypts of the mouse after in vivo administration of growth factors, Gut 36:864–873.

Rao, M.C., Orellana, S.A., Field, M., Robertson, D.C., and Giannella, R.A., 1981, Comparsion of the biological actions of three purified heat-stable enterotoxin: effect on ion transport and guanylate cyclase activity in rabbit ileum in vitro, Infect. Immun. 33:165–170.

Saeed, A.M. and Greenberg, R.N., 1985, Preparative Purification of *Escherichia coli* heat-stable enterotoxin, Analyt. Biochem. 151:431–437.

Saeed, A.M., McMillian, R., Huckelberry, V., Abernathy, R., and Greenberg, R.N., 1987, Specific receptor for *Escherichia coli* heat-stable enterotoxin (STa) may determine susceptibility of piglets to diarrheal disease, FEMS Microbiol. Lett. 43:247–251.

Schmidt, G.H., Winton, D.J., and Ponder, B.A., 1988, Development of the pattern of cell renewal in the crypt-villus unit of chimaeric mouse small intestine, Development 103:785–790.

Schulz, S., Green, C.K., Yuen, P.S., and Garbers, D.L., 1990, Guanylyl cyclase is a heat-stabe enterotoxin receptor, Cell 63:941–948.

Sears, C.L. and Kaper, J.B., 1996, Enteric bacterial toxins: mechanisms of action and linkage to intestinal secretion, Microbiol. Rev. 60:167–215.

Simmons, J.G., Hoyt, E.C., Westwick, J.K., Brenner, D.A., Pucilowska, J.B., and Lund, P.K., 1995, Insulin-like growth factor-I and epidermal growth factor interact to regulate growth and gene expression in IEC-6 intestinal epithelial cells, Molecular. Endocr. 9:1157–1165.

Staples, S.J., Asher, S.E., and Giannella, R.A., 1980, Purification and characteristics of heat-stable enterotoxin produced by a strain of *E. coli* pathogenic for man, J. Biol. Chem. 255:4716–4721.

Steeb, C.B., Trahair, J.F., and Read, L.C., 1995, Administration of insulin-like growth factor-I (IGF-I) peptides for three days stimulates proliferation of the small intestinal epithelium in rats, Gut 37:630–638.

Vaandrager, A.B., Schulz, S., De Jonge, H.R., and Garders, D.L., 1993, Guanylyl cyclase C is an *N*-linked Glycoprotein receptor that accounts for multiple heat-stable enterotoxin binding proteins in the intestine. J. Biol. Chem. 268:2174–2179.

Wada, A., Hirayama, T., Kitao, S., Fujisawa, J., Hidaka, Y., and Shimonishi, Y., 1994, Pig intestinal membrane-bound receptor (guanylyl cyclase) for heat-stable enterotoxin: cDNA cloning, functional expression, and characterization. Microbiol. Immunol. 38:535–541.

Ziegler, T.R., Almahfouz, A., Pedrini, M.T., and Smith, R.J., 1995, A comparsion of rat small intestinal insulin and insulin like growth factor I receptors during fasting and refeeding, Endocrinology 136:5148–5154.

10

REPRODUCTION OF LESIONS AND CLINICAL SIGNS WITH A CNF2-PRODUCING *ESCHERICHIA COLI* IN NEONATAL CALVES

Sigrid Van Bost and Jacques Mainil

University of Liège
Faculty of Veterinary Medicine
Laboratory of Bacteriology
Sart Tilman B43a
B-4000 Liège
Belgium

1. SUMMARY

CNF2-producing necrotoxigenic *E. coli* (NTEC2) are associated with diarrhoea and septicaemia in calves. We orally inoculated neonatal calves with a NTEC2 strain in order to reproduce clinical signs and lesions. We observed diarrhoea in each inoculated calf, bacteraemia (80%), the presence of CNF2+ bacteria in the lungs (80%) and in the liver (20%). The observed lesions were inflammation of the entire gut, hypertrophy of the mesenteric lymph nodes and hepatisation of the lungs. We were unable to detect characteristic lesions that are classical signs of septicaemia.

2. INTRODUCTION

Necrotoxigenic *Escherichia coli* (NTEC) produce cytotoxic necrotizing factor 1 (CNF1) or 2 (CNF2). NTEC1 have been isolated from cases of extraintestinal infections in humans (Caprioli et al., 1987), of diarrhoea in calves and pigs (Holland, 1990), of extraintestinal infections in cattle, pigs, goats, cats and dogs (Pohl et al., 1993) and of diarrhoea in rabbits and haemorrhagic colitis in horses (Ansuini et al., 1994). NTEC2 are generally restricted to ruminants with diarrhoea and/or septicaemia (DeRycke et al., 1990; Pohl et al., 1993; Derycke et al., 1987; Oswald et al., 1991). CNF are 110–115 kDa toxins either encoded by the chromosome (CNF1) (Falbo et al., 1992) or by a

Mechanisms in the Pathogenesis of Enteric Diseases 2, edited by Paul and Francis.
Kluwer Academic / Plenum Publishers, New York, 1999.

transferable F-like plasmid called Vir (Oswald et al., 1989; Smith, 1974). In vitro, CNF toxins induce on various eukaryotic cells lines a drastic reorganization of the microfilamental network into thick stress fibres. This phenomenon is accompanied by a block of cytokinesis, leading to the formation of giant multinucleated cells. This phenotype is associated with the ability of CNF toxin to induce a postranlational modification of the 21 kDa Rho GTP-binding protein which is involved in the regulation of microfilament network (Oswald et al., 1994; Schmidt et al., 1997). In vivo, CNF toxins induce necrosis in rabbit skin. Experimental infection of neonatal pigs with NTEC1 O88 induced an early enteritis, progressing to enterocolitis and bacteraemic spread to the lungs. Infection with NTEC1 O32 produced a milder but similar enterocolitis, also with bacterial colonisation of the lungs. The histopathological changes in both cases were characteristic of a toxemia (Wray et al., 1993). Intravenous injection of partially purified CNF1 toxin to lambs induced the development of severe clinical signs starting six hours after the inoculation, and consisted mainly in neurological signs and mucoid diarrhoea. The most striking lesions were oedema and haemorrhage in the central nervous system and foci of coagulation necrosis in the myocardium (De Rycke et al., 1990). In natural infection in rabbits, Asuini et al. (1994), observed post mortem enteritis mainly of the ileum and the caecum. In horses with dysentery, post mortem examination revealed a severe haemorrhagic colitis and caecitis (Ansuini et al., 1994). If we consider the adhesins associated with NTEC strains: most NTEC1 isolates hybridized with Pap probe and either with Sfa or Afa probes. In contrast, most NTEC2 strains hybridize with F17 and/or Afa probes (Mainil et al., 1997). Here, we describe the clinical signs and lesions obtained after an oral challenge in neonatal calves with a NTEC2 bovine isolate.

3. EXPERIMENTAL PROCEDURES AND RESULTS

NTEC2 strain B20A was isolated from the faeces of a calf with diarrhoea and belongs to serotype O15:K14. It was positive for: serum resistance, aerobactin production, ability to adhere to calf intestinal villi, and hybridization with F17A and CNF2 probes (Oswald et al., 1991). Six newborn Friesan calves received 300 ml of colostrum just after the birth. This colostrum was tested by agglutination for the absence of specific antibodies against the B20A strain. At six hours, 5 calves received 250 ml of saline containing 10^9 to 10^{12} bacteria and one calf received 250 ml of saline.

A faeces sample was taken each 4 hours post inoculation, diluted and platted on Gassner Agar medium. The plates were incubated overnight at 37°C. The number of CFU was counted and the colonies were blotted onto a filter in order to perform a colony hybridization (Mainil et al., 1990) with a CNF2 probe (Oswald et al., 1994). This allowed us to calculate the excretion rate of CNF2[+] bacteria. We noticed that the fecal excretion started 24–32 hours post inoculation and persisted until death (Table 1). The rate of excretion ranged from 10^7 CFU/ml to 10^{10} CFU/ml. Diarrhoea occurred in each calf inoculated with the NTEC2 B20A strain, but was absent in the control calf. Diarrhoea started 28–40 hours post inoculation and persisted until death (Table1). Therefore, there was a good correlation between fecal excretion of CNF2[+] bacteria and diarrhoea. We confirmed identity between the inoculated strain and the CNF2[+] bacteria recovered from faeces by pulse field gel electrophoresis (data not shown). The faeces were tested by ELISA for the presence of Enterotoxigenic *E. coli*, Cryptosporidium, Rota and Corona viruses. All the samples were negative. The calves were euthanasied

Table 1. Fecal excretion of NTEC2 B20A strain and diarrhoea appearance

Calves	Death hour	Diarrhoea appearance	Diarrhoea end	NTEC2 strains appearance in the faeces	NTEC2 strains disappearance in the faeces
7	36 Pi	28 Pi	36 Pi	24 Pi	36 Pi
8	74 Pi	28 Pi	74 Pi	28 Pi	74 Pi
9	39 Pi	28 Pi	39 Pi	24 Pi	39 Pi
10	45 Pi	40 Pi	45 Pi	28 Pi	45 Pi
11	57 Pi	32 Pi	57 Pi	32 Pi	57 Pi
control	45 Pi	—	—	—	—

between 36 and 74 hours post inoculation. Samples were taken from: the intestinal content of all parts of the gut, the mesenteric lymph nodes, the liver, the kidneys, the spleen, the lungs and from the heart blood. These samples were analysed for the presence of CNF2+ bacteria as described above. No CNF2$^+$ bacteria were isolated from the kidneys, spleen or mesenteric lymph nodes. By contrast, CNF2$^+$ bacteria were isolated from the small intestine (5/5) and colon (5/5), lungs (4/5), heart blood (4/5), and liver (1/5). The necropsy analysis revealed in each inoculated calf: inflammation of the entire intestine, hypertrophy of the mesenteric lymph nodes and a hepatisation of the cranial lobes of the lungs.

4. CONCLUSIONS

NTEC2 strains were associated with diarrhoea and/or septiceamia in calves. By oral inoculation of neonatal calves with a NTEC2 strain, we were able to consistently reproduce diarrhoea. The fecal excretion of the inoculated strain and diarrhoea correlated, and no other classical cause of diarrhoea (Enterotoxigenic *E. coli*, Rota and Corona -viruses) was detected. These observations allow us to conclude that the inoculated strain was probably the cause of the diarrhoea. Moreover, the uninoculated calf did not exhibit diarrhoea. The presence of CNF2-positive bacteria in the blood indicates that the calves developed bacteraemia, but there were no lesions characteristic of septicaemia. The presence of CNF2 positive bacteria in the lungs confirmed the observation made by Wray et al. (1993) that NTEC possesses a tropism for lungs. There was no correlation between the severity of the lesions and the inoculation or the euthanasia time. The absence of bacteria in the mesenteric lymph nodes indicates that the NTEC2 reach the blood directly and from there to the organs without passage through the lymphatic system. We conclude from these experiments that we have developed an in vivo model allowing for reproduction of diarrhoea, bacteraemia and bacterial invasion. This model will be useful for the study of the virulence factors of NTEC2 strains.

ACKNOWLEDGMENTS

This work was supported by the European Community (Grant FAIR3-CT96-1335).

REFERENCES

Ansuini, A., Candotti, P., Vecchi, G., Falbo, V., Minelli, F., and Caprioli, A., 1994, Necrotoxigenic *Escherichia coli* in rabbit and horses, Vet. rec., 134:608.

Caprioli, A., Falbo, V., Ruggeri, F.M., Baldassari, L., Bisicchia, R., Ippolito, G., Romoli, E., and Donelli, G., 1987, Cytotoxic necrotizing factor production by hemolytic strains of *Escherichia coli* causing extraintestinal infections. J. Clin. Microbiol., 25:146–149.

De Rycke, J., Guillot, J.F., and Boivin, R., 1987, Cytotoxins in non-enterotoxigenic strains of *Escherichia coli* isolated from feces of diarrheic calves, Vet. Microbiol., 15:137–157.

De Rycke, J., Gonzalez, E.A., Blanco, J., Oswald, E., BLanco, M., and Boivin, R., 1990, Evidence for two types of cytotxic necrotizing factor in human and animal clinical isolates of *Escherichia coli*, J. Clin. Microbiol., 28:694–699.

Falbo, V., Famigelietti, M., and Caprioli, A., 1992, Gene block encoding production of cytotoxic necrotizing factor 1 and haemolysin in *Escherichia coli* isolates from extraintestinal infection, Infect. Immun., 60:2182–2187.

Holland, R.E., 1990, Some infectious causes of diarrhoea in young farms animals, Clin. Microbiol. Rev., 3:345–375.

Mainil, J.G., Jacquemin, E., Kaeckenbeeck, A., and Pohl, P., 1993, Association between the effacing (*eae*) gene and theShiga-like toxin-encoding genes in *Eschrichia coli* isloates from cattle, Am. J. Vet., Res., 54:1064–1068.

Mainil, J.G., Jacquemin, E., Herault, F., and Oswald, E., 1997, Presence of pap-, sfa-, and afa- related sequences in necrotoxigenic *Escherichia coli* isolates from cattle: evidence for new variants of the AFA family, Can. J. Vet. Res., 61:193–199.

Oswald, E., De Rycke, J., Guillot, J.F., and Boivin, R., 1989, Cytotoxic effect of multinucleation in HeLa cell cultures associated with the presence of Vir plasmid in *Escherichia coli* strains, FEMS Microbiol. Lett., 58:95–100.

Oswald, E., De Rycke, J., Lintermans, P., Van Muylen, K., Mainil, J., Daube, G., and Pohl, P., 1991, Virulence factors associated with the cytotoxic nevrotizing factor type 2 in bovine diarrheic and septicaemic strains of *Escherichia coli*, J. Clin. Microbiol., 29:2522–2527.

Oswald, E., Pohl, P., Jacquemin, E., Lintermans, P., Van Muylen, K., O'Brien, A.D., and Mainil, J., 1994, Specific DNA probes to detect *Escherichia coli* strains producing CNF1 or CNF2, J. Med. Microbiol., 40:428–434.

Pohl, P., Mainil, J., Devriese, L., Haesebrouck, F., Broes, A., Lintermans, P., and Oswald, E., 1992, Escherichia coli productrices de la toxine cytotoxique nécrosante de type 1 (CNF1) isolées à partir de processus pathologiques chez des chiens et des chats, Ann. Med. Vet. 137:21–25.

Pohl, P., Oswald, E., Van Muylen, K., Jacquemin, E., Lintermans, P., and Mainil, J., 1993, *Escherichia coli* producing CNF1 and CNF2 cytotoxins in animals with different disorders, Vet. res., 24:311–315.

Schmidt, G., Sehr, P., Wilm, M., Selzer, J., Mann, M., and Aktories, K., 1997, Gln 63 of Rho is deaminated by *Escherichia coli* cytotoxic necrotizing factor-1, Nature, 387:725–729.

Smith, H.W., 1974, A search for transmissible pathogenic characters in invasive strains of *Escherichia coli*: the discovery of a plasmid-controlled lethal character closely associated, or identified with colicin V., J. Gen. Microbiol., 83:95–111.

Wray, C., Piercy, D.W.T., Carroll, P.J., and Cooley, W.A., 1993, Experimental infection of neonatal pigs with CNF toxin-producing strains of *Escherichia coli*, Res. Vet. Sc., 54:290–298.

11

THE LOCUS FOR ENTEROCYTE EFFACEMENT (LEE) OF ENTEROPATHOGENIC *ESCHERICHIA COLI* (EPEC) FROM DOGS AND CATS

Frédéric Goffaux, Bernard China, Laurence Janssen, Vinciane Pirson, and Jacques Mainil

Laboratory of Bacteriology
Faculty of Veterinary Medicine
University of Liège
Sart Tilman B43a
B-4000 Liège
Belgium

SUMMARY

Enteropathogenic *Escherichia coli* (EPEC) produce attaching and effacing lesions. The genes responsible for this lesion are clustered on the chromosome forming a 35.5 kilobase pathogenesis island called LEE. The LEE was identified, characterized and completely sequenced from the human EPEC strain E2348/69. The LEE carries genes coding for: a type III secretion system (genes *esc* and *sep*), the translocated intimin receptor (gene *tir*), the outer membrane protein intimin (gene *eae*) and the *E. coli* secreted proteins EspA, EspB, and EspD (genes *esp*). In addition to man and farm animals, EPEC are also isolated from dogs and cats. We studied structurally and functionally the LEE of dog and cat EPEC. First, we used four probes scattered along the LEE to identify the presence of a LEE in canine and feline EPEC isolates. Second, by PCR, we checked the presence of genes homologous to *eae*, *sep*, *esp*, and *tir* genes in these strains. Third, since the four types of *eae* and *tir* genes were described, we developed a multiplex PCR in order to determine the type of *eae* and *tir* genes present in each strain. Fourth, we determined by PCR the site of the LEE insertion on the chromosome. Fifth, we tested several of the canine EPEC in their capacity to induce attaching and effacing lesions in the rabbit intestinal loop assay. We can conclude from this study: first, that the a LEE-like structure is present in all tested strains and that it con-

Mechanisms in the Pathogenesis of Enteric Diseases 2, edited by Paul and Francis.
Kluwer Academic / Plenum Publishers, New York, 1999.

tains genes homologous to *esp*, *sep*, *tir*, and *eae* genes; second, that there is some preferential associations between the type of *eae* gene and the type of *tir* gene present in
a strain; third, that the majority of the tested strains contained a LEE located elsewhere
on the chromosome in comparison to the human EPEC strain E2348/69; and fourth
that dog EPEC were able to induce attaching and effacing lesions in rabbit ileal loop
assay.

INTRODUCTION

Enteropathogenic *E. coli* (EPEC) is responsible for sporadic outbreaks of
diarrhoea in day care centres and nurseries in developed countries, however it remains
a leading cause of diarrhoea among infants in the developing world. EPEC
forms small microcolonies on the surface of infected epithelial cells, followed by
intimate contact and localized degeneration of the epithelial brush border microvilli.
This histopathological characteristic is called attaching and effacing (AE) lesion
(Moon et al., 1983). The AE lesion is associated with the accumulation of highly
organized cytoskeletal components (actin, α-actinin, myosin light chain, ezrin, and talin)
in epithelial cells immediately beneath the adherent bacteria (Finlay et al., 1992),
leading to the formation of a pedestal-like structure (Knuton, 1994; Nataro and
Kaper, 1998).

In human EPEC strain E2348/69 from serotype O127, most of the genes
necessary for the AE lesion are clustered on a 35.5 kb chromosomal pathogenicity
island called LEE (Locus of Enterocyte Effacement) (McDaniel et al., 1995) that
is sufficient to confer AE activity in vitro when introduced into a non-pathogenic
E. coli strain (McDaniel et al., 1997). The LEE can be divided into three regions.
The left end of the LEE contains genes (*sepABCD*) that encode for a type III
secretion system responsible for the secretion of proteins EspA, EspB, EspD
(Jarvis et al., 1995) and Tir (Kenny et al., 1997). The central portion of the LEE
contains 2 genes (*eae*, *tir*) the products of which promote intimate attachment of
bacteria to host cells and organization of cytoskeletal actin beneath adherent bacteria.
The *eae* gene encodes a 94 kDa outer membrane protein, intimin, required for
intimate adherence (Jerse et al., 1990). The *tir* gene encodes the intimin receptor
which is translocated into the eucaryotic cytoplasm where it becomes phosphorylated and then incorporated into the host cell membrane (Kenny et al., 1998). The
right portion of the LEE contains 3 genes (*espA*, *espD*, *espB*) that encode proteins
that are essential for EPEC-mediated signal transduction events within the host
cell, including tyrosine phosphorylation of Tir, increasing of IP3 and calcium levels,
leading to the AE lesion formation (Donnenberg et al., 1993; Lai et al., 1996; Kenny
et al., 1996).

Infections with EPEC were also described in dogs (Broes et al., 1988; Janke et al.,
1989) and cats (Popischil et al., 1987). Ultrastructural attaching and effacing lesions
were observed in the small intestine and colon of the animals. A study conducted by
Drolet et al. (1994) showed that in 13 cases of enteric colibacillosis, 12 were associated
with EPEC. Thus, *E. coli* should be considered of causal significiance when investigating diarrheal disease in dogs, particulary in puppies.

In this paper our objective is to demonstrate the presence of a LEE-related
pathogenicity island in dog EPEC (DEPEC) and cat EPEC (CEPEC) strains, and to
study the potential pathogenicity of these strains.

Table 1. Main characteristics of the EPEC strains studied

Strains	Eae[a]	SLT 1[a]	SLT 2[a]	LEEA	LEEB	LEEC	LEED	LEE lenght (kb)	A/E phenotype	species
25211-A2	+	−	−	+	+	+	+	35	2/2	Dog
25314	+	−	−	+	+	+	+	41	ND	Dog
26881	+	−	−	+	+	+	+	35	ND	Dog
32106-2	+	−	−	+	+	+	+	41	ND	Dog
41735-2	+	−	−	+	+	+	+	38	1/3	Dog
43401-2	+	−	−	+	+	+	+	38	ND	Dog
43769-2	+	−	−	+	+	+	+	41	ND	Dog
44318-3	+	−	−	+	+	+	+	35	1/2	Dog
45337-2	+	−	−	+	+	+	+	35	1/2	Dog
35314-1	+	−	−	+	+	+	+	41	ND	Cat
43748-1	+	−	−	+	+	+	+	41	ND	Cat
43750-1	+	−	−	+	+	+	+	35	ND	Cat
E2348/69	+	−	−	+	+	+	+	35.5	ND	Human
RDEC-1	+	−	−	+	+	+	+	ND	4/4	Rabbit
HB101	−	−	−	−	−	−	−	−	0/4	

a: Mainil et al., 1994.
ND: not determined.

EXPERIMENTAL RESULTS

Presence of a LEE-Related Structure

First, we investigated the presence of a LEE-related structure in DEPEC and CEPEC. Nine DEPEC strains and 3 CEPEC strains were used in this study (Table 1). All strains were isolated in Belgium from animals with diarrhoea and/or enteritis. The human EPEC strain E2348/69, EHEC strain ATCC43888 (O157H7), and bovine EHEC strain 193 (O26) were included as positive controls, non pathogenic *E. coli* K-12 HB101 is incorporated as negative control. We tested the capacity of DEPEC and CEPEC to hybridize with the LEE probes in a colony hybridization assay (Mainl et al., 1994; Table 2). These probes were scattered along the LEE (McDaniel et al., 1995). The results indicated that all isolates were positive with the four LEE probes (Table 1).

Second, we tested the presence of a LEE-related structure by restriction of total DNA with *Sma*I enzyme which does not cut into the LEE (McDaniel and Kaper, 1997), pulse field gel electrophoresis (PFGE) and hybridizations with the LEE probes (Goffaux et al., 1997). Figure 1 shows that the probes hybridized with a unique fragment ranging from 35 to 41 kb in each isolate except from strain 44318-3 in which 1 fragment of 24 kb, hybridized with LEEA and LEEB probes and another fragment of 11 kb hybridized with LEEC and LEED probes. We conclude that the tested DEPEC and CEPEC strains possessed a LEE-related structure and that a *Sma*I site is present in the LEE of one DEPEC strain.

Table 2. Probes used in this study

Probes	Plasmids	Restriction Enzymes	Fragment Size (bp)	References
LEEA	pCVD453	*Mlu*I/*Eco*RI	2870	McDaniel et al., 1995
LEEB	pCVD461	*Eco*RI/*Sal*I/*Pvu*II	2948	McDaniel et al., 1995
LEEC	pCVD443	*Sal*I/*Stu*I	1050	McDaniel et al., 1995
LEED	pCVD460	*Sma*I/*Xba*I	2300	McDaniel et al., 1995

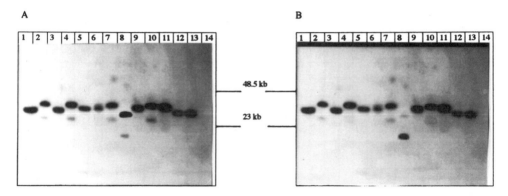

Figure 1. Hybridization on pulse field gel electrophoresis with LEE probes. The DNA of DEPEC and CEPEC strains was digested by *Sma*I and separated by PFGE, the gels were hybridized with LEEA and LEEB probes (panel A) and with LEEC and LEE D probes (Panel B). Lane 1: strain 25211-A2, lane 2: strain 25314, lane 3: strain 26881, lane 4: strain 32106-2, lane 5: strain 41735-2, lane 6: strain 43401-2, lane 7: strain 43769-2, lane 8: 44318-3, lane 9: 45337-23, lane 10: strain 35314-1, lane 11: strain 43748-1, lane 12: strain 43750-1, lane 13: strain E2348/69, lane 14: strain HB101.

Presence of LEE-Related Genes

We tested for the presence of genes related to the *sepABCD* and *espADB* genes by PCR amplification (China et al., 1996) of an internal fragment of each gene. The primers used and the length of the amplicons are listed in the Table 3. All strains gave an amplicon of the expected length for each PCR (data not show).

Associations between *eae* and *tir* Genes

In the LEE, we noted the presence of the *eae* gene encoding for the intimin protein and the *tir* gene encoding for the intimin receptor. The *eae* gene has been sequenced from the human EPEC strain E2348/69 (Jerse et al., 1990), from two human O157:H7 EHEC strains (Beebekhee et al., 1992; Yu and Kaper, 1992), from the Rabbit EPEC strain RDEC-1 (Abe et al., 1996), from the bovine O26 EHEC strain 193 (China et al., personal communication) and from the DEPEC strain 4221 (An et al., 1996). The alignment of all these sequences revealed the presence of constant and variable regions. We constructed primers based on a sequence from the constant part (B73) of the gene, and variable parts of the O127, O26 and O157:H7 *eae* alleals. The *tir* gene has been sequenced from the human EPEC strain E2348/69 (Eliott et al., 1998), from the human O157H7 EHEC strain EDL933 (Perna et al., 1998) and from an O26 and an O111 human EPEC strains (Paton et al., 1998). The sequence alignment revealed once again the presence of constant and variable regions. Therefore, we selected a primer (B139) in a constant part and primers in the variable parts of the O127, 0157 and O26/O111 strains. The primer sequences and the length of each amplicon are in Table 2. The results are presented in the Table 4. Comparing the results of the 2 multiplex PCRs we can see 3 types of associations: 2/12 are eae_{O127}-tir_{O127}, 2/12 are eae_{O26}-tir_{O26}, and 7/12 are eae_{O157}-tir_{O127}. In strain 44318-3 strain, we were unable to obtain an *eae* amplicon using our primers, indicating the presence of an other *eae* type in this strain.

Table 3. Primers used in this study

Genes	Primers and sequences	Size of the PCR product (bp)	References
3'LEE *SelC* O394	K255, 5'GGTTGAGTCGATTGATCTCTGG3' K260, 5'GAGCGAATATTCCGATATCTGGTT3' K261, 5'CCTGCAAATAAACACGGCGCAT3'	418 (K255–K260) 527 (K260–K261)	McDaniel et al., 1995
sepA	B127, 5'CTAACTTCTTTCCCCACA3' B128, 5'GCACTCACTTCAGCAACA3'	233	this study
sepB	F1, 5'ACAAGATAGAACCCAGTCAA3' F2, 5'CAATAGTCGTCGCCGTAAA3'	576	this study
sepC	F3, 5'ATACTCTCGCCTCGTTGCT3' F4, 5'CCATTACTTGCCATTGTCT3'	765	this study
sepD	F5, 5'ATGATTGTGACTGGCTAAC3' F6, 5'CTGATGAAGATGATTGCTC3'	375	this study
espA	Donne 99, 5'GCGAAAGCTCAACTTCCT3' Donne 100, 5'GCTGGCTATTATTGACCGTCGT3'	184	this study
espB	B60, 5'TGTTTTGAGCAGCACGAC3' B61, 5'ACAGATGAGATAGCACCAC3'	282	this study
espD	F7, 5'CGCTGGATTTACAACTGGT3' F8, 5'TGCTTTCTCTTCGGCTTTT3'	422	this study
eae	B73, 5'TACTGAGATTAAGGCTGATAA3' B74, 5'AGGAAGAGGGTTTTGTGTT3' B138, 5'GACCAGAAGAAGCATCCA3' B137, 5'TGTATGTCGCACTCTGATT3'	778 (B73–B74) 452 (B73–B138) 520 (B73–B137)	this study
tir	B139, 5'CRCCKCCAYTACCTTCACA3' IR4, 5'CGCTAACCTCCAAACCATT3' B141, 5'GTCGCAGTTTCAGTTTCAC3' B140, 5'GATTTTTCCCTCGCCACTA3'	342 (B139–TIR4) 781 (B139–B141) 560 (B139–B140)	this study

Table 4. PCR results

Strains	LEE location (bp)		Multiplex PCR	
	K255–K260	K260–K261	eae (pb)	tir (pb)
25211-A2	418	NA	452	342
25314	NA	527	778	342
26881	418	NA	452	342
32106-2	NA	527	778	342
41735-2	NA	527	520	560
43401-2	NA	527	520	560
43769-2	NA	527	778	342
44318-3	418	NA	NA	781
45337-2	NA	527	778	342
35314-1	NA	527	778	342
43748-1	NA	527	778	342
43750-1	NA	527	778	342
E2348/69	418	NA	452	342
ATCC43888	ND	ND	778	781
193	ND	ND	520	560
HB101	NA	527	ND	ND

NA: no amplification.
ND: not determined.

Location of the LEE

To investigate the insertion of the LEE on the chromosome, we used the triplex PCR (McDaniel et al., 1995) (Table 3). If the LEE is inserted between ORF O394 and the *selC* gene, the PCR reaction with primer K255–K260 gave a 418 bp amplicon, if the LEE was not inserted at this position, the PCR reaction with primers K260–K261 gave a 527 bp amplicon. The results of the PCR are presented in Table 4. A 418 bp amplicon was obtained with 3 isolates and a 527 bp amplicon with 9 isolates. Thus, in 25% of the AEEC canine strains, the LEE is inserted between the ORF O394 and *selC* gene, and in 75%, elsewhere.

Ligated Intestinal Loop Assay in Rabbits

Four DEPEC strains, which were associated with diarrhea and/or enteritis, were tested in the intestinal loop assay for their capacity to produce attaching and effacing lesions in vivo (China et al., 1997). Each isolate was tested in at least 2 different animals, and the positive control strain RDEC-1 and the negative control strain *E. coli* K-12 HB101 were tested in rabbits. The results are presented in Table 3. Each isolate was positive in at least one of the loops that was inoculated. The RDEC-1 strain was positive in all loops, and the *E. coli* laboratory strain HB101 was negative in all loops. AE lesions were observed histopathologically, and confirmed ultrastructurally in all loops inoculated with canine isolates, and the RDEC-1 strain.

CONCLUSIONS

In this work, we showed the presence in DEPEC and CEPEC strains, of a pathogenesis island related to the LEE of human EPEC. This genetic homology was confirmed by hybridization using four probes scattered along the LEE by PCR using primers deduced from the human EPEC strain E2348/69 LEE sequence. We conclude that the LEE of DEPEC and CEPEC strains possesses genes related to *eae*, *esp*, *esc*, and *tir* genes. However by using multiplex PCR, we showed that, although related, the *eae* and *tir* genes of DEPEC and CEPEC were sometimes different from the corresponding genes of the EPEC E2348/69 strain. Surprisingly, the association between the intimin gene and the intimin gene receptor are mainly heterologous. Seven of 12 strains had an eae_{O157} gene associated with a tir_{O127} gene. However, homologous combinations were also present: eae_{O127} with tir_{O127}, and eae_{O26} with tir_{O26}. These results raise the question of the complementary regions between the intimin and its receptor. Interestingly, the LEE in (7/9) DEPEC and (3/3) CEPEC strains is located elsewhere on the chromosome in comparison with the location of the LEE in the human EPEC strain E2348/69. This is consistent with our observations of bovine strains (Goffaux et al., 1997). There is a good correlation between this characteristic and the fact that the hybridizing fragment in PFGE was longer than 35 kb (except for strain 43750-1), indicating that the difference in length could be due to a difference in the position of *Sma*I sites flanking the LEE. Finally, we conclude from in vivo experimentation that the LEE of the four tested DEPEC strains were functional since these strains were able to induce attaching and effacing lesions in the rabbit ileal loop assay.

ACKNOWLEDGMENTS

Frédéric Goffaux is a fellow of the FRIA (Fonds de la Recherche appliquée à l'Industrie et à l'Agriculture). This work was financially supported by the "Ministère des classes moyennes et de l'agriculture, direction recherche et développement." We thank Philippe Stordeur, Etienne Jacquemin, and Hélène Boucher for their technical assistance during *in vivo* experiments.

REFERENCES

Abe, A., Kenny, B., Stein, M., and Finlay, B.B., 1997, Characterization of two virulence proteins secreted by rabbit enteropathogenic *Escherichia coli*, EspA and EspB, whose maximal expression is sensitive to host body temperature, Infect. Immun., 65:3547–3555.

Agin, T.S., Cantey, J.R., Boeedeker, E.C., and Wolf, M.K., 1996, Characterization of the *eaeA* gene from rabbit enteropathogenic *Escherichia coli* RDEC-1 and comparison to other *eaeA* genes from bacteria that cause attaching-afacing lesions, FEMS Microbiol. Lett., 14:249–258.

An, H., Fairbrother, J.M., Dubreuil, D., and Harel, J., 1997, Cloning and characterization of the *eae* gene from a dog attaching and effacing *Escherichia coli* strain 4221, FEMS Microbiol. Lett., 148:239–245.

Beebakhee, G., Louie, M., De Azavedo, J., and Brunton, J., 1992, Cloning and nucleotide sequence of the *eae* gene homologue from enterohemorrhagic *Escherichia coli* serotype O157:H7. FEMS Microbiol. Lett., 91:63–68.

Broes, A., Drolet, R., Fairbrother, J.M., and Johnson, W.M., 1988, Natural infection with attaching and effacing *Escherichia coli* in a diarrheic puppy, Can. J. Vet. Res., 52:280–282.

China, B., Pirson, V., and Mainil, J., 1996, Typing of bovine attaching and effacing *Escherichia coli* by multiplex in vitro amplification of virulence-associated genes, Appl. Environ. Microbiol., 62:3462–3465.

China, B., Pirson, V., Jacquemin, E., Pohl, P., and Mainil, J.G., 1997, Pathotypes of bovine verotoxigenic *Escherichia coli* isolates producing attaching/Effacing (AE) lesions in the ligated inbtestinal loop assay in rabbits, In Mechanisms in the pathogenesis of enteric diseases, Editors: Paul, P.S., Francis, D.H., and Benfield, D.A., Adv. Exp. Med. Biol. 412, pp. 311–316.

Donnenberg, M.S., Yu, J., and Kaper, J.B., 1993, A second chromosomal gene necessary for intimate attachment of enteropahtogenic *Escherichia coli* to epithelial cells, J. Bacteriol., 175:4670–4680.

Drolet, R., Fairbrother, J.M., Harel, J., and Helie, P., 1994, Attaching and effacing and enterotoxigenic *Escherichia coli* associated with enteric colibacillosis in the dog, Can. J. Vet. Res., 31:591–594.

Elliott, S.J., Wainwright, L.A., McDaniel, T.K., Deng, Y.K., Lai, L.C., McNamara, B.P., Donnenberg, M.S., and Kaper, J.B., 1998, The complete sequence of the locus of enterocyte effacement (LEE) from enteropathogenic *Escherichia coli* E2348/69, Mol. Microbiol., 28:1–4.

Finlay, B.B., Rosenshine, I., Donnenberg, M.S., and Kaper, J.B., 1992, Cytoskeletal composition of attaching and effacing lesions associated with enteropatogenic *Escherichia coli* adherence to HeLa cells, Infect. Immun., 60:2541–2543.

Goffaux, F., Mainil, J., Pirson, V., Charlier, G., Pohl, P., Jacquemin, E., and China, B., 1997, Bovine attaching and effacing *Escherichia coli* possess a pathogenesis island related to the LEE of the human enteropathogenic *E. coli* strain E2348/69, FEMS Microbiol. Lett., 154:415–421.

Janke, B.H., Francis, D.H., Collins, J.E., Libal, M.C., Zeman, D.H., and Johnson, D.D., 1989, Attaching and effacing *Escherichia coli* infections in calves, pigs, lambs and dogs, J. Vet. Diagn. Invest., 1:6–11.

Jarvis, K.G., Giron, J.A., Jerse, A.E., McDaniel, T.K., Donnenberg, M.S., and Kaper, J.B., 1995, Enteropathogenic *Escherichia coli* contains a putative type III secretion system necessary for the export of proteins involved in attaching and effacing lesion formation. Proc. Natl. Acad. Sci. USA, 92:7996–8000.

Jerse, A.E., Yu, J., Tall, B.D., and Kaper, J.B., 1990, A genetic locus of enteropathogenic *Escherichia coli* necessary for the production of ataching and effacing lesions on tissue culture cells. Proc. Natl. Acad. Sci. USA, 87:7839–7843.

Kenny, B., Lai, L.-C., Finlay, B.B., and Donnenberg, M.S., 1996, EspA, a protein secreted by enteropathogenic *Escherichia coli* is required to induces in epithelial epithelial cells. Mol. Microbiol., 20:313–323.

Kenny, B., DeVinney, R., Stein, M., Reinscheid, D.J., Frey, E.A., and Finlay, B.B., 1997, Enteropathogenic *E. coli* (EPEC) transfers its receptor for intimate adherence into mammalian cells, Cell, 91:511–520.

Knutton, S., Rosenshine, I., Pallen, M.J., Nisan, I., Neves, B.C., Bain, C., Wolff, C., Dougan, G., and Frankel, G., 1998, A novel EspA-associated surface organelle of enteropathogenic *Escherichia coli*; involved in protein translocation into epithelial cells. EMBO J., 17:2166–2176.

Knutton, S., Attaching and Effacing *E. coli*. In: *Escherichia coli* in domestic animals and humans, Editor: Gyles, C.L., 1994, CAB International, Wallingford, UK, pp. 567–591.

Lai, L.C., Wainwright, L.A., Stone, K.D., and Donnenberg, M.S., 1997, A third secreted protein that is encoded by the enteropazthogenic *Escherichia coli* pathogenicity island is required for transduction of signals and for attaching and effacing activities in host cells. Infect. Immun., 65:2211–2217.

Mainil, J.G., Jacquemin, E., Bez, S., Pohl, P., and Kaeckenbeeck, A., 1994, La détection, au moyen de sondes génétiques, de souches potentiellement attachantes et effaçantes d'*Escherichia coli* (AEEC) isolées de veaux, de porcelets et de carnivores. In: biotechnologies du diagnostic et de la prévention des maladies animales, Editor: AUPELF-UREF, John Libbey Eurotext, Paris, France, pp. 73–79.

McDaniel, T.K., Jarvis, G., Donnenberg, M.S., and Kaper, J.B., 1995, A genetic locus of enterocyte effacement conserved among diverse enterobacterial pathogens. Proc. Natl. Acad. Sci. USA, 92:1664–1668.

McDaniel, T.K. and Kaper, J.B., 1997, A cloned pathogenicity island from enteropathogenic *Escherichia coli* confers the attaching and effacing phenotype on E. coli K-12, Mol. Microbiol., 23:399–407.

Moon, H.W., Whipp, S.C., Argenzio, R.A., Levine, M.M., and Gianella, R.A., 1983, Attaching and effacing activities of rabbit and human enteropathogenic *Escherichia coli* in pig and rabbit intestines. Infect. Immun., 53:1340–1351.

Nataro, J.P. and Kaper, J.B., 1998, Diarrheagic *Escherichia coli*. Clin. Microbiol. Rev., 11:142–201.

Paton, A.W., Manning, P.A., Woodrow, M.C., and Paton J.C., 1998, The translocated intimin receptor (Tir) of shiga toxigenic *Escherichia coli* isolates belonging to serotype O26, O111, and O157 react with sera from patients with hemolytic-uremic syndrome and exhibit marked sequence heterogeneity. Genbank acession number AF070067–AF070068–AF070069.

Perna, N., Mayhew, G.F., Posfai, G., Elliot, S., Donnenberg, M.S., Kaper, J.B., and Blattner, F.R., 1998, Molecular evolution of a pathogenicity island from enterohemorrhagic *Escherichia coli* O157:H7. Infect. Immun., 66:3810–3817.

Popischil, A., Mainil, J.G., Baljer, G., and Moon, H.W., 1987, Attaching and effacing bacteria in the intestines of calves and cats with diarrhea, Vet. Path., 24:330–334.

Yu, J. and Kaper, J.B., 1992, Cloning and characterization of the *eae* gene of enterohaemorrhagic *Escherichia coli* O157:H7. Mol. Microbiol., 6:411–471.

12

AGE-DEPENDENT VARIATION IN THE DENSITY AND AFFINITY OF *ESCHERICHIA COLI* HEAT-STABLE ENTEROTOXIN RECEPTORS IN MICE

Ahmad M. Al-Majali,[1] J. Paul Robinson,[2] Elikplimi K. Asem,[2] Carlton Lamar,[2] M. James Freeman,[1] and A. Mahdi Saeed[1]*

Departments of Veterinary Pathobiology[1] and
Basic Medical Sciences[2]
School of Veterinary Medicine
Purdue University
West Lafayette, Indiana 47907

1. SUMMARY

Enterotoxigenic strains of *Escherichia coli* that produce heat-stable enterotoxin (STa), are a major cause of diarrheal disease worldwide. Resistance to diarrheal disease in human infants and newborn animals has been attributed to a gradual turnover in the intestinal brush border membrane receptors to bacterial pili. In this study, we demonstrated age-dependent variation in the density and affinity of the mouse enterocyte receptors specific for STa. Flow cytometry and radiolabeled-STa (^{125}I-STa) assays were used as more reliable quantitative measures for the characterization of STa-enterocyte receptor interaction. These assays indicated a stronger interaction of STa with its putative receptor on the enterocytes of the 2-day-old suckling mice than with enterocytes from 1-week, 2-week and 2-month-old mice. Scatchard plot analysis of ^{125}I-STa-receptor interaction suggested that STa-receptors exist at a higher number on enterocytes from the 2-day-old mice than enterocytes of the older mice. Additionally, receptors from the 2-day-old mice had a greater affinity for STa ligand than receptors from the older mice. Density of STa receptors on enterocytes and their affinity to STa may determine the extent of binding and severity of secretory response. This may further explain the increased susceptibility of newborn animals and human infants to STa-mediated diarrheal disease.

Mechanisms in the Pathogenesis of Enteric Diseases 2, edited by Paul and Francis.
Kluwer Academic / Plenum Publishers, New York, 1999.

2. INTRODUCTION

Secretory diarrhea caused by enterotoxigenic *Escherichia coli* (ETEC) is a major cause of death among human infants and young animals in the developing countries (Dreyfus et al., 1984; Saeed et al., 1987; Vaandrager et al., 1993). Virulence factors that enable ETEC strains to cause diarrheal disease during the first days of life include specific surface fimbriae, which mediate bacterial adherence to intestinal epithelial cells, and enterotoxins that stimulate intestinal secretion (Butler and Clarke, 1994; Jaso-Friedmann et al., 1992; Sack, 1980). It was found that colonization by ETEC can be blocked either by lack of fimbrial receptors, or presence of receptor analogs in the mucous layer that inhibit binding to intestinal cells suggesting a key role of ETEC fimbriae in host specificity and age susceptibility in pigs (Dean, 1990). ETEC produce different types of enterotoxins; heat-labile enterotoxin (LT) and two types of heat-stable enterotoxins (STa and STb) (Saeed and Greenberg, 1985; Sears and Kaper, 1996). STa-mediated diarrhea is more common and more severe in young animals and human infants (Cohen et al., 1986; 1988; Rao et al., 1981; Saeed et al., 1987). STa is a cysteine-rich, nonimmunogenic, 18- or 19-amino acid peptide with a molecular weight of 2 kDa (Butler and Clarke, 1994; Sears and Kaper, 1996). STa has been found to increase guanylate cyclase activity and guanosine $3',5'$-cyclic monophosphate (cGMP) concentration in the mammalian small intestinal cells (Guandalini et al., 1982; Guerrant et al., 1980). The sequence of events which ends in stimulation of intestinal fluid secretion and diarrhea is initiated by STa binding to a specific receptor located on the brush border membrane of the intestinal epithelial cells of the host (Giannella et al., 1983; Jaso-Friedmann et al., 1992). STa receptor is believed to be part of the extracellular motif of the brush border-associated guanylyl cyclase (Schulz et al., 1990; Vaandrager et al., 1993; Wada et al., 1994). The STa/receptor binding has been studied in human, pig and rat intestine. In all of these species, an increase in brush border membrane-STa receptor density was observed in the immature intestine (Cohen et al., 1986; 1988; Jaso-Friedmann et al., 1992). This coincides with the period of increased susceptibility to STa-induced diarrheal disease that occurs in early life of humans and animals. Stevens et al. (1971), have described two periods of increased porcine responsiveness to STa; during the first week of life and directly after weaning. It is not clear whether the susceptibility to ETEC-STa changes with age and if this change results from alterations in the density and/or affinity of the enterocytes receptors that are specific for this enterotoxin. The development of age-dependent resistance against ETEC diarrheal diseases was observed in more than one species of animals. Moon and Whipp (1970) found that STb is capable of inducing secretion in 7-day-old pigs but not in 7-week-old ones. Previous studies on the effect of age on the interaction between STa and its putative receptor revealed that immature rat jejunum was much more sensitive to the secretory effect of STa than adult jejunum. In this study, we hypothesized that the susceptibility of the 2-day-old mice that are used in the suckling mouse assay of ETEC-STa is modulated by an increased number of STa receptors on their enterocytes, and that the affinity of these receptors to the STa toxin may be age-dependent. Currently, the suckling mouse model is the only reliable bioassay for ETEC-STa. Flow cytometry, ^{125}I-STa affinity binding and indirect immunofluorescence assays were utilized to characterize the interaction of ETEC-STa with its putative receptor on enterocytes of different age-groups of mice.

3. MATERIALS AND METHODS

3.1. STa Purification

STa was produced and purified to homogeneity using the methods described by Staples et al. (1980) and modified by Saeed and Greenberg (1985).

3.2. Experimental Animals

Four different age groups (2-day, 1-week, 2-week, and 2-month-old) of Swiss Webster mice were used in this experiment (8–10 mice in each group). The mouse room had 13–15 complete air changes per hour and was maintained at $22 \pm 1°C$ temperature with $45 \pm 2\%$ relative humidity and a 12/12-h light/dark cycle. Mice were euthanized by ether anesthesia followed by cervical dislocation, and single cell suspensions of enterocytes were prepared from each group as described below.

3.3. Isolation of Suckling Mouse Enterocytes

Enterocytes were isolated as described previously (Al-Majali et al., 1998). The population of cells harvested was monitored by periodic wet mount examination through the whole procedure to assess the quantity and quality of the isolated enterocytes. Cell counts and cell viability were determined by dye-exclusion using 0.2% trypan blue. Only cell suspensions that contained over 80% viable cells were used for indirect immunofluorescence, flow cytometric analysis and ^{125}I-STa binding assay.

3.4. Indirect Immunofluorescence Assay

Intestinal cryostat sections were incubated with 50 μl (100 μg/ml of 10 mM PBS) of HPLC-purified STa for 45 minute at 37°C. After washing three times with PBS (pH 7.4), slides were incubated at 37°C for 45 minute with 50 μl of 1:10 diluted anti-STa antibody produced in rabbit. Slides were washed three times in PBS and reincubated with 50 μl of 1:100 diluted anti-rabbit-IgG-FITC-conjugated antibody (KPL, Gaithersburg, MD). After a 45-minute incubation, slides were rinsed in PBS and examined using a Nikon labophot epi-fluorescence microscope.

3.5. Flow Cytometry Analysis

Enterocytes were prepared for staining by three additional washes with PBS, pH 7.2, containing 0.5% BSA. In a volume of 100 μl, 10^5 enterocytes in PBS-BSA were incubated with 50 μl of HPLC purified STa (10 μg/ml of 10 mM PBS) for 45 minute at 37°C. After washing three times in PBS-BSA, enterocytes were resuspended in 100 μl of PBS-BSA. Fifty-microliter of STa-specific antiserum produced in rabbits was diluted 1:10 in PBS, added to the enterocyte suspension and incubated for 30 minute at 4°C. Cells were washed three times with PBS-BSA and resuspended in 100 μl of PBS-BSA. Fifty-microliter of goat anti-rabbit-IgG-FITC-conjugated antibody (KPL, Gaithersburg, MD) diluted 1:100 in PBS was added to the enterocyte suspension and incubated for 30 minutes on ice. Cells were washed three times with PBS-BSA, resuspended in 1.0 ml of PBS, and kept on ice until flow cytometric analysis was performed. As a negative control, similar samples were incubated only with the secondary FITC-conjugated antibody and used to determine the threshold of specific staining. Flow cytometric analysis was performed using the Epics ELITE flow cytometer (Coulter Electronics, Hileah, FL.). FITC-stained cells were excited by using 15 mW of 488 nm argon laser light. Calibration beads were run and the mean fluorescent intensity was set at a fixed value, which was maintained throughout the experiment.

3.6. STa Iodination

HPLC-purified STa was radioiodinated in a reaction mixture that contained the following: STa, 100 µg; 0.2 M sodium phosphate (pH 7.2), 45 µl; one Iodo-bead® (Pierce, Rockford, IL); Na-^{125}I (NEN, Boston, MA), 1.0 mCi; and 2% D-glucose, 25 µl. After 15 minutes incubation at room temperature, radiolabeled STa (^{125}I-STa) was separated from free iodine using a Sep-Pack C-18 cartridge column (Waters Associates, Milford, MA). The column was pre-washed with 10 ml 100% methanol and equilibrated with 10 ml distilled water. Stepwise elution of the ^{125}I-STa was performed with (i) 10 ml of 0.1% trifluoroacetic acid (TFA) in 30% methanol (HPLC grade), (ii) 10 ml of 0.1% TFA in 60% methanol eluted, and (iii) 10 ml of 0.1% TFA in 100% methanol.

3.7. Binding Assay

Reaction mixtures containing isolated mice entrocytes (2×10^3), PBS-BSA and ^{125}I-STa (20–640 nM) were incubated in a final volume of 200 µl for 40 minute at 37°C in a shaking water bath. Unbound ^{125}I-STa was removed from bound ^{125}I-STa by vacuum filtration (Millipore Corp., Bedford, MA), using 1-µm, 2.5 cm GF/B glass filters (Whatman, Maidstone, England). Total binding was measured in a reaction mixture that did not contain the unlabeled STa, whereas nonspecific binding was measured in a reaction mixture that contained the labeled STa including 1000-fold excess of unlabeled STa. Specific binding was calculated by subtracting non-specific binding from the total binding. All experimental points were determined in duplicate. Specific binding data were used to calculate the apparent dissociation constants (K_d) and the maximum number of STa receptors (B_{max}) associated with enterocytes (Scatchard, 1949).

4. RESULTS

4.1. Indirect Immunofluorescence Assay

Indirect immunofluorescence study of enterocytes from STa-susceptible mice revealed the localization of intensely stained areas mostly at the brush border membrane region. Cryostat sections obtained from small intestine of 2-day-old suckling mice showed an intensely fluorescent brush border membrane after treatment with rabbit anti-STa and anti-rabbit-IgG-FITC-conjugated antibodies (Fig. 1). Some fluorescence was found in some focal areas inside the mucosa of the intestine. Fluorescence intensities were relatively low in the intestinal sections and enterocyte smears obtained from 1-week and 2-week-old mice when compared with that of the 2-day-old suckling mice suggesting that fluorescence intensity is inversely related to age.

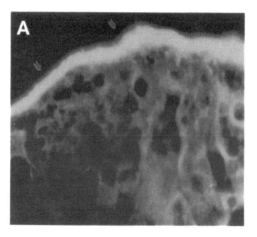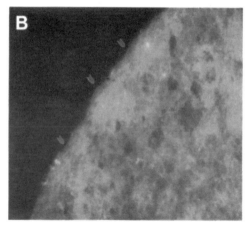

Figure 1. Immunofluorescence staining of STa toxin in cryostat sections of mice small intestine. A: 2-day-old suckling mouse intestinal section incubated with STa and anit-STa-Rabbit IgG serum and stained with FITC-conjugated anti-rabbit IgG antibodies; B: Control, 2-day-old suckling mouse intestinal section incubated only with STa and stained by FITC-conjugated anti-rabbit IgG antibodies. (×1000).

4.2. Flow Cytometry Analysis

The binding of STa to its putative receptor was studied using flow cytometric analysis. A histogram showing significantly increased fluorescence intensity was associated with the 2-day-old suckling mice enterocytes that were stained with rabbit anti-STa and anti-rabbit-IgG-FITC-conjugated antibodies. Only weak fluorescence was demonstrated in similarly prepared and processed samples from the 1-week and 2-week-old mice. No fluorescence was observed on processed enterocytes from any age groups when no STa was added. The staining results of freshly isolated enterocytes from different age groups of suckling mice are shown in Fig. 2.

4.3. Effect of ^{125}I-STa Concentration on Binding

Binding assays with enterocytes from each age group were performed to characterize the association of STa with its putative receptor on the enterocyte surface. The binding of ^{125}I-STa to enterocytes from each group of mice was saturable, and reached a plateau (Fig. 3). The specific binding of ^{125}I-STa to enterocytes from 2-day-old mice was about 2-fold higher than the specific binding of ^{125}I-STa to enterocytes obtained from 1-, 2-week, and 2-month old mice. Non-specific binding in the 2-day-old group enterocytes accounted for only 4–8% of total binding whereas non-specific binding for enterocytes from the 1-week, 2-week, and 2-month old mice accounted for 40–50% of the total binding.

4.4. Stoichiometry of ^{125}I-STa Binding to the Different Age Group of Mice Enterocytes

Scatchard analysis of specific binding data suggest the existence of a single class of STa receptors associated with enterocytes from different age groups. Calculation of dissociation constants (K_d) and maximum number of receptors (B_{max}) suggested higher

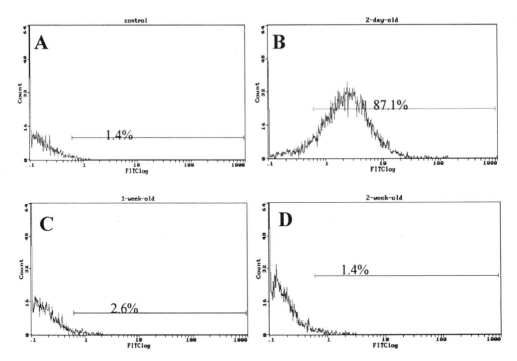

Figure 2. Representative flow cytometric histograms from different age groups of mice. A: control, no STa toxin was added; B: Enterocytes from 2-day-old mice; C: Enterocytes from 1-week-old mice; D: 2-week-old mice. Enterocytes where incubated with STa, rabbit anti-STa serum, and stained with anti-rabbit-IgG-FITC conjugated antibodies. Similar trends were obtained upon repeating the experiment.

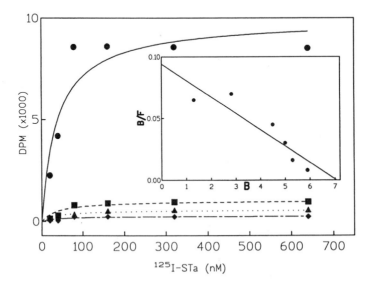

Figure 3. Specific binding of ^{125}I-STa to enterocytes obtained from different age groups of mice in the presence of increasing concentrations of ^{125}I-STa. ●——●, enterocytes from 2-day-old suckling mice; ■---■, enterocytes from 1-week-old suckling mice; ▲·····▲, enterocytes from 2-week-old mice; and ◆—·—◆, enterocytes from adult (2-month-old) mice. Nonspecific binding was determined in incubation mixtures containing ^{125}I-STa and a 1000-fold excess of unlabeled STa. Similar trends were obtained upon repeating the experiment. Inset represents Scatchard plot for the 2-day-old enterocytes. Scatchard plot analyses for the specific binding data of the different age groups are shown in Table 1.

Table 1. Binding properties of ^{125}I-STa to enterocytes from mice of different age groups[a]

Mouse age group	Specific binding (%)[b]	Dissociation constant (nM)	STa receptor density (nM/mg protein)
2-day-old	94	75	7.2
1-week-old	72	125	0.30
2-week-old	62	1430	0.36
2-month-old	60	1111	0.40

[a] Similar trends were obtained upon repeating the experiment.
[b] Each number represents the average of 6 readings.

affinity and receptor density for STa in the 2-day-old suckling mice enterocytes than in other age groups. STa-receptor density of the 2-day-old suckling mice was 20-fold higher than that of the 1-week, 2-week-, and 2-month-old mice (Table 1). The dissociation constant of STa receptor of enterocytes obtained from 2-day-old suckling mice (75 nM) was 10-fold lower than that obtained from 2-week and 2-month-old mice. The K_d of the 1-week-old suckling mice (125 nM) was 2-fold higher than that of the 2-day-old suckling mice. ^{125}I-STa binding properties are shown in Table 1.

5. DISCUSSION

The age-dependent resistance to diarrheal disease caused by enterotoxigenic *Escherichia coli* (ETEC) was first reported in pigs. Moon and Whipp (1970), found that some strains of ETEC cause secretory diarrhea only in neonatal pigs under two weeks old, whereas, other strains have the ability to cause diarrhea in neonatal and older pigs. Enterotoxins are among the most important virulence factor of ETEC and are considered the immediate mediator of diarrhea (Cohen et al., 1988; Sears and Kaper, 1996). High doses of STa were found to affect the secretory response in ligated intestinal loops, and addition of STb to STa-treated loops increased this secretory response. Although differences may exist in the sensitivity of neonatal and adult hosts to bacterial enterotoxins, little is known about changes of enterotoxin receptor affinity and density in the first weeks after birth.

In this study, the presence of STa receptors on enterocytes obtained from mice of different age groups was demonstrated using flow cytometry and indirect immunofluorescence assays. The absence of fluorescence in the control group, where no toxin was added, suggested a specific interaction between STa and its putative receptor. The significant increase in the fluorescence intensity in the 2-day-old suckling mice enterocytes, which were treated with STa, rabbit anti-STa, and anti-rabbit-IgG-FITC conjugated antibodies, must have been due to an increase in either the receptor number or the affinity of STa to these receptors (Fig. 3). Similar results were obtained using indirect immunofluorescence staining (Fig. 1). For further investigation of STa-receptor stoichiometry, ^{125}I-STa binding affinity to STa-receptors on the mice-enterocytes was performed. The ^{125}I-STa binding affinity data suggested that a significantly higher number of STa receptors was present on the enterocytes of the 2-day-old mice group than older mice (Fig. 3). The number of the STa receptors on the enterocytes of the 1-week, 2-week, and 2-month-old mice was significantly lower than that of the 2-day-old mice (Table 1). Unlike previous reports in pigs (Jaso-Friedmann et al., 1992), our data suggests an increase in the STa receptor affinity in the 2-day-old suckling mice (Table 1). This age-dependent affinity of STa receptors may be due to conformational or structural changes in the extracellular domain of the guanylate cyclase protein. Further investigation is needed to elucidate this age-dependent affinity. Binding of ^{125}I-STa to mice intestinal cells was shown to be rapid, specific, saturable, temperature dependent, and belongs to a single class of receptors. It is unclear why STa receptors exist in a larger number on enterocytes from neonatal animals. It is possible that the STa receptor functions as a receptor for growth promoting peptide(s) and that an increased number of receptors for this peptide would be needed in the intestine of the neonate. It is noteworthy that, recently, we studied the effect of dietary insulin on the response of suckling mice enterocytes to STa. Insulin was found to up-regulate this response (Al-Majali et al., 1998). It is likely that multiple factors contribute to the increased susceptibility of newborn animals to ETEC. This predilection might be variably expressed on the basis of permissive host factors, including brush border membrane changes that may be induced by dietary antigens, stress, or by environmental factors. The high susceptibility to ETEC might be augmented or more fully expressed in response to host or environmental factors. In addition, this report describes the use of flow cytometry to study the interaction of STa with its putative receptor. Conventional fluorescent microscopy analysis results only in inaccurate estimates of fluorescence intensity due to the scoring protocol used (++++; for high fluorescent intensity, +; for relatively low fluorescent intensity). Using flow cytometry, studying the STa/receptor interaction was possible through accurate determination of the intensity of fluorescence on enterocytes of the different age groups of suckling mice. In summary, we have demonstrated using indirect flow cytometry, immunofluorescence, and ^{125}I-STa binding assays that, in suckling mice, STa-receptor numbers and affinity are age-dependent. STa-receptor numbers and affinity were higher in the 2-day-old mice suckling mice than older mice. These results may further explain the increased susceptibility of immature and young animals to STa-mediated diarrheal disease. This model will be utilized in future studies for further investigations of the mechanism of STa-mediated diarrheal disease in humans and animals.

REFERENCES

Al-Majali, A., Asem, E., Lamar, C., Robinson, J.P., Freeman, M.J., and Saeed, A.M., 1998, Effect of dietary insulin on the response of suckling mice enterocytes to *Escherichia coli* heat-stable enterotoxin, Vet. Res. 29 (In Press).

Butler, D.G. and Clarke, R.C., 1994, Diarrhea and dysentery in calves, In: *Escherichia coli* in domestic animals and humans, Editor: Gyles, C.L., CAB International, Walingford, UK, pp. 91–116.

Cohen, M.B., Guarino, A., Shukla, R., and Giannella, R.A., 1988, Age-related differences in receptors for the *Escherichia coli* heat-stable enterotoxin in the small and large intestine of children, Gastroenterology 94:367–373.

Cohen, M.B., Moyer, M.S., Luttrell, M., and Giannella, R.A., 1986, The immature rat small intestine exhibits an increased sensitivity and response to *Escherichia coli* heat-stable enterotoxin, Pediatr. Res. 20:555–560.

Dreyfus, L.A., Jaso-Friedmann, L., and Robertson, D.C., 1984, Characterization of the mechanism of action of *Escherichia coli* heat-stable enterotoxin, Infect. Immun. 44:493–501.

Giannella, R.A., Luttrell, M., and Thompson, M.R., 1983, Binding of *Escherichia coli* heat-stable enterotoxin to receptors on rat intestinal cells, Am. J. Physiol. 245:G492–G498.

Guandalini, S., Rao, M.C., Smith, P.L., and Field, M., 1982, cGMP modulation of ileal ion transport: invitro effects of *Escherichia coli* heat-stable entrotoxin, Am. J. Physiol. 243:G36–G41.

Guerrant, R.L., Hughes, J.M., Chang, B., Robertson, D.C., and Murad, F., 1980, Activation of intestinal Guanylate cyclase by heat-stable enetrotoxin of *Escherichia coli*: studies of tisuue specificity, potential receptors, and intermediates. J. Infect. Dis. 142:220–228.

Jaso-Friedmann, L., Dreyfus, L.A., Whipp, S.C., and Robertson, D.C., 1992, Effects of age on activation of procine intestinal guanylate cyclase and binding of *Escherichia coli* heat-stable enterotoxin (STa) to procine intestinal cells and brush border membrane. Am. J. Vet. Res. 53:2251–2258.

Moon, H.W. and Whipp, S.C., 1970, Development of resistance with age by swine intestine to effect of enterotoxigenic *Escherichia coli*. J. Infect. Dis. 122:220–223.

Rao, M.C., Orellana, S.A., Field, M., Robertson, D.C., and Giannella, R.A., 1981, Comparsion of the biological actions of three purified heat-stable enterotoxin: effect on ion transport and guanylate cyclase activity in rabbit ileum in vitro, Infect. Immun. 33:165–170.

Sack, R.B., 1980, Enterotoxigenic *Escherichia coli*: identification and characterization, J. Infect. Dis. 142:279–286.

Saeed, A.M. and Greenberg, R.N., 1985, Preparative Purification of *Escherichia coli* heat-stable enterotoxin, Analyt. Biochem. 151:431–437.

Saeed, A.M., McMillian, R., Huckelberry, V., Abernathy, R., and Greenberg, R.N., 1987, Specific receptor for *Escherichia coli* heat-stable enterotoxin (STa) may determine susceptibility of piglets to diarrheal disease, FEMS Microbiol. lett. 43:247–251.

Scatchard, G., 1949, The attractions of proteins for small molecules and ions. Ann. NY. Acad. Sci. 51:660–672.

Schulz, S., Green, C.K., Yuen, P.S., and Garbers, D.L., 1990, Guanylyl cyclase is a heat-stabe enterotoxin receptor, Cell 63:941–948.

Sears, C.L. and Kaper, J.B., 1996, Enteric bacterial toxins: Mechanisms of action and linkage to intestinal secretion, Microbiol. Rev. 60:167–215.

Staples, S.J., Asher, S.E., and Giannella, R.A., 1980, Purification and characteristics of heat-stable enterotoxin produced by a strain of E. coli pathogenic for man, J. Biol. Chem. 255:4716–4721.

Stevens, J.B., Gyles, G.A., and Barnum, D.A., 1971, Production of diarrhea in pigs in response to *Escherichia coli* enterotoxin, Am. J. Vet. Res. 33:220–223.

Vaandrager, A.B., Schulz, S., De Jonge, H.R., and Garders, D.L., 1993, Guanylyl cyclase C is an *N*-linked Glycoprotein receptor that accounts for multiple heat-stable enterotoxin binding proteins in the intestine. J. Biol. Chem. 268:2174–2179.

Wada, A., Hirayama, T., Kitao, S., Fujisawa, J., Hidaka, Y., and Shimonishi, Y., 1994, Pig intestinal membrane-bound receptor (guanylyl cyclase) for heat-stable enterotoxin: cDNA cloning, functional expression, and characterization. Microbiol. Immunol. 38:535–541.

13

K88 ADHESINS OF ENTEROTOXIGENIC *ESCHERICHIA COLI* AND THEIR PORCINE ENTEROCYTE RECEPTORS

David H. Francis, Alan K. Erickson, and Philippe A. Grange

The Department of Veterinary Science
South Dakota State University
Brookings, South Dakota
U.S.A., 57007-1396

1. SUMMARY

The three antigenic variants of the K88 fimbrial adhesin (K88ab, K88ac, and K88ad) of enterotoxigenic *Escherichia coli* (ETEC) each exhibit unique specificity with regard to their hemagglutination characteristics. The variants are also unique in the specificity of their binding to the brush borders of enterocytes isolated from pigs with different genetic backgrounds. Diversity in enterocyte binding specificity suggests the existence of several K88 receptors, expressed individually or in various combinations on porcine enterocytes. Three candidate receptors have been identified that may explain the adhesion of K88 fimbrial variants to various porcine enterocytes. These receptors are an intestinal mucin-type sialoglycoprotein (IMTGP), an intestinal transferrin (GP74), and an intestinal neutral glycosphingolipid (IGLad). The IMTGP binds K88ab and K88ac, but not K88ad. The GP74 binds K88ab, but not K88ac or K88ad, and the IGLad binds K88ad, but not K88ab or K88ac. Each of the candidate receptors has been found in brush borders that are adhesive for the fimbriae that bind the respective receptor. They have not been found in brush borders that are not adhesive for those same fimbriae. The presence of IMTGP was highly correlated with susceptibility of neonatal gnotobiotic pigs to ETEC expressing K88ab or K88ac.

2. INTRODUCTION

Enterotoxigenic *Escherichia coli* (ETEC) is a major cause of diarrhea and death in neonatal and newly weaned pigs (Wilson and Francis, 1988; Moon and Bunn, 1993).

Mechanisms in the Pathogenesis of Enteric Diseases 2, edited by Paul and Francis.
Kluwer Academic / Plenum Publishers, New York, 1999.

Strains that produce the K88 (F4) fimbriae account for about half of ETEC infections in pigs (Moon and Bunn, 1993). The fimbriae bind to enterocyte brush borders, mediating bacterial colonization and facilitating the production of diarrhea by allowing elaboration of bacterial enterotoxins in close proximity to the epithelial cell membrane. As an early event in the colonization of the small intestine by ETEC, fimbrial attachment to receptors on enterocyte brush borders is a critical juncture in the pathogenesis of colibacillosis. If the animal is to prevent the development of disease, it will be by interdicting this event. This may be done through innate resistance, which is exhibited as failure to express the receptors to which K88 fimbriae bind, or through acquired immunity, which is exhibited in the production of antibodies that block the binding of K88 fimbriae to their receptors on enterocyte brush borders. The importance of the fimbrial adhesin/enterocyte receptor interaction to the outcome of infection makes study of this interaction essential to an understanding of pathogenesis of diarrhea caused ETEC.

The historical importance of K88[+] ETEC as a swine pathogen is underscored by evidence of a coevolutionary relationship between development of fimbrial variants and receptors to which they bind on porcine enterocytes. The benefit of disease resistance appears to have driven selection for K88 receptor modification in the pig population. Such selection by the host appears to have resulted in selection for modified adhesion specificity by the pathogen to exploit the host population made resistant by selection for receptor modification. Selection for structural modification by both the host and the pathogen has ultimately resulted in diversity in both fimbrial adhesins and K88 receptors.

There are three antigenic variants of K88 fimbriae: K88ab, K88ac, and K88ad (Mooi and de Graaf, 1978; Guinee and Jansen, 1979; Gaastra and Amstru-Pedersen, 1986). The structural genes for the fimbriae have been sequenced. Differences in sequence are confined to the gene encoding the major fimbrial protein subunit, *FaeG*, indicating that antigenic diversity is the result of mutational changes in this gene (Bakker et al., 1992; Foged et al., 1986; Gaastra et al., 1981; Gaastra et al., 1983; Josephsen et al., 1984). The Fab fragments of monoclonal antibodies to variant-specific epitopes of K88 adhesins block fimbrial adhesion to receptor-containing porcine enterocytes, whereas Fab fragments of monoclonal antibodies to conserved epitopes do not block fimbrial adhesin binding to receptor-containing porcine enterocytes (Talib, 1994; Sun et al., 1997). These observations strongly suggest a relationship between antigenic diversification and receptor selection.

3. K88 ADHESIN PHENOTYPES AMONG PIGS

Existence of phenotypic diversity in pigs with regard to susceptibility and resistance to K88[+] ETEC was first reported nearly 25 years ago by Rutter, Sellwood and their colleagues (Rutter et al., 1975; Sellwood et al., 1975). These investigators demonstrated that bacteria expressing K88 fimbriae bound to isolated enterocytes of some, but not all pigs. The ability for piglet enterocytes to support adherence of K88[+] *E. coli* was found to be inherited in a simple Mendelian fashion as a dominant trait. Further, fimbrial binding was found to correlate with susceptibility of pigs to K88[+] *E. coli* infection. Thus, susceptibility to enterotoxigenic colibacillosis caused by K88[+] *E. coli* was shown to be an inherited characteristic. Using the *in vitro* brush border adherence assay reported by Sellwood et al. (1975) and utilizing *E. coli* expressing each of the three K88

Table 1. Number (%) of animals of each adhesion phenotype among neonatal and weanling (3–5 week-old) pigs

Age Group	No. Pigs	A	B	C	D	E	F
Neonate	46	25 (54)	0 (0)	2 (4)	19 (41)	0 (0)	0 (0)
Weanling[a]	96	41 (43)	5 (5)	6 (6)	11 (11)	27 (28)	6 (6)

[a]from Baker et al., 1997.

antigenic variants, other investigators later identified as many as 5 phenotypes of pigs relative to patterns of K88 fimbrial adhesion to enterocyte brush borders (Bijlsma et al., 1982; Rapacz and Hasler-Rapacz, 1986). These adhesion patterns were designated by Bijlsma et al. (1982) as: A (binds K88ab, K88ac, and K88ad); B (binds K88ab and K88ac); C (binds K88ab and K88ad); D (binds K88ad) and E (binds no K88 variant fimbriae). These phenotypic characterization studies were done by investigators examining only one herd of pigs in each case. We extended these studies by examining 3 to 5 week-old pigs from many herds and 4 pure breeds for a much wider genetic base (Baker et al., 1997). In so doing, we identified one additional phenotype (F, binds K88ab only) and determined the prevalence of pigs of each phenotype. We found that nearly one-half of the pigs examined (45%) produced brush borders that bound all three K88 variants, almost 20% produced brush borders that bound no K88 variants, and the remainder of pigs produced brush borders that bound one, or two, but not all K88 variants (Table 1). In subsequent studies using pigs less than one week old from several herds, we identified only three phenotypes among 46 pigs: A, C and D (Francis, personal observations, Table 1). The differences in phenotypes observed in neonatal and 3–5 week old pigs suggests that the phenotypes of some pigs may change as the pigs get older. This assumption is supported by the work of Hu et al. (1993), who reported that the binding of K88ad to brush borders of pigs of the D phenotype ceased by about 16 weeks of age. While K88ad binding is clearly not lost in all pigs with age, it appears to be extinguished in some pigs as they mature. If ability to bind K88ad is lost from brush borders, pigs of phenotype A would become phenotype B, pigs of phenotype C would become phenotype F, and pigs of phenotype D would become phenotype E. These changes occurring in some, but not all pigs would explain the emergence of 6 phenotypes as pigs mature.

4. K88 RECEPTORS ON PORCINE ENTEROCYTES

Our interest in the identification and characterization of the K88 adhesion phenotypes of pigs stemmed from the widely held assumption that correlation made by Rutter et al. (1975) between brush border binding, and piglet susceptibility to ETEC would hold for all pig phenotypes and all K88 variant fimbriae. Identification of the resistance factor(s), and the gene(s) encoding it (them) would make possible, the identification and selective breeding of pigs that are resistant to K88+ ETEC-induced disease.

Presence of diversity among pigs with regard to K88 fimbrial binding has facilitated our efforts to identify porcine K88 adhesin receptors. In attempting to identify these receptors, we have assumed that differences in adhesiveness of intestinal brush borders from pigs of each of the 6 K88 variant binding phenotypes are due to the presence of K88 variant receptors on those brush borders. Further, we have assumed that individual or combinations of receptors to which one or more K88 variants bind define the adhesive properties of the phenotype. We have used the following criteria as a guide in the identification of candidate receptors for K88 fimbriae of porcine brush borders: 1) The receptor must display specificity for the particular K88 fimbrial adhesin variant; 2) The receptor must be detectable exclusively in brush borders phenotyped as adhesive for that particular K88 fimbrial adhesin variant; and 3) The receptor must be expressed in multiple animals of the same adhesive phenotype (Billey et al., 1998).

While many research groups have identified brush border, or mucin molecules that bind one or more of the K88 variants, we are only aware of three candidate K88 receptors that fulfill the criteria established above. These candidate receptors in chronological order of their identity are intestinal mucin-type sialoglycoproteins (IMTGPs; Erickson et al., 1992), an intestinal transferrin (GP74; Grange and Mouricout, 1996), and an intestinal neutral glycosphingolipid (IGLad; Grange et al., 1999). The IMTGPs bind K88ab and K88ac, but not K88ad (Billey et al., 1998). They typically appear in Western blots of sodium dodecyl sulfate polyacrylamide electrophoretic gels (SDS-PAGE) as broad bands with molecular masses in the range of 210 to 230 kDa (IMTGP-1), and 240 to 300 kDa (IMTGP-2), respectively (Erickson et al., 1992). These two K88 adhesin receptors have similar amino acid compositions, reactivities with lectins, elution characteristics by gel filtration and hydroxyapatite chromatography, and susceptibility to neuraminidase (Erickson et al., 1994; Grange et al., 1998). The IMTGPs have been found in brush borders from many, but not all pigs whose enterocytes exhibit phenotypic adhesin binding pattern A and all pigs whose enterocytes exhibit phenotypic adhesin binding pattern B (Billey et al., 1998). Carbohydrate structural analysis of IMTGPs indicated that the receptors contain the sugars Gal, Glc, Man, Fuc, GalNAc, GlcNAc, and NeuAc (Grange et al., 1998). Treatment of IMTGPs with the neuraminidase which removes terminal sialic acid residues had no effect on K88ac adhesin binding, but caused an upshift in the position of IMTGP bands in Western bolts of SDS-PAGE gels. Treatment of IMTGPs with β-galactosidase caused a similar effect. However, sequential treatment with neuraminidase and β-galactosidase decreased binding of K88ac to 11% of the control in ELISA tests and to extinction in Western blots. These results indicate that the receptors contain both sialic acid and β-linked galactosyl residues and that the presence of sialic acid residues prevents the removal of many of the galactose residues by β-galactosidase treatment. In addition, galactose residues that are exposed by treatment of IMTGPs with neuraminidase are essential in recognition of receptors by the K88ac adhesin (Grange et al., 1998).

Grange and Mouricout (1996) identified an enterocyte membrane associated isoform of transferrin that binds K88ab, but not K88ac or K88ad. This enterocyte transferrin (GP74) was found in brush borders exhibiting adhesion pattern A, but not in brush borders exhibiting adhesion pattern E. Its presence in brush borders from pigs of other adhesive phenotypes has not been determined. Carbohydrate composition analysis of GP74 indicated that it contains GlcNc, Man, Gal, NeuAc and Fuc.

An intestinal brush border neutral glycosphingolipid, which we have designated IGLad binds K88ad, but not K88ab or K88ac. Carbohydrate composition analysis of partially purified IGLad identified Gal, Glc, and GlcNAc, and GalNAc. Preliminary characterization experiments using lectins showed that IGLad contains the terminal glycanic structure, Galβ1-4GlcNAc. Removal of terminal β-linked galactose residues from IGLad decreased the recognition of IGLad by the K88ad adhesin, indicating that terminal β-linked galactose is an essential component of the K88ad adhesion recognition site of

Table 2. Carbohydrate composition of candidate K88 receptors

Receptor	Gal	GlcNAc	Glc	NeuAc	GalNAc	Man	Fuc
IMTGP-1[a]	39%	9%	4%	20%	18%	7%	4%
IMTGP-2[a]	26%	9%	24%	14%	7%	18%	2%
GP74[b]	23%	30%	0%	11%	0%	29%	7%
IGLad[c]	47%	16%	31%	0%	6%	0%	0%

[a] from Grange et al., 1998.
[b] from Grange and Mouricout, 1996.
[c] from Grange et al., 1999.

IGLad. Studies with purified glycosphingolipid standards demonstrated that K88ad adhesin binds to neolactotetraosylceramide (nLc$_4$Cer;Galβ1-4GlcNAcβ1-3Galβ-4Glcβ1-1Cer), lactotriosylceramide (Lc$_3$Cer; GlcNAcβ1-3Galβ1-4Glcβ1-1Cer) and lactototetraosylceramide (Lc$_4$Cer; Galβ1-3GlcNAcβ1-3Galβ1-4Glcβ1-Cer). Based on these observations, IGLad appears to be nLc$_4$Cer. IGLad has been found in brush borders exhibiting adhesion pattern A or D, but not in brush borders exhibiting adhesion pattern E (Grange et al., 1999).

Comparison of the carbohydrate compositions of IMTGP-1, IMTGP-2, GP74 and IGLad indicate that all contain Gal and GlcNAc, and that no other sugar is shared by all the candidate receptors (Table 2). This observation supports the assumption that Gal is critical in receptor recognition by K88 fimbriae. Unique characteristics of receptors that account for specificity differences in their recognition remain to be determined.

5. BIOLOGICAL RELEVANCE OF K88 RECEPTORS

The availability of piglets whose enterocytes express the candidate K88 receptors in various combinations has allowed us to test the biological relevance of identified K88 receptors. It has also enabled us to determine the significance of the piglet phenotypes identified by the binding of K88$^+$ ETEC to isolated enterocyte brush borders (Francis et al., 1998). Thirty-one neonatal gnotobiotic piglets were inoculated with either K88ab$^+$, or K88ac$^+$ ETEC and observed for clinical signs of disease, including diarrhea, dehydration, anorexia, and lethargy. Animals were euthanized when they became moribund. Thirteen of the pigs developed severe diarrhea, became dehydrated and died, or became moribund. Another pig became severely lethargic, but not dehydrated. Of these 14 pigs that became severely ill, 12 expressed IMTGP. None of the 17 pigs that failed to become severely ill expressed IMTGP. Adherent bacteria were observed in multiple intestinal tissue sections from 11/12 piglets that expressed IMTGP, but in only one section from 1/19 piglets that did not express IMTGP. Bacteria concentrations were significantly higher in the intestines of pigs expressing IMTGP than in pigs not expressing that receptor (Table 3). These observations strongly suggest that IMTGP is a biological receptor for K88ab$^+$ and K88ac$^+$ ETEC.

Interestingly, of the 17 pigs that did not become severely ill and did not express IMTGP, 8 (47%) had brush borders that supported the adherence of large numbers (14 ± 4/brush border vesicle) of K88ab$^+$ and K88ac$^+$ *E. coli* (Francis et al., 1998). This suggests the existence of another receptor besides IMTGP that can bind K88ac (that receptor may also bind K88ab and K88ad; see Billey et al., 1998 for discussion). However,

Table 3. Indicators of illness or microbial colonization in IMTGP⁺ and IMTGP⁻ gnotobiotic piglets challenged with K88ab⁺, or K88ac⁺ ETEC[a]

Observation or Measure	IMTGP⁺ piglets (Phenotype A)	IMTGP⁻ piglets (Phenotype A, C, and D)
Severe dehydration and lethargy	12[b]/12	2/19
Adherent bacteria	11/12	1[c]/19
Bacteria/gram jejunum (Mean ± S.D.)	$1.1 \times 10^9 \pm 6.4 \times 10^8$	$4.7 \times 10^7 \pm 1.3 \times 10^{8\text{d}}$

[a] from Francis et al., 1998.
[b] one pig was lethargic, but not severely dehydrated.
[c] only one tissue section from one pig.
[d] significantly less that value for IMTGP⁺ pigs, $P = 8 \times 10^{-8}$, unpaired Student's T-Test.

that receptor does not appear to support colonization of ETEC. Therefore, it is not likely biologically relevant to disease. The poor correlation in this study between bacterial adherence to brush borders and manifestation of clinical illness suggests that the brush border adherence assay is not as good of an indicator of piglet susceptibility as previously presumed. It is of interest that Rutter et al. (1975) reported that 9% of the pigs in their study had brush borders that supported adherence of K88⁺ *E. coli*, but which were not susceptible to K88⁺ ETEC. Thus, even these early investigators observed imperfect correlation between brush border adherence of K88⁺ *E. coli* and piglet susceptibility.

We also conducted studies to determine whether expression of IGLad could be correlated with susceptibility to K88ad⁺ ETEC. While all pigs tested expressed IGLad, few if any developed severe diarrhea or became dehydrated (Francis, personal observations). Further, the concentration of bacteria in the small intestines of these pigs was considerably less that observed in IMTGP⁺ pigs challenged with K88ab⁺, or K88ac⁺ ETEC. Despite expression of similar virulence determinants (LT, STb, hemolysin), the K88ad⁺ ETEC was markedly less virulent than the K88ab⁺ and K88ac⁺ ETEC strains described above. This observation raises doubts regarding the biological relevance of the receptors recognized by K88ad, including IGLad. The size and length of a receptor may be critical to its function under natural conditions in the small intestine. The IMTGP is a large molecule whose protein backbone is made rigid by numerous N- and O-glycans. As a consequence of this configuration, it likely projects through the glycocalyx and is highly accessible to K88ab⁺, and K88ac⁺ *E. coli*. The IGLad is a much smaller molecule and does not project through the glycocalyx. Thus, it may not be readily accessible to K88ad⁺ *E. coli*. It is possible that IGLad only binds K88ad⁺ *E. coli* under in vitro conditions because much of the glycocalyx is removed from brush borders by shear forces during the grinding and washing required for their preparation. Because K88ad appears not to facilitate development of diarrheal disease, function of this K88 variant is uncertain. Perhaps the fimbria serves a purpose other than facilitating rapid proliferation of *E.* coli in the small intestines, such as enabling the bacterium to sustain permanent residence in the colon. The inability of K88ad⁺ ETEC to cause severe diarrhea in gnotobiotic pigs may explain why such organisms are so rarely identified in colibacillosis. Interestingly, ETEC expressing K88ab is also rarely identified in association with naturally occurring colibacillosis, yet such a strain was shown to be highly virulent to gnotobiotic pigs. The selective advantage of K88ac⁺ that allows ETEC that express it to overwhelmingly dominate over strains expressing the other K88 variants remains to be determined.

REFERENCES

Baker, D.R., Billey, L.O., and Francis, D.H., 1997, Distribution of K88 *Escherichia coli*-adhesive and nonadhesive phenotypes among pigs of four breeds, Vet. Microbiol. 54:123–132.

Bakker, D., Willemsen, P.T.J., Simons, L.H., van Zjderveld, F.G., and F.K. de Graaf, F.K., 1992, Characterization of the antigenic and adhesive properties of FaeG, the major subunit of K88 fimbriae, Mol. Microbiol. 6:247–255.

Bijlsma, I.G.W., de Nijs, A., van der Meer, C., and Frik, J.F., 1982, Different pig phenotypes affect adherence of *Escherichia coli* to jejunal brush borders by K88ab, K88ac, and K88ad antigen, Infect. Immun. 37:891–894.

Billey, L.O., Erickson, A.K., and Francis, D.H., 1998, Multiple receptors on porcine intestinal epithelial cells for the three variants of *Escherichia coli* K88 fimbrial adhesin, Vet. Microbiol. 59:203–212.

Erickson, A.K., Baker, D.R., Bosworth, B.T., Casey, T.A., Benfield, D.A., and Francis, D.H., 1994, Characterization of porcine intestinal epithelial receptors for the K88ac fimbrial adhesin of *Escherichia coli* as mucin-type sialoglycoproteins, Infect Immune 62:5404–5410.

Erickson, A.K., Willgohs, J.A., McFarland, S.Y., Benfield, D.A., and Francis, D.H., 1992, Identification of two porcine brush border glycoproteins that bind the K88ac adhesin of *Escherichia coli* and correlation of these binding glycoproteins with the adhesive porcine phenotype, Infect. Immun. 60:983–988.

Foged, N.T., Klemm, P., Elling, F., Jorsal, S.E., Zeuthen, J., 1986, Monoclonal antibodies to K88ab, K88ac, and K88ad fimbriae from enterotoxigenic *Escherichia coli*. Microb. Pathog. 1:57–69.

Francis, D.H., Grange, P.A., Zeman, D.H., Baker, D.R., Sun, R., and Erickson, A.K., 1998, Expression of mucin-type glycoprotein K88 receptors strongly correlates with piglet susceptibility to K88+ enterotoxigenic *Escherichia coli*, but adhesion of this bacterium to brush borders does not, Infect. Immun. 66:4050–4055.

Gaastra, W. and Amstru-Pedersen, P., 1986, Serologic variants of the K88 antigen, In: Protein-carbohydrate interactions in biological systems, Editors: Lark, D.L. and Normark, S., Academic Press Inc., London, UK, pp. 95–102.

Gaastra, W., Klemm, P., and de Graaf, F.K., 1983, The nucleotide sequence of the K88ad protein subunit of porcine enterotoxigenic *Escherichia coli*, FEMS Microbiol. Lett. 18:177–183.

Gaastra, W., Mooi, F.R., Stuitje, A.R., and de Graaf, F.K., 1981, The nucleotide sequence of the gene encoding the K88ab protein subunit of porcine enterotoxigenic *Escherichia coli*, FEMS Microbiol. Lett. 12:41–46.

Grange, P.A., Erickson, A.K., Anderson, T.J., and Francis, D.H., 1998, Characterization of the carbohydrate moiety of intestinal mucin-type sialoglycoprotein receptors for the K88ac adhesin of *Escherichia coli*, Infect. Immun. 66:1613–1621.

Grange, P.A., Erickson, A.K., Levery S.B., and Francis, D.H., 1999, Identification of an intestinal neutral glycosphingolipid as a phenotype-specific receptor for the K88ad fimbrial adhesion of *Escherichia coli*, Infect. and Immun. 67: In press.

Grange, P.A. and Mouricout, M.A., 1996, Transferrin associated with the porcine intestinal mucosal is a receptor specific for K88ab fimbriae of *Escherichia coli*, Infect. Immun. 64:606–610.

Guinee, P.A.M. and Jansen, W.H., 1979, Behavior of *Escherichia coli* K antigens K88ab, K88ac, and K88ad in immunoelectrophoresis, double diffusion, and hemagglutination, Infect. Immun. 23:700–705.

Hu, Z.L., Hasler-Rapacz, J., Huang S.C., and Rapacz, J., 1993. Studies in swine on inheritance and variation in expression of small intestinal receptors mediating adhesion of the K88 enteropathogenic *Escherichia coli* variants, J. Heredity 84:157–165.

Josephsen, J., Hansen, F., de Graaf, F.K., and Gaastra, W., 1984, The nucleotide sequence of the K88ac fimbriae of porcine enterotoxigenic *Escherichia coli*. FEMS Microbiol. Lett. 25:301–306.

Mooi, F.R. and de Graaf, FK., 1978, Isolation and characterization of K88 antigen, FEMS Microbiol. Lett. 5:17–20.

Mooi, F.R. and de Graaf, F.K., 1985, Molecular biology of fimbriae of enterotoxigenic *Escherichia coli*, Curr. Top. Microbiol. Immunol. 118:119–138.

Moon, H.W. and Bunn, T.O., 1993, Vaccines for preventing enterotoxigenic *Escherichia coli* infections in farm animals. Vaccine, 11:213–220.

Rapacz, J. and Hasler-Rapacz, J., 1986, Polymorphism and inheritance of swine small intestinal receptors mediating adhesion of three serological variants of *Escherichia coli*-producing K88 pilus antigen, Animal Genetics 17:305–321.

Rutter, J.M., Burrows M.R., Sellwood R., and Gibbons R.A., 1975, A genetic basis for resistance to enteric disease caused by *E. coli*, Nature (London) 257:135–136.

Sellwood, R., Gibbons, R.A., Jones, G.W., and Rutter, J.M., 1975, Adhesion of enteropathogenic *Escherichia coli* to pig intestinal brush borders: The existence of two pig phenotypes. J. Med. Microbiol. 8:405–411.

Sun, R., Anderson, T.J., Erickson, A.K., and Francis, D.H., 1997, The variable domains of *Escherichia coli* K88ac fimbriae are involved in receptor binding, Abstract, Conf. Research Workers in Animal Diseases, Chicago, IL.

Talib, S.M., 1994, Role of conserved and variable domains of *Escherichia coli* K88 adhesins in porcine colibacillosis, Masters Thesis, South Dakota State University.

Wilson, R.A. and Francis, D.H., 1986, Fimbriae and enterotoxins associated with *E. coli* serotypes isolated from clinical cases of porcine colibacillosis, Am. J. Vet. Res. 47:213–217.

14

EDEMA DISEASE AS A MODEL FOR SYSTEMIC DISEASE INDUCED BY SHIGA TOXIN-PRODUCING *E. COLI*

Nancy A. Cornick,[1] Ilze Matise,[1] James E. Samuel,[2] Brad T. Bosworth,[3#] and Harley W. Moon[1]

Veterinary Medical Research Institute
Iowa State University, Ames, Iowa[1]
Department Medical Microbiology and Immunology
College of Medicine
Texas A&M University
College Station, Texas[2]
and Enteric Diseases and Food Safety Research Unit
National Animal Disease Center
USDA-ARS, Ames, Iowa[3]

1. SUMMARY

Edema disease (ED) is a naturally occurring disease of weaned pigs caused by host adapted strains of *E. coli* that produce Shiga toxin (STEC). We determined the temporal and quantitative relationships between intestinal colonization by STEC, levels of Shiga toxin (Stx2e) in the gut, in the blood, and clinical manifestations of ED. Bacterial colonization (10^8 CFU/cm ileum) was highest 4 days post inoculation (pi) in animals that did not develop clinical disease and 6 days pi in animals with clinical signs of ED. The mean time for the development of clinical signs of ED was 6 days pi (range 4–10). Average peak titers of Stx2e in the ileum were 1:16,384 in asymptomatic animals and 1:32,768 in clinical animals. Titers of Stx2e in the feces reflected the toxin titers in the ileum but were lower. Intestinal titers of Stx2e and the density of bacterial colonization were predictive of clinical ED for a group of animals but not for individuals. Approximately 50% of the pigs that had Stx2e titers of $\geq$1:4096 and a bacterial density

---

[#] Present address: Pig Improvement Company, Franklin, KY

Mechanisms in the Pathogenesis of Enteric Diseases 2, edited by Paul and Francis.
Kluwer Academic / Plenum Publishers, New York, 1999.

of $\geq 10^6$ CFU/cm in their ileum, had clinical ED. Pigs that had intestinal Stx2e titers <1 : 4096 were asymptomatic. Stx2e was detected in the red cell fraction of blood from some of the pigs with clinical ED and in some that were asymptomatic. Stx2e was not detected in the serum of any animals. ED may be a useful model for predicting the temporal and quantitative relationships between bacterial colonization, Stx levels in the gut and blood and systemic disease for STEC in other species.

2. INTRODUCTION

Shiga toxin-producing *E. coli* (STEC) cause gastrointestinal disease in people. In the majority of patients the symptoms last several days to a week and then resolve. However, some 5–10% of patients (particularly children and elderly) develop a systemic disease known as hemolytic uremic syndrome (HUS) (Griffin et al., 1988; Tarr, 1995). A minority of patients with HUS also have neurologic sequelae (Tarr, 1995). The majority of epidemic outbreaks of STEC in the United States are caused by *E. coli* O157:H7. However, many serotypes of STEC have been associated with sporadic outbreaks of disease both in the United States and worldwide (Bonnet et al., 1998; Huppertz et al., 1996; Paton et al., 1996; Tarr and Neill, 1996; USDHHS, 1995). Shiga toxin and intimin, an outer membrane protein, are two of the known virulence factors produced by STEC. Many strains of *E. coli* O157:H7 also have a large plasmid. However, neither the plasmid or intimin are required by all strains for virulence (de Azavedo et al., 1994; Dytoc et al., 1994; Willshaw et al., 1992).

Edema disease is a disease that occurs in post weaning pigs and is caused by host adapted strains of STEC (Smith and Halls, 1968). These *E. coli* produce a variant of Shiga toxin, Stx2e and adhere to the porcine small intestine by F18 fimbriae (Bertschinger et al., 1990; Marques et al., 1987). There are both subclinical (asymptomatic) and clinical manifestations of the disease. Pigs with subclinical disease often have necrosis in the arterioles of the intestinal tract and brain and a decreased weight gain (Kausche et al., 1992). The hallmarks of clinical disease are neurologic impairment, sudden death and gross edema of the eyelids, intestinal tract and mesentery and microscopic arteriolar necrosis (Bertschinger and Gyles, 1994; Smith and Halls, 1968). Edema disease is an attractive model to study STEC induced disease for several reasons. First, it is a naturally occurring STEC disease of pigs that primarily effects young animals. Second, there is generally a prodromal phase of diarrhea, although in edema disease this is caused by a heat stable enterotoxin. Thirdly, the neurologic signs of clinical edema disease are caused by systemic toxemia (MacLeod et al., 1991), which is also thought to occur in human patients prior to the appearance of HUS (Tarr, 1995). While much is known regarding the pathogensis of STEC disease, little is known about the dynamics of bacterial growth and toxin production during STEC infection. In this study we determined the temporal and quantitative relationships between initial STEC exposure and: the colonization of the intestinal tract, the appearance of toxin in the intestinal tract and feces, the appearance of Shiga toxin in the blood and the onset of clinical signs.

3. EXPERIMENTAL DESIGN

3.1. Primary Study

Fifty 3 week-old pigs were orally inoculated with 10^{10} CFU of *E. coli* strain S1191 which produces Stx2e, heat stable enterotoxin STb and F18 fimbriae (Bertschinger et al., 1990). Control pigs were inoculated with a nonpathogenic strain of *E. coli.* Pigs were euthanized when advanced neurologic signs of edema disease were apparent. In addition, randomly selected, asymptomatic principals were necropsied at intervals post inoculation (pi). Blood was drawn just prior to euthanasia to test for the presence of Stx2e. At necropsy sections of ileum and colon were collected for bacteriologic counts and ileal, rectal and colonic contents were collected for toxin assay. Individual fecal samples were collected from all of the principals on days 1–10 and assayed for Stx2e. All of the positive blood samples and at least one positive intestinal sample from each animal were neutralized using bovine polyclonal antibody to Stx2 (Tesh et al., 1993).

3.2. Secondary Study

In another set of experiments 20 principals and 9 controls were challenged and observed as described above. Blood samples were collected at the onset of clinical signs to monitor Shiga toxemia. In addition, 10/20 principals were bled on days 3 and 7 pi.

4. RESULTS

4.1. Primary Study

Nine of the principal pigs exhibited clinical signs of edema disease including neurological disturbances, ataxia, or became moribund and were euthanized. Sudden death occurred in an additional 7 pigs. The onset of clinical signs ranged from 4–10 days pi with the majority of pigs (14/16) exhibiting clinical disease on days 5–7 pi. The 34 remaining principals were asymptomatic throughout the study. None of the control pigs showed any signs of edema disease or died.

In randomly selected, asymptomatic principals bacterial colonization of the ileum peaked on day 4 pi with a mean value of 1.6×10^8 CFU/cm (Fig. 1). The peak ileal colonization of pigs with clinical edema disease occurred on day 6 pi. The peak bacterial count of these pigs was 2.4×10^8 CFU/cm. Titers of Shiga toxin in the ileal content paralleled the bacterial colonization and peaked at 1:16,384 (day 4) and 1:32,768 (day 6) for asymptomatic and clinical pigs, respectively. Shiga toxin was not detected in the ileal content of control pigs.

Shiga toxin was detected in the feces of each of the principal pigs by day 1 pi (Fig. 2). Fecal titers of Shiga toxin reflected the toxin titers in the ileum but tended to be lower. The mean fecal toxin titer of pigs with clinical edema disease was significantly higher than that of asymptomatic principals ($p < 0.05$). The fecal toxin titers of individual pigs varied widely in both clinical and asymptomatic principals, and were not predictive for the development of clinical edema disease in individual animals (Table 1). For example, pig 727 had fecal titers of Shiga toxin of 1:131,072 for several days and did not ever show signs of clinical edema disease. In contrast, pig 625 had a fecal toxin titer of 1:4096 on day 5 pi and presented with clinical edema disease on day 7 pi. Fecal toxin titers were predictive for a group of animals at a high risk for developing clinical disease. Indeed, 16/34 animals (47%) that had peak fecal toxin titers of ≥1:4096 developed clinical disease. None of the animals that had peak fecal toxin titers of <1:4096 showed signs of clinical edema disease. Shiga toxin was not detected in the feces of the control pigs.

Shiga toxin was detected in the red blood cell fraction of 5/7 pigs with clinical

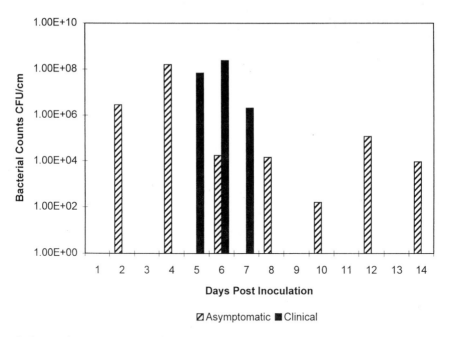

Figure 1. Geometric mean colony forming units of strain S1191 in the ileum of randomly selected asymptomatic principals (n = 3 pigs/day on days 2–10 and 2 pigs/day on days 12–14) and clinical principals (n = 3 pigs/day).

edema disease. The mean toxin titer in the blood of these 5 animals was 1:64. Toxin was not detected in the blood of 18 asymptomatic principals or from controls. Shiga toxin was also not detected in the serum of any animals tested.

4.2. Secondary Study

Eight of 20 principals developed clinical edema disease. Shiga toxin was detected in the red blood cell fraction from 5/8 of these. The mean toxin titer from these 5 clinical pigs was 1:74. Two asymptomatic pigs also had detectable Stx in their blood. Of these two, one became moribund a day later but the other pig remained asymptomatic throughout the study. This pig had a toxin titer of 1:32.

5. DISCUSSION

Our data indicated that fecal titers of Shiga toxin were reflective of intestinal toxin titers and were predictive of clinical disease for a population of pigs (Fig. 2), but not for individual animals (Table 1). Fecal toxin titers identified a group of pigs at high risk for developing clinical edema disease. Approximately 50% of the pigs that had peak fecal toxin titers of ≥1:4096 had clinical disease. If these data are reflective of human disease caused by STEC, then monitoring fecal levels of Shiga toxin may be of prognostic value. Past studies have not indicated a prognostic value for free Stx in the feces, however, many of these samples were collected late in the course of the infection and sequential samples were not obtained (Karmali et al., 1985; Ramotar et al., 1995). Early

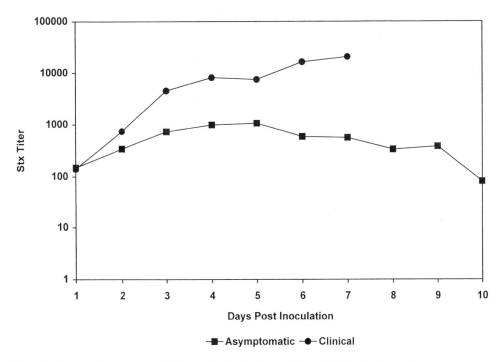

Figure 2. Geometric mean titer of Shiga toxin in the feces of pigs with clinical edema disease and asymptomatic principals.

fecal samples greatly increase the probability of recovering *E. coli* O157:H7 (Griffin et al., 1988; Spika et al., 1986; Tarr et al., 1990; Wells et al., 1983). Our data also indicate that the numbers of STEC colonizing the intestinal tract decrease several orders of magnitude after the first few days of infection (Fig. 1).

To our knowledge this is the first report of Stx2e being detected in the blood of pigs with clinical edema disease. This is further evidence that toxin is delivered from the gut to the site of systemic tissue damage by the blood (Boyd et al., 1993; Marques et al., 1987; Waddell and Gyles, 1995). Our ability to detect Stx2e from red blood cells and not from serum is supported by reports of both in vitro (Waddell et al., 1998) and in vivo (Boyd et al., 1993) binding of Stx2e to pig erythrocytes. Vero cell toxicity has been reported from the serum of gnotobiotic pigs infected with strains of

Table 1. Fecal titers of Shiga toxin from selected pigs following inoculation with strain S1191

Pig	Status	Days Post Inoculation									
		1	2	3	4	5	6	7	8	9	10
727	Asymptomatic	NT[a]	128	131,072	8,192	65,536	131,072	131,072	32,768	8192	128
629	Asymptomatic	256	4096	2,048	4,096	32,768	16,384	16,384	1,024	NT	NT
74	Asymptomatic	256	128	128	512	2,048	128	128	128	64	NT
625	Clinical	128	64	512	1,024	4,096	512	1,024[b]			
62	Clinical	64	4096	4,096	8,192[b]						
720	Clinical	128	128	131,072	131,072	32,768	65,536[b]				

[a] Not tested.
[b] Died or euthanized with clinical edema disease.

enterohemorrhagic *E. coli* (Tzipori et al., 1987; Tzipori et al., 1988). Detectable Stx was also reported from the concentrated serum of mice infected with STEC (Kurioka et al., 1998). Our detection of Stx in the blood of an asymptomatic principal implies that systemic toxemia is not always fatal and suggests that host susceptibility may play an important role in moderating the effects of systemic toxemia. None of the pigs in this study had detectable neutralizing antibody to Stx2e prior to challenge. In our experience, pigs with edema disease (both clinical and asymptomatic) seldom develop neutralizing antibody to Stx2e (Bosworth et al., 1996; Gordon et al., 1992; Kausche et al., 1992).

This study demonstrated that fecal titers of Shiga toxin reflected intestinal toxin levels and could be used to define a group of animals that were at an increased risk of developing clinical edema disease. However, fecal toxin titers could not be used to predict the development of systemic disease for individual animals. The correlation of clinical disease and detectable Shiga toxin in the peripheral blood documents the occurrence of systemic toxemia in the pathogensis of STEC disease. Edema disease may be a useful model to study other diseases induced by intestinal infection with STEC and systemic toxemia.

ACKNOWLEDGMENTS

We thank Sheridan Booher, Sophia Franck, Matthew Mettenberg, and Dawn Wiarda for technical support. This work was supported by NIH grant AI41328 and the Frank K. Ramsey endowment.

REFERENCES

Bertschinger, H.U., Bachmann, M., Mettler, C., Pospischil, A., Schraner, E.M., Stamm, M., Sydler, T., and Wild, P. 1990. Adhesive fimbriae produced in vivo by *Escherichia coli* O139:K12(B):H1 associated with enterotoxaemia in pigs. Vet. Microbiol. 25:267–281.

Bertschinger, H.U. and Gyles, C.L. 1994. Oedema disease of pigs. In: *Escherichia coli* in Domestic Animals and Humans, Editor: Gyles, C., Wallingford, CAB International, pp. 193–220.

Bonnet, R., Souweine, B., Gauthier, G., Rich, C., Livrelli, V., Sirot, J., Joly, B., and Forestier, C. 1998. Non-O157:H7 Stx2-producing *Escherichia coli* strains associated with sporadic cases of hemolytic uremic syndrome in adults. J. Clin. Microbiol. 36:1777–1780.

Bosworth, B.T., Samuel, J.E., Moon, H.W., O'Brien, A.D., Gordon, V.M., and Whipp, S.C. 1996. Vaccination with genetically modified Shiga-like toxin IIe prevents edema disease in swine. Infect. Immun. 64:55–60.

Boyd, B., Tyrrell, G., Maloney, M., Gyles, C., Brunton, J., and Lingwood, C. 1993. Alteration of the glycolipid binding specificity of the pig edema toxin from globotetraosyl to globotriaosyl ceramide alters in vivo tissue targeting and results in a verotoxin I-like disease in pigs. J. Exp. Med. 177:1745–1753.

de Azavedo, J., McWhirter, E., Louie, M., and Brunton, J. 1994. *EAE* negative Verotoxin-producing *Escherichia coli* associated with hemolytic uremic syndrome and hemorrhagic colitis. In: Recent Advances in Verocytotoxin-producing *Escherichia coli* Infections, Editors: Karmali, M. and Goglio, A., Elsevier, Amsterdam, pp. 265–268.

Dytoc, M.T., Ismaili, A., Philpott, D.J., Soni, R., Brunton, J.L., and Sherman, P.M. 1994. Distinct binding properties of *eaeA*-negative verocytotoxin-producing *Escherichia coli* of serotype O113:H21. Infect. Immun. 62:3494–3505.

Gordon, V.M., Whipp, S.C., Moon, H.W., O'Brien, A.D., and Samuel, J.E. 1992. An enzymatic mutant of Shiga-like toxin II variant is a vaccine candidate for edema disease of swine. Infect. Immun. 60:485–490.

Griffin, P.M., Ostroff, S.M., Tauxe, R.V., Greene, K.D., Wells, J.G., Lewis, J.H., and Blake, P.A. 1988. Illness associated with *Escherichia coli* O157:H7 infections. Ann. Intern. Med. 109:705–712.

Huppertz, H., Busch, D., Schmidt, H., Aleksic, S., and Karch, H. 1996. Diarrhea in young children associated with *Escherichia coli* non-O157 organisms that produce Shiga-like toxin. J. Pediatr. 128:341–346.

Karmali, M., Petric, M., Lim, C., Fleming, P., Arbus, G., and Lior, H. 1985. The association between idiopathic hemolytic uremic syndrome and infection by verotoxin-producing *Escherichia coli*. J. Infect. Dis. 151:775–782.

Kausche, F.M., Dean, E.A., Arp, L.H., Samuel, J.E., and Moon, H.W. 1992. An experimental model for sub-clinical edema disease (*Escherichia coli* enterotoxemia) manifest as vascular necrosis in pigs. Amer. J. Vet. Res. 53:281–287.

Kurioka, T., Yunou, Y., and Kita, E. 1998. Enhancement of susceptibility to Shiga toxin-producing *Escherichia coli* O157:H7 by protein calorie malnutrition in mice. Infect. Immun. 66:1726–1734.

MacLeod, D.L., Gyles, C.L., and Wilcock, B.P. 1991. Reproduction of edema disease of swine with purified Shiga-like toxin II variant. Vet. Pathol. 28:66–73.

Marques, L.R.M., Peiris, J.S.M., Cryz, S.J., and O'Brien, A.D. 1987. *Escherichia coli* strains isolated from pigs with edema disease produce a variant of Shiga-like toxin II. FEMS Microbiol. Lett. 44:33–38.

Paton, A.W., Ratcliff, R.M., Doyle, R.M., Seymour-Murray, J., Davos, D., Lanser, J.A., and Paton, J.C. 1996. Molecular microbiological investigation of an outbreak of hemolytic uremic syndrome caused by dry fermented sausage contaminated with Shiga-like toxin-producing *Escherichia coli*. J. Clin. Microbiol. 34:1622–1627.

Ramotar, K., Henderson, E., Szumski, R., and Louie, T.J. 1995. Impact of free verotoxin testing on epidemiology of diarrhea caused by verotoxin-producing *Escherichia coli*. J. Clin. Microbiol. 33:1114–1120.

Smith, H.W. and Halls, S. 1968. The production of oedema disease and diarrhoea in weaned pigs by the oral administration of *Escherichia coli*: factors that influence the course of the experimental disease. J. Med. Microbiol. 1:45–59.

Spika, J.S., Parsons, J.E., Nordenberg, D., Wells, J.G., Gunn, R.A., and Blake, P.A. 1986. Hemolytic uremic syndrome and diarrhea associated with *Escherichia coli* O157:H7 in a day care center. J. Pediatr. 109:287–291.

Tarr, P.I. 1995. *Escherichia coli* O157:H7: clinical diagnostic, and epidemiological aspects of human infection. Clin. Infect. Dis. 20:1–10.

Tarr, P.I. and Neill, M.A. 1996. Perspective: The problem of non-O157:H7 Shiga toxin (Verotoxin)-producing *Escherichia coli*. J. Infect. Dis. 174:1136–1139.

Tarr, P.I., Neill, M.A., Clausen, C.R., Watkins, S.L., Christie, D.L., and Hickman, R.O. 1990. *Escherichia coli* O157:H7 and the hemolytic uremic syndrome: importance of early cultures in establishing the etiology. J. Infect. Dis. 162:553–556.

Tesh, V., Burris, J., Owens, J., Gordon, V., Waldolkowski, E., O'Brien, A.D., and Samuel, J. 1993. Comparison of the relative toxicities of Shiga-like toxins type I and type II for mice. Infect. Immun. 61:3392–3402.

Tzipori, S., Karch, H., Wachsmuth, K.I., Robins-Browne, R.M., O'Brien, A.D., Lior, H., Cohen, M.L., Smithers, J., and Levine, M.M. 1987. Role of a 60-megadalton plasmid and Shiga-like toxins in the pathogensis of infection caused by enterohemorrhagic *Escherichia coli* O157:H7 in gnotobiotic piglets. Infect. Immun. 55:3117–3125.

Tzipori, S., Wachsmuth, K.I., Smithers, J., and Jackson, C. 1988. Studies in gnotobiotic piglets on non-O157:H7 *Escherichia coli* serotypes isolated from patients with hemorrhagic colitis. Gasterenterology 94:590–597.

USDHHS. 1995. Outbreak of acute gastroenteritis attributable to *Escherichia coli* serotype O104:H21. Morbid. Mortal. Weekly Rep. 44 (27).

Waddell, T.E., Coomber, B.L., and Gyles, C.L. 1998. Localization of potential binding sites for the edema disease verotoxin (VT2e) in pigs. Can. J. Vet. Res. 62:81–86.

Waddell, T.E. and Gyles, C.L. 1995. Sodium deoxycholate facilitates systemic absorption of verotoxin 2e from pig intestine. Infect. Immun. 63:4953–4956.

Wells, J.G., Davis, B.R., Wachsmuth, I.K., Riley, L.W., Remis, R.S., Sokolow, R., and Morris, G.K. 1983. Laboratory investigation of hemorrhagic colitis outbreaks associated with a rare *Escherichia coli* serotype. J. Clin. Microbiol. 18:512–520.

Willshaw, G.A., Scotland, S.M., Smith, H.R., and Rowe, B. 1992. Properties of Verocytotoxin-producing *Escherichia coli* of human origin of O serogroups other than O157. J. Infect. Dis. 166:797–802.

15

ULTRASTRUCTURE AND DNA FRAGMENTATION ANALYSIS OF ARTERIOLES IN SWINE INFECTED WITH SHIGA TOXIN-PRODUCING *ESCHERICHIA COLI*

Ilze Matise,[1] Theerapol Sirinarumitr,[1]* Brad T. Bosworth,[2#] and Harley W. Moon[1]

[1] Veterinary Medical Research Institute
Iowa State University
Ames, Iowa 50011
[2] Enteric Diseases and Food Safety Research Unit
National Animal Disease Center
USDA/ARS, Ames, Iowa, 50010

SUMMARY

Shiga toxins (Stx) produced by *E. coli* are potent cytotoxins that affect the vascular system. In humans, systemic toxemia causes renal glomerular damage manifested as hemolytic uremic syndrome. In swine, Stx-producing *E. coli* (STEC) cause edema disease that is characterized microscopically by segmental arteriolar smooth muscle cell (SMC) lesions. Our objectives were to characterize ultrastructurally and by TUNEL the type of death (apoptosis or necrosis) that occurs in SMCs during edema disease. Increased DNA fragmentation consistent with apoptosis was detected by TUNEL in arterioles of challenged pigs 14–15 days post inoculation. Ultrastructurally 3 grades of SMC lesions were distinguished: 1) Partial loss of SMCs, intercellular space filled with granular cellular debris admixed with membrane bound vacuoles; 2) Complete loss of SMCs; only granular cellular debris and clear vacuoles remained within basement

* Present address: Veterinary Pathology, Kasetsart University, Nakorn-Pathom 73140, Thailand
# Present address: Pig Improvement Company, Franklin, KY, 42134

Mechanisms in the Pathogenesis of Enteric Diseases 2, edited by Paul and Francis.
Kluwer Academic / Plenum Publishers, New York, 1999.

membrane; 3) Inflammation of media; SMCs replaced by a rim of cellular debris located in the periphery of vessel wall. The most common lesion detected was grade 1 (9 ilea and 4 brains). We did not find apoptotic nuclear changes in SMCs or apoptotic inclusion bodies within resident cells. Our study indicates, that (1) Stx produced during edema disease does not cause SMC apoptosis 14–15 dpi; (2) SMCs undergo an array of changes from degeneration to necrosis.

1. INTRODUCTION

Shiga toxin-producing E. coli (STEC) are human and animal enteric pathogens that also are capable of causing systemic vascular damage (Karmali et al., 1985; Griffin and Tauxe, 1991). Numerous studies suggest that systemic complications result from either direct or indirect vascular toxicity of Stx (Obrig et al., 1988; Tesh et al., 1991; Kaplan, 1994; Obrig et al., 1994).

In human medicine, STEC is the major cause of hemolytic uremic syndrome (HUS) in children (Brotman et al., 1995; Tarr, 1995). In animals, such as pigs and mice, these organisms cause central nervous system (CNS) disturbances (Francis et al., 1989; Wadolkowski et al., 1990; Dykstra et al., 1993; Bertschinger and Gyles, 1994). The microscopic lesion of HUS is thrombotic microangiopathy predominantly affecting the microvasculature of the kidney and brain. The lesions are characterized by endothelial cell (EC) swelling and detachment from basement membrane, subendothelial fibrin deposits and thrombi (Richardson et al., 1988; Habib, 1992). Although the lesions are characterized, the pathogenesis of these lesions is not clear. It is well known, however, that the cytotoxic mechanism of Stx in cell cultures is the inhibition of protein synthesis (O'Brien and Holmes, 1987; O'Brien et al., 1992).

Stx is cytotoxic to EC in vitro and two types of cell death, namely necrosis and apoptosis, can be induced depending on the culture conditions (Louise and Obrig, 1991; Tesh et al., 1991; Louise and Obrig, 1995). Necrosis is induced upon EC incubation with Stx and the EC sensitivity to Stx can be increased by pre-incubation with cytokines such as tumor necrosis factor α (TNF-α). Under these conditions some 20–30% of EC undergo apoptosis (Obrig, 1998).

In HUS patients the predominant EC changes are swelling and detachment from the basement membrane. It is not clear, however, whether EC loss is via necrosis or apoptosis during natural STEC infections. Increased local or systemic production of pro-apoptotic cytokines, such as TNF-α and interleukin-1β, occurs occasionally in HUS patients (Karpman et al., 1995; Lopez et al., 1995; Tesh, 1998). Usually inflammation is not a component of the thrombotic lesion, and the absence of it suggests that EC death may occur through apoptosis. However, consistent neutrophilia and increased numbers of neutrophils were found within the kidneys of the HUS children in a recent study of HUS with a diarrheal prodrome (Inward et al., 1997). Karpman et al. studied the morphology of the renal cortical tissue from several children with postenteropathic HUS (Karpman et al., 1998). They reported thrombosis of glomerular blood vessels and necrosis of tubular epithelial cells. By TUNEL staining (a method that identifies DNA fragmentation characteristic of apoptosis), they identified numerous positive nuclei of tubular epithelial cells and fewer positive cells in glomeruli.

Swine edema disease is an attractive model to determine whether Stx-associated vascular lesions are due to apoptosis or necrosis. A microscopic hallmark of subclinical edema disease is a vascular lesion commonly referred to as arteriolar necrosis

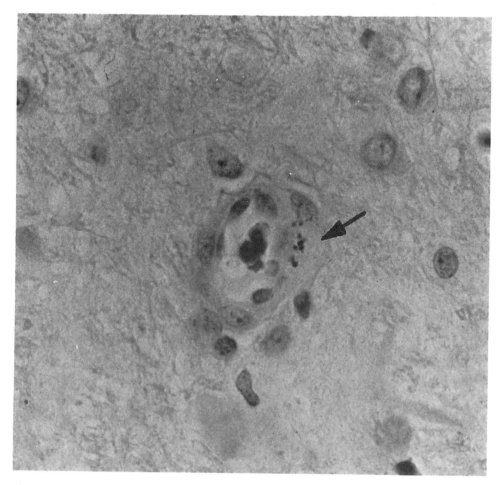

Figure 1. Histologic section of brain stem from a pig. Arteriole with segmental changes of media character-ized by karyorrhectic nuclear remnants of smooth muscle cells (arrow).

(Bertschinger and Gyles, 1994). This lesion is often found in the brain stem and sub-mucosa of the gastrointestinal tract of infected pigs. It is characterized by segmental areas with karyorrhectic and pyknotic changes in smooth muscle cells (SMC) and the absence of inflammation (Fig. 1) (Kausche et al., 1992; Bertschinger and Gyles, 1994). These are typical features of both, apoptosis and necrosis. Our objectives were to deter-mine the type of SMCs death that occurs in edema disease, in the vascular lesion com-monly referred to as arteriolar necrosis.

2. MATERIALS AND METHODS

2.1. Bacterial Strains and Animal Challenge

Three week old piglets were challenged with 10^{10} colony forming units of strain S1191 orally. This is a characteristic edema disease *E. coli* strain that produces F18ab fimbriae, heat stable enterotoxin and Stx2e. Control animals were challenged with a non-pathogenic *E. coli* strain 123. Animals were observed 2× daily throughout experiment for neurological disturbances or subcutaneous edema indicative of edema disease. Animals were euthanized by intravenous administration of barbituates. Samples were collected 14–15 days post inoculation (dpi) from subclinical principals, i.e., S1191 infected animals that did not exhibit clinical signs at any time during the experiment.

2.2. TUNEL

Ileum (1 m proximal of ileocecal valve) and brain stem were collected from 10 principals and 5 controls. Tissues were fixed in 10% neutral buffered formalin, sections embedded in paraffin and sectioned for hematoxylin and eosin (H&E) stain and TUNEL (terminal deoxynucleotidyl transferase(TdT)-mediated X-dUTP nick end labeling) stain. An ApopTag kit (Oncor, Gaitherburg, MD) was used for TUNEL assay according to the manufacturer's instructions.

H&E sections were evaluated for the presence of an arteriolar lesion characterized by SMC death. A section was considered positive if two or more arterioles of the ileal submucosa or brain stem were affected. TUNEL stained sections were evaluated qualitatively and quantitatively. Section was considered to be positive if two or more arterioles/section contained labeled SMCs (qualitative scoring). For quantitative evaluation, the number of positive arterioles was expressed as a percent of the total number of arterioles in the section. Quantitative scoring was done for 9/10 brains and ilea of subclinical principals and all controls.

2.3. Transmission Electron Microscopy (TEM)

At the end of the experiment, animals were sedated with sodium pentobarbital intravenously until a deep anesthetic state was attained. Ileal samples were collected 1 meter proximal to ileocecal junction and immersed immediately in gluteraldehyde solution. Animals were euthanized with an injection of barbituates and brain stem was collected from some of the pigs. Samples were processed further for TEM by post fixation with osmium in Na Cacodylate buffer followed by dehydration in acetone and embedding in plastic.

Eleven ileal samples and 6 brain samples collected from principals of 2 experiments contained arteriolar lesions that were characterized ultrastructurally. Additionally, ileal arterioles of 5 control animals (14 dpi) and brain stem arterioles of 3 control animals (12 dpi) were characterized ultrastructurally.

3. RESULTS

3.1. TUNEL

Four of the 10 brain and 6/10 ileal samples were positive for DNA fragmentation in arteriolar SMCs. Six of these TUNEL positive samples also had detectable arteriolar lesions in H&E stained sections. An additional brain sample was positive for arteriolar lesions in H&E but was negative for TUNEL staining.

Figure 2 shows the proportion of TUNEL positive arterioles. Arteriolar lesion positive principals had more TUNEL positive arterioles than did the principals without

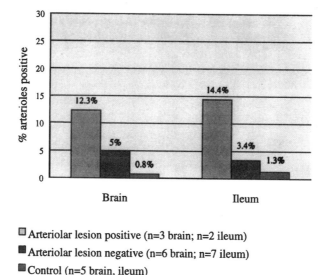

Arteriolar lesion positive (n=3 brain; n=2 ileum)
Arteriolar lesion negative (n=6 brain; n=7 ileum)
Control (n=5 brain, ileum)

Figure 2. TUNEL positive arterioles in control pigs and pigs with or without arteriolar lesions (H&E) following challenge with Shiga toxin-producing *E. coli*.

the lesions (12–14% versus 3–5%). None of the 5 control animals had detectable arteriolar lesions, however, background arteriolar TUNEL labeling was detected in 1–2% of arterioles of control tissues.

In summary, these results show that increased DNA fragmentation occurred in STEC challenged principals.

3.2. TEM

Changes in arterioles were present in SMCs and in ECs of principals. SMC changes were not seen in arterioles of control animals, however, an arteriole with segmental EC necrosis was detected in the ileum of one control animal.

Arteriolar SMC lesions were present in 9/11 ilea and in 4/6 brains. Three grades of SMC lesions were distinguished. Grade 1 lesions were characterized by partial loss of SMCs and focal aggregates of cellular debris within intercellular spaces (Figs. 3 and 4). Cellular debris included membrane bound vacuoles, and granular debris indicative of lytic necrosis. Remaining SMCs had limited degenerative changes. There was moderate thickening of basement membranes. Sometimes SMC with dark condensed cytoplasm indicative of coagulation necrosis were recognized. Grade 2 lesions were characterized by complete loss of SMCs with only clear vacuoles and granular cellular debris remaining between basement membranes. Grade 3 lesions were characterized by marked expansion of the tunica media by monocytes, lymphocytes and neutrophils, distortion of the vascular wall by marked fibrin accumulation. Numerous karyorrhectic and pyknotic nuclei were present within media and SMCs were replaced by a rim of cellular debris located in periphery of the vessel wall. Occasionally erythrocytes were observed intramurally or perivascularly in the arterioles of all grades. The lesion most commonly observed was grade 1 (9/11 ilea and 4/6 brains). Grade 2 and grade 3 lesions were present in the ileal arterioles of 3/11 animals. We did not find apoptotic nuclear

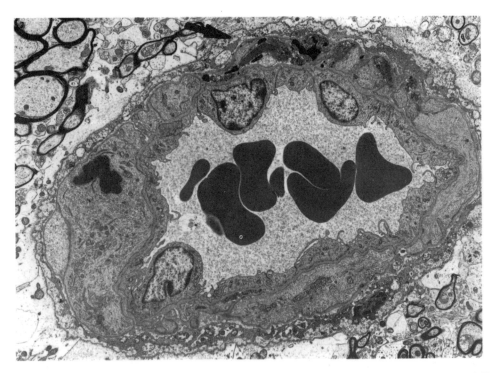

Figure 3. TEM of an arteriole in the brain stem of pig 15 days post infection with S1191. Focal area of disrupted smooth muscle cells (arrow) is covered by unaffected endothelial cells.

changes in SMCs or apoptotic inclusion bodies within the resident cells in arterioles from either organ from any of the pigs.

Degenerative and necrotic EC changes also occurred in arterioles from 5/11 ilea and 4/6 brains from the principals. These were characterized by irregular and discontinuous plasma membranes, cytoplasmic condensation, and nuclear condensation with chromatin clumping and margination.

4. DISCUSSION

This study focused on the lesions that occur in arterioles of subclinically affected pigs 14–15 days after the exposure to STEC. Increased DNA fragmentation consistent with apoptosis was detected by TUNEL in arterioles of principals. These results tended to correlate with the arteriolar lesion status determined by H&E. The significance of this finding, however, is not clear since it is recognized that limited DNA fragmentation may also occur during cell death by necrosis (Gold et al., 1994; Migheli et al., 1995; Yasuda et al., 1995). Ultrastructural morphologic changes observed in SMCs of arterioles were consistent with necrotic changes (more often cytolytic and occasionally coagulative). Therefore we conclude that the histologic lesions detected in subclinical edema disease at 14–15 days post exposure was the result of necrosis rather than apoptosis.

We now know from other experiments (manuscript in preparation by N. Cornick)

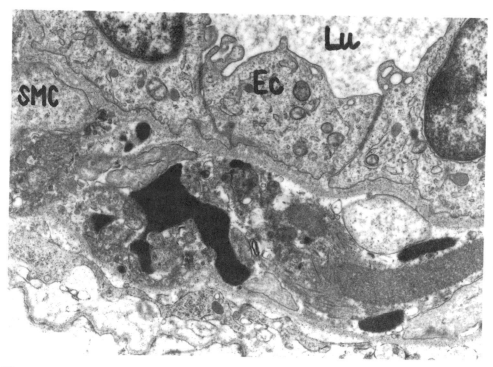

Figure 4. Higher magnification of segmental necrosis shown in Figure. 3. Media contains necrotic cellular debris, membrane bound vacuoles, and nuclear remnants. Basement membranes are thickened and tight junctions between endothelial cells are accentuated. Lu = lumen, Ec = endothelial cell, SMC = smooth muscle cell.

that the earliest occurrence of detectable lesions (in H&E) in subclinical principals is 12 days post exposure. However, we do not know what ultrastructural changes precede SMC necrosis. It seems probable that EC injury precedes SMC injury and/or that EC injury is repaired quicker than SMC injury. Ultrastructurally, swelling and vacuolation of arteriolar ECs is common and SMC necrosis occurs less frequently during early stages (2–7 dpi) of edema disease (Methiyapun et al., 1984). In vitro Stx studies show that cytotoxic dose and cellular response differs depending on cell types. It is likely that SMC response to Stx is different from the EC response. For example, mesangial cells are a subset of SMCs and Van Setten et al. indicates that in vitro exposure of human renal mesangial cells to Stx caused the inhibition of protein synthesis but not cell death as seen with ECs (Van Setten et al., 1997).

In this study, we encountered the limitations of TUNEL assay as an indicator of apoptosis and concluded that ultrastructural analysis is a valuable method for distinguishing the type of cell death that occurs in vivo. Other researchers studying vascular SMC death have reported a similar disagreement between TUNEL and TEM results. Bobryshev et al. used both TUNEL and TEM to determine the type of cell death that occurs in atheromatous plaque by TUNEL and by TEM (Bobryshev et al., 1997). By the TUNEL method, they found 9–40% TUNEL positive cells within the plaque, the majority of which were SMCs (75%). Upon ultrastructural evaluation they found intimal cells with condensed chromatin and convoluted cell surfaces, but no cells with typical morphologic expression of apoptosis were detected.

ACKNOWLEDGMENTS

This work was financed by the NIH grant AI41328. We thank N. Cornick for productive discussions and N. Cheville for advice with the interpretation of micrographs. This work would have not be possible without the electron microscopy expertise of J. Stasko and J. Olsen and the strong lab support of S. Booher, M. Mettenberg, D. Wiarda, and S. Frank.

REFERENCES

Bertschinger, H.U. and Gyles, C.L., 1994, Oedema disease of pigs, In: *Escherichia coli* in Domestic Animals and Humans, Ed.: Gyles, C., CAB International, Wallingford, pp. 193–219.

Bobryshev, Y.V., Babaev, V.R., Lord, R.S., and Watanabe, T., 1997, Cell death in atheromatous plaque of the carotid artery occurs through necrosis rather than apoptosis, In Vivo. 11:441–452.

Brotman, M., Gianella, R.A., Alm, C.P.F., Bauman, H., Bennet, A.R., Black, R.E., Bruhn, M., Cohen, M.B., Gorbach, S.L., Kaper, J.B., Roberts, M.R., Staneck, J.L., Taylor, S., and Troutt, H.F., 1995, Consensus conference statement: *Escherichia coli* O157:H7 infections—an emerging national health crisis, July 11–13-1994, Gastroenterology. 108:1923–1934.

Dykstra, S.A., Moxley, R.A., Janke, B.H., Nelson, E.A., and Francis, D.H., 1993, Clinical signs and lesions in gnotobiotic pigs inoculated with Shiga-like toxin I from *Escherichia coli*, Vet. Pathol. 30:410–417.

Francis, D.H., Moxley, R.A., and Andraos, C.Y., 1989, Edema disease-like brain lesions in gnotobiotic piglets infected with *Escherichia coli* serotype O157:H7, Infect. Immun. 57:1339–1342.

Gold, R., Schmied, M., Giegerich, G., Breitschopf, H., Hartung, H.P., Toyka, K.V., and Lassman, H., 1994, Differentiation between cellular apoptosis and necrosis by the combined use of *in situ* tailing and nick translation techniques, Lab. Invest. 71:219–225.

Griffin, P.M. and Tauxe, R.V., 1991, The epidemiology of infections caused by *Escherichia coli* O157:H7, other enterohemorrhagic *E. coli*, and the associated hemolytic uremic syndrome, Epidem. Rev. 13:60–98.

Habib, R., 1992, Pathology of the hemolytic uremic syndrome, In: Hemolytic-Uremic Syndrome and Thrombotic Thrombocytopenic Purpura, Ed.: Kaplan, B.S., Trompeter, R.S., and Moake, J.L., Marcel Dekker, Inc., New York, pp. 315–353.

Kaplan, B.S., 1994, Clinical and pathophysiological aspects of the hemolytic uremic syndrome, In: Recent Advances in Verocytotoxin-producing *Escherichia coli* Infections, Ed.: Karmali, M. and Goglio, A., Elsevier, Amsterdam, pp. 301–304.

Karmali, M.A., Petric, M., Lim, C., Fleming, P.C., Arbus, G.S., and Lior, H., 1985, The association between idiopathic hemolytic-uremic syndrome and infection by verotoxin-producing *Escherchia coli*, J. Infect. Dis. 151:775–782.

Karpman, D., Andreasson, A., Thysell, H., Kaplan, B.S., and Svanborg, C., 1995, Cytokines in childhood hemolytic uremic syndrome and thrombotic thrombocytopenic purpura, Pediatr. Nephrol. 9:694–699.

Karpman, D., Hakansson, A., Perez, M.R., Isaksson, C., Carlemalm, E., Caprioli, A., and Svanborg, C., 1998, Apoptosis of renal cortical cells in the hemolytic-uremic syndrome: in vivo and in vitro studies, Infect. Immun. 66:636–644.

Kausche, F.M., Dean, E.A., Arp, L.H., Samuel, J.E., and Moon, H.W., 1992, An experimental model for subclinical edema disease (*Escherichia coli* enterotoxemia) manifest as vascular necrosis in pigs, Amer. J. Vet. Res. 53:281–287.

Lopez, E.L., Contrini, M.M., Devoto, S., De Rosa, M.F., Grafia, M.G., Genero, M.H., Canepa, C., Gomez, H.F., and Cleary, T.G., 1995, Tumor necrosis factor concentrations in hemolytic uremic syndrome patients and children with bloody diarrhea in Argentina, Pediatr. Infect. Dis. J. 14:594–598.

Louise, C.B. and Obrig, T.G., 1991, Shiga toxin-associated hemolytic-uremic syndrome: combined cytotoxic effects of Shiga toxin, interleukin-1β, and tumor necrosis factor alpha on human vascular endothelial cell in vitro, Infect. Immun. 59:4173–4179.

Louise, C.B. and Obrig, T.G., 1995, Specific interaction of *Escherichia coli* O157:H7—derived Shiga-like toxin II with human renal endothelial cells, J. Infect. Dis. 172:1397–1401.

Methiyapun, S., Pohlenz, J.F.L., and Bertschinger, H.U., 1984, Ultrastructure of the intestinal mucosa in pigs experimentally inoculated with an edema disease-producing strain of *Escherichia coli* (O139:K12:H1), Vet. Pathol. 21:516–520.

Migheli, A., Attanasio, A., and Schiffer, D., 1995, Ultrastructural detection of DNA strand breaks in apoptotic neural cells by *in situ* end-labeling techniques, J. Pathol. 176:27–35.

O'Brien, A.D. and Holmes, R.K., 1987, Shiga and Shiga-like toxins, Microbiol. Rev. 51:206–220.

O'Brien, A.D., Tesh, V.L., Donohue-Rolfe, A., Jackson, M.P., Olsnes, S., Sandvig, K., Lindberg, A.A., and Keush, G.T., 1992, Shiga toxin: biochemistry, genetics, mode of action, and role in pathogenesis, Curr. Top. Microbiol. Immunol. 180:65–94.

Obrig, T.G., 1998, Interaction of Shiga toxins with endothelial cells, In: *Escherichia coli* O157:H7 and Other Shiga toxin-Producing *E. coli* Strains, Ed.: Kaper, J.B. and O'Brien, A.D., ASM Press, Washington, DC, pp. 303–311.

Obrig, T.G., Del Vecchio, P.J., Brown, J.E., Moran, T.P., Rowland, B.M., Judge, T.K., and Rothman, S.W., 1988, Direct cytotoxic action of Shiga toxin on human vascular endothelial cells, Infect. Immun. 56:2373–2378.

Obrig, T.G., Louise, C.B., Lingwood, C.A., Daniel, T.O., Kaye, S.A., Boyd, B., and Jackson, M.P., 1994, Shiga toxin-endothelial cell interactions, In: Recent Advances in Verocytotoxin-producing *Escherichia coli* Infections, Ed.: Karmali, M.A. and Goglio, A.G., Elsevier, Amsterdam, pp. 317–324.

Richardson, S.E., Karmali, M.A., Becker, L.E., and Smith, C.R., 1988, The histopathology of the hemolytic uremic syndrome associated with verocytotoxin-producing *Escherichia coli* infections, Hum. Pathol. 19:1102–1108.

Tarr, P.I., 1995, *Escherichia coli* O157:H7: clinical diagnostic, and epidemiological aspects of human infection, Clin. Infect. Dis. 20:1–10.

Tesh, V.L., 1998, Cytokine response to Shiga toxin, In: *Escherichia coli* O157:H7 and Other Shiga Toxin-Producing *E. coli* Strains, Ed.: Kaper, J.B. and O'Brien, A.D., ASM Press, Washington, DC, pp. 226–235.

Tesh, V.L., Samuel, J.E., Perera, L.P., Sharefkin, J.B., and O'Brien, A.D., 1991, Evaluation of the role of Shiga and Shiga-like toxin in mediating direct damage to human vascular endothelial cells, J. Infect. Dis. 164:344–352.

Van Setten, P.A., van Hinsberg, V.W., van den Heuvel, L.P., van der Velden, T.J., van de Kar, N.C., Krebbers, R.J., Karmali, M.A., and Monnens, L.A., 1997, Verocytotoxin inhibits mitogenesis and protein synthesis in purified human glomerular mesangial cells without affecting cell viability: evidence for two distinct mechanisms, J. Am. Soc. Nephrol. 8:1877–1888.

Wadolkowski, E.A., Burris, J.A., and O'Brien, A.D., 1990, Mouse model for colonization and disease caused by enterohemorrhagic *Escherichia coli* O157:H7, Infect. Immun. 58:2438–2445.

Yasuda, M., Umemura, S., Osamura, R.Y., Kenjo, T., and Tsutsumi, Y., 1995, Apoptotic cells in the human endometrium and placental villi: pitfalls applying TUNEL method, Arch. Histol. Cytol. 58:185–190.

16

PATHOGENESIS OF *ESCHERICHIA COLI* O157:H7 IN WEANED CALVES

Evelyn A. Dean-Nystrom,[1] Brad T. Bosworth,[1†] and Harley W. Moon[2]

Enteric Diseases and Food Safety, USDA
Agricultural Research Service
National Animal Disease Center
Ames, Iowa 50010[1]
Veterinary Medical Research Institute
College of Veterinary Pathology
Iowa State University
Ames, Iowa 50011[2]

1. SUMMARY

Cattle are an important reservoir of Shiga toxin-producing *Escherichia coli* O157:H7 and other enterohemorrhagic *E. coli* (EHEC) that cause diarrhea, hemorrhagic colitis, and hemorrhagic uremic syndrome in humans. One strategy for reducing human foodborne EHEC infections is to reduce the levels of EHEC in cattle. Bovine O157:H7 infection models will facilitate identification of virulence factors involved in bovine infections. O157:H7 cause severe diarrhea and attaching and effacing (A/E) mucosal lesions in colostrum-deprived neonatal (< 2 h) calves. We hypothesized that O157:H7 also cause A/E lesions in older calves, but these were not detected in earlier studies because intestinal levels of O157:H7 were too low (<10^6 CFU/g of tissue) for detection of focally distributed microscopic lesions. Weaned 3- to 4-month-old calves were fasted 48 h, inoculated via stomach tube with 10^{10} CFU of O157:H7 or nonpathogenic *E. coli*, necropsied 4 d pi and examined histologically. Calves inoculated with O157:H7 had higher intestinal levels of inoculated *E. coli* than control animals. The rectum was the major site of colonization. A/E lesions were seen in the rectum and cecum of calves with high levels of O157:H7. Weaned calves, like neonatal calves, are susceptible to intestinal damage induced by EHEC O157:H7. The rectum and cecum

†Current address: 3033 Nashville Road, Franklin, KY 42134

Mechanisms in the Pathogenesis of Enteric Diseases 2, edited by Paul and Francis.
Kluwer Academic / Plenum Publishers, New York, 1999.

may be principal sites of EHEC O157:H7 colonization during the carrier-shedder state in cattle.

2. INTRODUCTION

Cattle are an important reservoir of Shiga toxin-producing *Escherichia coli* O157:H7 and other enterohemorrhagic *E. coli* (EHEC) that cause diarrhea, hemorrhagic colitis, and hemorrhagic uremic syndrome in humans (Griffin and Tauxe, 1991; Su and Brandt, 1995; Whipp et al., 1994). In the United States, EHEC O157:H7 disease in humans has occurred as a consequence of ingestion of cattle products, especially improperly cooked ground hamburger and raw milk. Both dairy and beef cattle are asymptomatically infected with EHEC O157:H7 and non-O157:H7 EHEC and are a reservoir for these strains (Griffin and Tauxe, 1991).

One strategy for reducing the incidence of human foodborne EHEC infections in humans is to reduce the levels of EHEC in cattle. We are using bovine models of O157:H7 infection to identify the site and mechanisms of EHEC O157:H7 infections in cattle. Our ultimate goal is to identify ways to prevent cattle from becoming infected with EHEC O157:H7. This will reduce cattle-to-human transmission of EHEC O157:H7.

We have shown that EHEC O157:H7 bacteria cause acute disease in neonatal calves (Dean-Nystrom et al., 1997; Dean-Nystrom et al., 1998). Colostrum-deprived neonatal (<12-h-old) calves develop severe, sometimes fatal, diarrhea and have attaching and effacing (A/E) lesions in the large and small intestines as early as 18h after inoculation with EHEC O157:H7. A/E lesions are consistently seen by histologic staining in intestinal tissues that contain at least $10^6 \log_{10}$ CFU of EHEC O157:H7 bacteria per gram of tissue, but are rarely found in tissues with fewer bacteria (Dean-Nystrom et al., 1998). The neonatal calf EHEC O157:H7 infection model is useful for studying virulence factors required for acute bovine infections, but is less suitable for identifying factors involved in asymptomatic EHEC O157:H7 infections in cattle.

3. EXPERIMENTAL DESIGN AND PROCEDURE

We are developing a weaned calf model of EHEC O157:H7 infections to study virulence factors that promote intestinal colonization and fecal shedding in cattle. Earlier studies have shown that weaned calves remain clinically healthy, but are colonized and shed variable numbers of EHEC O157:H7 for variable periods after they are experimentally infected with EHEC O157:H7 (Cray and Moon, 1995). We hypothesized that O157:H7 cause A/E lesions in older calves like they do in neonatal calves, but these were not detected in earlier studies because intestinal levels of O157:H7 at necropsy were too low (i.e., $<10^6$ CFU per gram of tissue) for focally distributed microscopic lesions to be detected. Since fasted ruminants shed higher numbers of *E. coli* and other enteric pathogens than do well-fed animals (Rasmussen et al., 1993), we fasted three 4-month-old weaned calves for 48h prior to inoculation with EHEC O157:H7 to increase intestinal levels of EHEC O157:H7 at necropsy. Fasted calves were inoculated via stomach tube with 10^{10} CFU of EHEC O157:H7 (9 calves) or nonpathogenic *E. coli* control strain (3 calves), necropsied at 4d postinoculation, and examined histologically.

4. RESULTS

Nine of nine calves inoculated with EHEC O157:H7 and two of three calves inoculated with control *E. coli* developed watery diarrhea by 18 h and 3 d after inoculation, respectively. However, five calves infected with EHEC O157:H7 and both of the diarrheic control calves had coccidia (based on histology). The occurrence of diarrhea in calves inoculated with O157:H7 two days earlier than in control calves may be evidence that EHEC O157:H7 contributes to diarrhea in some weaned calves.

At 4 days postinoculation, higher numbers of inoculated bacteria were recovered from the intestines of weaned calves inoculated with EHEC O157:H7 than from the control calves (Table 1). Multifocal A/E bacterial lesions were found in the rectum of three calves inoculated with EHEC O157:H7 and also in the cecum of two of these calves. These A/E lesions were similar to those in neonatal calves (Fig. 1). However, the extent of intestinal damage in the rectums and ceca of weaned calves infected with EHEC O157:H7 was less than that in similarly infected neonatal calves. No A/E bacteria were found in the spiral colon or ileum of any of the O157:H7-infected calves or in any site in control calves. The A/E bacteria were identified as O157:H7 *E. coli* by immunoperoxidase staining with anti-O157:H7 serum (Dean-Nystrom et al., 1997).

The calves that had A/E bacteria had higher numbers of EHEC O157:H7 bacteria in the rectum and cecum than did the calves in which no lesions were found. A/E bacteria were found in the three calves that had greater than 10^6 CFU of EHEC O157:H7/g of rectal tissue, but not in those with lower counts. Two of the three calves with rectal lesions that had greater than 10^5 CFU of EHEC O157:H7/g of cecal tissue also had A/E bacteria in the cecum. Coccidia were seen in the intestinal mucosa of two of the three calves that had A/E bacteria.

5. DISCUSSION

These studies clearly demonstrate that weaned calves, like neonatal calves, are colonized by EHEC O157:H7 (i.e., have higher intestinal levels of inoculated bacteria at 4 days postinoculation than do calves inoculated with a nonpathogenic control *E. coli* strain) and are susceptible to intestinal damage induced by EHEC O157:H7. High

Table 1. CFU of *E. coli* per gram of tissue or feces in necropsy samples from weaned calves 4 days after inoculation with EHEC O157:H7 strain 86-24 (n = 9) (McKee et al., 1995) or a nonpathogenic *E coli* O43:H28 control strain 123 (n = 3) (Moon et al., 1968). Samples from which no inoculated bacteria were recovered were recorded as 1×10^3

E. coli strain	Log₁₀ CFU/g of tissue of inoculated bacteria (*range*)				
	Ileum	Cecum	Spiral Colon	Rectum	Feces
O157:H7	3.2	4.5	4.6	4.9	5.6
	(*3–5.0*)	(*3.3–5.8*)	(*4.0–5.6*)	(*3–7.0*)	(*3.1–7.3*)
Control	3	3.4	3	3.5	4.2
	(*3*)	(*3–4.2*)	(*3*)	(*3–4.5*)	(*3–5.9*)

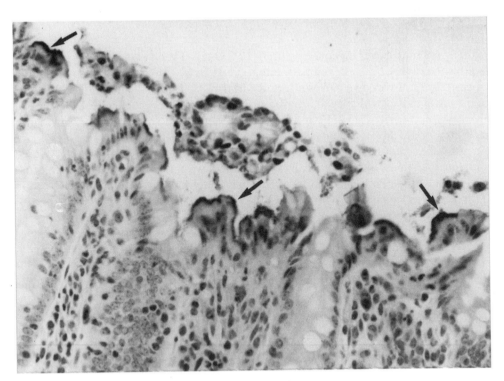

Figure 1. Immunoperoxidase-stained section of weaned calf rectum 4 days after inoculation with EHEC O157:H7 strain 86-24 (McKee et al., 1995). There are scattered colonies of A/E EHEC O157:H7 (dark patches, indicated by arrows) on the intestinal mucosa.

bacterial counts and A/E lesions were found only in the rectum and cecum and only in some of the calves inoculated with EHEC O157:H7. We speculate that the rectum and cecum may be the principal sites of EHEC O157:H7 colonization during the carrier-shedder state in cattle. We are using the weaned calf model to identify virulence factors that promote colonization of the lower large intestines of cattle by EHEC O157:H7 bacteria and to identify interventions that prevent EHEC O157:H7 infections and transmission in cattle.

ACKNOWLEDGMENTS

We thank M. I. Inbody, N. C. Lyon, R. W. Morgan, R. A. Schneider, and J. A. Stasko for technical assistance and J. Laufer for providing veterinary services and performing necropsies.

REFERENCES

Cray, W. C., Jr. and Moon, H. W., 1995, Experimental infection of calves and adult cattle with *Escherichia coli* O157:H7, Appl. Environ. Microbiol. 61:1586–90.
Dean-Nystrom, E. A., Bosworth, B. T., Cray, W. C., Jr., and Moon, H. W., 1997, Pathogenicity of *Escherichia coli* O157:H7 in the intestines of neonatal calves, Infect. Immun. 65:1842–1848.

Dean-Nystrom, E.A., Bosworth, B.T., Moon, H.W., and O'Brien, A.D., 1998, *Escherichia coli* O157:H7 requires intimin for enteropathogenicity in calves, Infect. Immun. 66:4560–4563.

Griffin, P.M. and Tauxe, R.V., 1991, The epidemiology of infections caused by *Escherichia coli* O157:H7, other enterohemorrhagic *E. coli* and the associated hemolytic uremic syndrome, Epidemiol. Rev. 13:60–98.

McKee, M.L., Melton-Celsa, A.R., Moxley, R.A., Francis, D.H., and O'Brien, A.D., 1995, Enterohemorrhagic *Escherichia coli* O157:H7 requires intimin to colonize the gnotobiotic pig intestine and to adhere to HEp-2 cells, Infect. Immun. 63:3739–3744.

Moon, H.W., Sorensen, D.K., and Sautter, J.H., 1968, Experimental enteric colibacillosis in piglets, Can. J. Comp. Med. 32:493–497.

Su, C. and Brandt L.J., 1995, *Escherichia coli* O157:H7 infection in humans, Ann. Intern. Med 123:698–714.

Whipp, S.C., Rasmussen, M.A., and Cray, W.C., Jr., 1994, Animals as a source of *Escherichia coli* pathogenic for human beings, J. Am. Vet. Med. Assoc. 204:1168–1175.

17

DISTRIBUTION OF A NOVEL LOCUS CALLED PAA (PORCINE ATTACHING AND EFFACING ASSOCIATED) AMONG ENTERIC *ESCHERICHIA COLI*

Hongyan An, John M. Fairbrother, Clarisse Desautels, and Josée Harel*

Groupe de recherche sur les maladies infectieuses du porc
Université de Montréal
Faculté de médecine vétérinaire
C. P. 5000, Saint-Hyacinthe
Québec, Canada J2S 7C6

1. SUMMARY

Using Tn*phoA* transposon insertion mutagenesis, we found a porcine EPEC (PEPEC) mutant demonstrating as inability to induce AE lesions. The insertion was identified in a gene designated *paa* (porcine attaching and effacing associated). The distribution of *paa* in PEPEC O45 strains revealed that it was associated with presence of the *eae* and its AE phenotype *in vivo*. On examination of enteric *E. coli* isolates from humans and various animal species, a strong correlation with the presence of *paa* was found in EHEC O157:H7 and O26, and dog, rabbit, and pig *eae*-positive isolates, and to a lesser extent in human EPEC *eae*-positive isolates. Also, among porcine ETEC isolates, a strong association was found with the presence of LT encoded genes. In contrast, *paa* sequence was rarely found in enteric *E. coli* isolates lacking ETEC and AEEC virulence determinants. Thus, our results suggest that Paa could play a role in the AE mechanism and other mechanisms of enteric disease.

*Corresponding author: Josée Harel, Telephone: (450) 773-8521 ext. 8233, Fax: (450) 778-8108, e-mail: harelj@ere.umontreal.ca

Mechanisms in the Pathogenesis of Enteric Diseases 2, edited by Paul and Francis.
Kluwer Academic / Plenum Publishers, New York, 1999.

2. INTRODUCTION

Attaching and effacing *Escherichia coli* (AEEC) represent a group of isolates involved in enteric infections of man and animals (Levine, 1987). Naturally occuring AEEC have been identified in postweaning diarrhea (PWD) by light microscopy and subsequent by experimental inoculated piglets (Janke et al., 1989; Hélie et al., 1991; Zhu et al., 1994). *E. coli* serogroup O45 strains are often isolated from cases of PWD in pigs and are mostly able to induce attaching and effacing (AE) lesions *in vivo* and *in vitro*. This AE phenomenom is characterized by intimate bacteria adherence and the cell membrane, with effacement of target brush borders and disruption of the underlying cytoskeleton (Helie et al., 1991; Zhu et al., 1994; 1995). These histopathologic changes are indistinguishable from those produced by enteropathogenic *E. coli* (EPEC) (Moon et al., 1983).

A chromosomal gene cluster (35-kb) necessary for the production of the AE lesion has been identified as a pathogenicity island termed the locus of enterocyte effacement or the "LEE" region (McDaniel et al., 1995; McDaniel and Kaper, 1997). The LEE region encodes a type III secretion system (Jarvis et al., 1995) and several *E. coli*-secreted proteins, including EspA, EspB, EspD, and Tir (Kenny et al., 1996; Donnenberg et al., 1993; Lai et al., 1997; Kenny et al., 1997), which are required for intimate attachment and AE lesion formation (Donnenberg et al., 1997). The LEE region also encodes intimin (Jerse et al., 1990), an outer membrane protein adhesin (Frankel et al., 1994) that mediates intimate EPEC-host cell interaction. Recently, Kenny et al. (1997) have shown that an intimin receptor, Tir, is a bacterial protein translocated onto the surface of infected target cells and that the intimin-Tir interaction triggers the organization of polymerized actin into a cup-like pedestal beneath the attached EPEC bacterium.

E. coli causes diarrhea in swine, from the newborn to the postweaning period (Taylor, 1989; Zhu et al., 1994). Our early reports showed that AE lesions in naturally occurring postweaning diarrhea cases were associated with the presence of *E. coli* isolates of serogroup O45 (Hélie et al., 1991; Zhu et al., 1994). These *E. coli* were named porcine EPEC, or PEPEC. The AE capacity of PEPEC isolates both *in vivo* in experimentally inoculated piglets and *in vitro* in ileal loop explants was associated with the presence of the *eae* gene and expression of the Eae protein (Zhu et al., 1994; 1995).

Recently, we have created a bank of Tn*phoA* mutants in PEPEC strain 1390 and screened for the loss of their capacity to induce the typical histopathological AE lesions in pig intestinal ileal explants. In this previous study, one mutant M155 did not induce AE lesions. The Tn*phoA* insertion was shown to reside in a gene called *paa* (for porcine AE associated) gene (An, 1998). The importance of *paa* among enteric *E. coli* was studied by examining the distribution of *paa* among enteric *E. coli* isolated from human and animals.

3. MATERIALS AND METHODS

3.1. Bacterial Strains

In total, 385 *E. coli* isolates were examined in this study. The strains from animals cases had been isolated at Faculté de Médecine Vétérinaire, Saint-Hyacinthe, Québec,

Canada. Strains from human cases had been kindly provided by Wendy Johnson, LSPQ and F. Caya. They were serotyped with rabbit antisera for the *E. coli* O serogroups (Zhu et al., 1994). These strains were stored on Dorset agar until this study began. In this study, twenty-one *eae* positive VTEC isolates belonging to O157 (n = 14) and O26 (n = 2) serogroups, twelve human *eae* positive EPEC isolates belonging to O26 (n = 1), O111 (n = 2), O55 (n = 1), and O18 (n = 1) serogroups, and 106 *eae* positive and 123 *eae* negative *E. coli* intestinal isolates from humans, rabbits, dogs, and pigs, the latter mostly belonging to the O45 serogroup. All isolates in Table 1 were negative on colony hybridization for verotoxin (VT), and enterotoxins STa, STb, and LT genes with the exception of VTEC isolates which were VT positive (Fairbrother 1998, unpublished data). A total of 88 isolates in Table 2 were identified as toxigenic isolates and 32 non ETEC were positive for either VT2 or extraintestinal virulence factors Pap/CNF.

The *paa* gene was cloned from wild-type pathogenic *E. coli* strain 1390 (serogroup O45) that was isolated from a 4-week-old pig with postweaning diarrhea. O45 strain 1390 induces typical AE lesions both *in vitro* and *in vivo* (Zhu et al., 1994; Zhu et al., 1995), contains sequences homologous to *eae*, and expresses a 97 kDa Eae protein (Zhu et al., 1994; Zhu et al., 1995).

3.2. Colony Hybridization

E. coli strains were spotted onto Luria-Bertani agar and incubated for 4 to 5 h at 37°C. Colonies were then transferred to Whatman 3MM filter paper 451 (Whatman, Inc., Clifton, N.J.). The filters were processed, hybridized, and revealed by autoradiography as described previously (Zhu et al., 1994). Gene probes for various virulence factors were either derived from recombinant plasmids or generated by PCR as described previously (Zhu et al., 1994). The *paa* probe was a 350 bp PCR fragment derived from the 5' end of the *paa* gene (accession number U82533). A 790 bp *eae* probe derived from the *eae* gene of a EPEC strain was generated by PCR (Beaudry et al., 1996). Probes were radiolabelled with [α-^{32}P]CTP as described previously (Beaudry et al., 1996).

4. RESULTS

4.1. Distribution of *paa* among Different AE *E. coli*

Using the colony hybridization test, we examined the relationship between the presence of the *paa* and *eae* genes in *E. coli* isolates from human and animals. Overall the *paa* related sequences were detected in 74% of *eae* positive isolates of enteric *E. coli*. In contrast, none of the 167 *eae* negative *E. coli* isolates from human, dogs, or pigs were *paa* positive. The correlation between *paa* and *eae* in EHEC O157 and dog isolates were observed as 100% and 87%, respectively, whereas a lower proportion in pig O45, rabbit, and EPEC isolates were found as 63%, 71%, and 25%, respectively.

Homologous sequences of the *paa* gene were identified in 15 isolates out of 24 *eae* positive PEPEC strains, of which 21 were AE positive *in vivo* or *ex vivo* as tested proeviously (Zhu et al., 1994) (Table 1).

Also, on examination of porcine ETEC isolates, it has been found that homologous sequences of the *paa* gene were strongly associated with the presence of the LT

Table 1. Relationship between the presence of the *paa* and *eae* genes in intestinal *E. coli* isolates from humans and animals

Isolate origin[a]		No. of isolates				
		Total	*eae*	*paa*	*paa/eae*	*paa/eae* (%)
Human	VTEC (O157)	14	14	14	14/14	100
	VTEC (others)	7	7	5	5/7	71
	VTEC	3	0	0	0/0	0
	EPEC[b]	12	12	3	3/12	25
	Others	27	2	0	0/2	0
Rabbit		23	21	15	15/21	71
Dog		23	15	13	13/15	87
Pig	O45	33	24[c]	15	15/24	63
	Non O45	123	0	5	0/0	0

[a]Isolates were from the feces or intestinal contents of individuals with diarrhea and were negative by gene probe for VT, STa, STb, and LT with the exception of the EHEC isolates which were VT positive.
[b]Belonging to serogroup O26, O111, O55, or O18.
[c]All except 3 *eae*[+] isolates were AE positive when examined in pig ileal explant culture and in experimentally inoculated piglets (Zhu et al., 1994; 1995).

encoded genes (Table 2). In contrast, *paa* sequence was rarely found in enteric *E. coli* isolates lacking ETEC and AEEC virulence determinants.

5. DISCUSSION

The *paa* gene was initially found by transposon mutagenesis in a PEPEC strain 1390 (An, 1998). The PEPEC *paa*⁻ mutant exhibited an inability to induce AE lesions. *paa* is a gene encoding for a secreted protein of 27.6 kDa. Significantly, the amino acid sequence of the Paa shares 49% identity to an accessory colonization factor AcfC of *Vibrio cholerae*. Although the *paa* gene is important for the AE activity of the PEPEC O45 strain 1390 since a mutation abolishes the AE activity, its role in the pathogenicity of PEPEC strains has not yet been elucidated.

The distribution of *paa* in the PEPEC O45 strains revealed that not only *eae* but also *paa* is associated with many O45 strains that were shown to produce typical AE in both experimental inoculation of gnotobiotic piglets and *in vitro* ileal segments (Table 1). The presence of *paa* and *eae* sequences in the porcine O45 strains is highly

Table 2. Relationship between the presence of the *paa* and various toxin genes in toxigenic isolates from pigs

Isolate groups	Pathotype	Total	*paa* (+)	*paa* (−)	*paa* (+) %
ETEC	STa	3	3	0	100
	STa-STb	16	2	14	12.5
	STa-STb-LT	13	13	0	100
	STa-STb-VT2	1	0	1	0
	STa-VT2	3	0	3	0
	STb	15	0	15	0
	STb-LT	37	20	17	54.1
Non ETEC	VT2	6	0	6	0
	Pap/CNF	26	0	26	0
Negative control		123	5	118	4

correlated with the AE phenotype as all 15 *paa* positive, *eae* positive O45 isolates were AE positive. However, the observation that three *eae* positive but *paa* negative porcine O45 strains were AE negative provides further evidence for the importance of the *paa* gene in the AE activity of porcine O45 strains.

The correlation between the presence of the *paa* and *eae* genes among the isolates from humans and different animal species was also studied. Our results suggest that the *paa* gene may have a more important role in the AE activity of EHEC and dog isolates but to a lower extent in rabbit, pig O45, and human EPEC isolates. On the other hand, these finding could be due to a lower homology between the *paa* probe and the related sequences in isolates of these species. The presence of a functionally related but less homologous gene present in the *paa* negative isolates, thus, can not be ruled out. Alternatively, the presence of the *paa* gene could reflect some differences in the mechanisms of AE activity and/or the development of diarrhea in isolates from different animal species and pathotypes such as the EHEC and EPEC.

We also found a correlation between the *paa* and LT encoded genes. LT is an important virulence factor in the development of ETEC diarrhea in pigs. Our results suggest that the *paa* gene could have role in development of enteric disease.

ACKNOWLEDGMENTS

This work was supported in part by the Medical Research Council of Canada grant MT11720 and the Fonds pour la Formation des Chercheurs et l'Aide à la Recherche du Québec (FCAR) grant 0214.

REFERENCES

An, H., 1998, Genetic analysis of virulence determinants of attaching and effacing *Escherichia coli* strains isolated from pigs and dog, Ph.D. thesis, Université de Montréal, 192 p.

Beaudry, M., Zhu, C., Fairbrother, J.M., and Harel, J., 1996, Genotypic and phenotypic characterization of *Escherichia coli* isolates from dogs manifesting attaching and effacing lesions, J. Clin. Microbiol. 34:144–148.

Donnenberg, M.S., and Kaper, J.B., 1993, A second chromosomal gene necessary for initimate attachment of enteropathogenic *Escherichia coli* to epithelial cells, J. Bacteriol. 175:4670–4680.

Donnenberg, M.S., Kaper, J.B., and Finlay, B.B., 1997, Interactions between enteropathogenic *Escherichia coli* and host epithelial cells, Trends in Microbiol. 5:109–114.

Frankel, G., Candy, D.C.A., Everest, P., and Dougan, G., 1994, Characterization of the C-terminal domains of intimin-like proteins of enteropathogenic and enterohemorrhagic *Escherichia coli*, *Citrobacter freundii*, and *Hafnia alvei*, Infect. Immun. 62:1835–1842.

Hélie, P., Morin, M., Jacques, M., and Fairbrother, J.M., 1991, Experimental infection of newborn pigs with an attaching and effacing *Escherichia coli* O45:K "E65" strain, Infect. Immun. 59:814–821.

Janke, B.H., Francis, D.H., Collins, J.E., Libal, M.C., Zeman, D.H., and Johnson, D.D., 1989, Attaching and effacing *E. coli* infections in calves, pigs, lambs, and dogs, J. Vet. Diag. Invest. 1:6–11.

Jarvis, K.G., Giron, J.A., Jerse, A.E., McDaniel, T.K., Donnenberg, M.S., and Kaper, J.B., 1995, Enteropathogenic *Escherichia coli* contains a specialized secretion system necessary for the export of proteins involved in attaching and effacing lesion formation, Proc. Natl. Aca. Sci. USA. 92:7996–8000.

Jerse, A.E., Yu, J., Tall, B.D., and Kaper, J.B., 1990, A genetic locus of enteropathogenic *Escherichia coli* necessary for the production of attaching and effacing lesions on tissue culture cells, Proc. Natl. Acad. Sci. USA. 87:7839–7843.

Kenny, B., Lai, L., Finlay, B.B., and Donnenberg, M.S., 1996, EspA, a protein secreted by enteropathogenic *Escherichia coli*, is required to induce signals in epithelial cells, Mol. Microbiol. 20:313–323.

Kenny, B., Abe, A., Stein, M., and Finlay, B.B., 1997, Enteropathogenic *Escherichia coli* protein secretion is induced in response to conditions similar to those in the gastrointestinal tract, Infect. Immun. 65:2606–2612.

Lai, L.C., Wainwright, L.A., Stone, K.D., and Donnenberg, M.S., 1997, A third secreted protein that is encoded by the enteropathogenic *Escherichia coli* pathogenicity island is required for transduction of signals and for attaching and effacing activities in host cells, Infect. Immun. 65:2211–2217.

Levine, M.M. and Edelman, R., 1984, Enteropathogenic *Escherichia coli* of classic serotypes associated with infant diarrhea: epidemiology and pathogenesis, Epidemiol. Rev. 6:31–51.

McDaniel, T.K., Jarvis, K.G., Donnenberg, M.S., and Kaper, J.B., 1995, A genetic locus of enterocyte effacement conserved among diverse enterobacterial pathogens, Proc. Natl. Acad. Sci. USA. 92:1664–1668.

Moon, H.W., Whipp, S.C., Argenizio, R.A., Levine, M.M., and Giannella, R.A., 1983, Attaching and effacing activities of rabbit and human enteropathogenic *Escherichia coli* in pig and rabbit intestines, Infect. Immun. 41:1340–1351.

Taylor, D.J., 1989, Colibacillosis in Pig diseases. pp. 86–97, Editor: Taylor, D.J., The Burlington Press Ltd., Forxton, Cambridge.

Zhu, C., Harel, J., Jacques, M., Desautels, C., Donnenberg, M.S., Beaudry, M., and Fairbrother, J.M., 1994, Virulence properties and attaching-effacing activity of *Escherichia coli* O45 from swine postweaning diarrhea, Infect. Immun. 62:4153–4159.

Zhu, C., Harel, J., Jacques, M., and Fairbrother, J.M., 1995, Interaction with pig ileal explants of *Escherichia coli* O45 isolates from swine with post-weaning diarrhea., Can. J. Vet. Res. 59:118–123.

18

POTENTIATION OF THE EFFECTIVENESS OF LACTOBACILLUS CASEI IN THE PREVENTION OF *E. COLI* INDUCED DIARRHEA IN CONVENTIONAL AND GNOTOBIOTIC PIGS

Alojz Bomba,[1] Radomíra Nemcová,[1] Soňa Gancarčíková,[1] Róbert Herich,[1] and Rudolf Kaštel[2]

[1] Research Institute of Experimental Veterinary Medicine
Hlinkova 1/A, 040 01 Košice
Slovak Republic
[2] University of Veterinary Medicine
Komenského 73, 040 01 Košice
Slovak Republic

SUMMARY

The influence of preventive administration of *Lactobacillus casei subsp. casei* and maltodextrin KMS X-70 on *Escherichia coli* 08: K88 adhesion in the gastrointestinal tract of 11 conventional and 6 gnotobiotic piglets was investigated. The preventive administration of *L. casei* alone had almost no inhibitory effect on the adherence of *E. coli* to the jejunal mucosa of gnotobiotic and conventional piglets while the lactobacilli administered together with maltodextrin decreased the number of *E. coli* colonising jejunal mucosa of gnotobiotic piglets by 1 logarithm ($4.95 \log 10/cm^2$) in comparison with the control group ($5.96 \log 10/cm^2$). *L. casei* administered in combination with maltodextrin decreased the number of *E. coli* colonising the jejunum of conventional piglets by more than two and half logarithm ($4.75 \log 10/cm^2$, $p < 0.05$) in comparison with the control ($7.42 \log 10/cm^2$). The inhibitory effect of *Lactobacillus casei* and maltodextrin KMS X-70 on the adhesion of *E. coli* to the intestinal mucosa of conventional and gnotobiotic pigs was probably mediated by *Lactobacillus*—produced antibacterial substances and stimulation of imunity.

Mechanisms in the Pathogenesis of Enteric Diseases 2, edited by Paul and Francis.
Kluwer Academic / Plenum Publishers, New York, 1999.

1. INTRODUCTION

Gastrointestinal diseases have been the major cause of morbidity and mortality in piglets at an early stage of life. Enterotoxigenic *Escherichia coli* are frequently identified as causative agents of diarrhoeal diseases of infectious etiology in piglets (Fairbrother, 1993). Administration of probiotics is one of the effective methods of prevention of gastrointestinal diseases in the young of farm animals (Bomba et al., 1997). Lactobacilli are the most frequently used microorganisms for probiotic purposes (Fuller, 1989; Jonsson and Conway, 1992).

The information about the effectiveness of probiotics in the prevention of gastrointestinal diseases in the young under practical conditions are often controversial which results in the requirement for marked increase in their effectiveness. The progress in the development of more effective probiotics is conditional upon further intensive research oriented on the explanation of the mechanism of their effect. Each microorganism can interact with other microorganisms by means of one or several mechanisms which can be expressed with varying intensity. Therefore a complex study of the mechanism of effect of each respective microorganism intended for probiotic purposes is inevitable. Such an approach can lead to an explanation of the mono- or polyfactorial character of the mechanisms studied. This is a starting point for potentation of the effectiveness of probiotics which can be achieved either by intensifying one of the mechanisms or extending the scale of mechanisms of the respective probiotic.

The effectiveness of probiotics can be increased in 3 ways: by gene manipulation, by combining several strains of microorganisms or combining probiotics with synergistically acting components. From the practical point of view the last method is the most suitable one. It uses synergistic effects of autochtonous microflora and natural substances. The pathogenicity of *E. coli* is conditional on two factors: the ability to produce enterotoxin and the presence of colonization factors enabling the carrier to colonize the mucosa of the small intestine (Bertschinger et al., 1972; Jones and Rutter, 1972; Smith and Gyles, 1970). The aim of the present study was to investigate the influence of preventive administration of *Lactobacillus casei* and maltodextrin KMS X-70 on *E. coli* adhesion in the gastrointestinal tract of conventional and gnotobiotic piglets.

2. MATERIALS AND METHODS

2.1. Animals and Nutrition

Altogether, two experiments were carried out. The first experiment was conducted on 6 germ—free piglets and the second one on 11 conventional piglets. The piglets were divided into 3 groups, E, L, and M, in both experiments. In the first experiment, gnotobiotic piglets were fed dried whole milk (PMV, Hradec Králové, Czech Republic) four times a day, ad libitum. In the second experiment, conventional piglets had ad libitum access to a maternal milk.

2.2. Inoculation of Pigs and Administration of Maltodextrin

Piglets of all groups in each of the experiments were inoculated with *Escherichia coli* 08: K88 at the age of 5 days. During the experiments, the piglets of groups L and

M were inoculated daily with *Lactobacillus casei subsp. casei*. In addition to that, maltodextrin KMS X-70 (JEP CEREPA, Červená Řečice, Czech Republic) was administered to the piglets of group M in each of the experiments. The *Lactobacillus casei* strain was selected from 81 strains which were isolated from the gut contents of healthy suckling piglets, 7–14 days old, on the basis of the most pronounced in vitro inhibitory effect against enterotoxigenic *E. coli*. The *E. coli* inoculum contained 1×10^5 germs in 1 ml and the *L. casei* inoculum 1×10^8 germs in 1 ml volume. Inocula were administered to animals once a day at a dose of 2 ml. Maltodextrin KMS X-70 was administered to piglets once a day at a dose of 1 g in the first experiment. In the second experiment, maltodextrin KMS X-70 was administered to the piglets four times per day at a dose 0.3 g.

2.3. Biological Material and Chemical Analyses

Samples of blood were taken from piglets at the age of 7 days. Pigs of all groups were slaughtered at the age of 7 days, i.e. 2 days after *E. coli* inoculation. Immediately after slaughter samples were obtained of the jejunum, ileum and colon (10 cm^2) and their contents. Tissue samples were taken into 0.15 M PBS (ph 7.2), cooled to 4°C for 30 minutes, then the tissue samples were washed 3 times and homogenized in the homogenizators under 5000 rotations. Selective Rogosa agar and Mc Conkey agar were used to culture Lactobacillus and *E. coli* counts, respectively.

pH was measured by pH meter (LP Prague, Czech Republic). The concentration of lactic and acetic acids in the intestinal content was determined by capillary isotachophoresis on a capillary isotachophoresis analyzer (Radioecological Institute, Košice, Slovakia). Hydrochloric acid 0.001 mmol/l (pH 4.25) and capronic acid 5 mmol/l (pH 4.5) were used as conducting and finishing electrolytes, respectively. Number of leukocytes in the blood was determined using common haematological methods. A MSHP test (microsphaeric haematological particles test, manufactured by ARTIM Prague, Czech Republic) was used to determine the phagocytic activity of leukocytes in the blood. Phagocytic activity of leukocytes was determined by the method of Toman and Pšikal (1985). Heparinized blood was incubated with MSHP particles at 37°C for 60 minutes. MSHP particles were in vitro phagocyted by leukocytes. Phagocytic activity (FA) of leukocytes was estimated as the percentage of phagocyting leukocytes from the whole number of leukocytes. The index of phagocytic activity (IFA) was determined as average number of MSHP particles phagocyted by one potential phagocyte. The t-test was employed for statistical evaluation.

3. RESULTS

In the first experiment, the counts of *E. coli* 08: K88 adhered to the jejunal and ileal mucosa of 7 day old gnotobiotic pigs reached 5.96 and 6.67 log 10/cm^2 in the group E, 5.94 and 6.31 log 10/cm^2 in the group L, 4.95 and 6.27 log 10/cm^2 in the group M, respectively (Fig. 1). The pH values of the content of jejunum and ileum were 6.55 and 6.26 in the group E, 6.65 and 6.63 in the group L, 6.23 and 5.92 in the group M, respectively. The concentration of lactic acid in the jejunum and ileum was 29.96 and 72.33 mmol/l in the group E, 29.04 and 62.40 mmol/l in the group L, 39.0 and 37.60 mmol/l in the group M, respectively. The concentration of acetic acid in the jejunum and ileum was 23.4 and 46.7 mmol/l in the group E, 21.10 and 35.50 mmol/l in the group L, 24.0

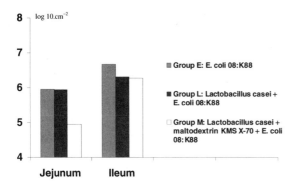

Figure 1. The numbers of *E. coli* 08: K88 adhered to the jejunal and ileal mucosa in 7 days old gnotobiotic pigs after administration of *Lactobacillus casei* and maltodextrin KMS X-70.

and 21.0 mmol/l in the group M, respectively. The differences between groups were insignificant.

In the second experiment, the numbers of total *E. coli* adhered to the jejunal, ileal, and colonic mucosa of 7 day old conventional pigs reached 7.42, 7.41, and 7.33 $\log 10/cm^2$ in the group E, 7.05, 7.65, and 7.34 $\log 10/cm^2$ in the group L, 4.75, 7.48, and 6.92 $\log 10/cm^2$ in the group M, respectively. The number of *E. coli* adhered to jejunal mucosa was significantly lower ($p < 0.05$) in the piglets of group M in comparison with the group E. The pH values of the content of jejunum and ileum were 6.40 and 6.94 in the group E, 6.57 and 7.44 in the group L, 6.21 and 7.44 in the group M, respectively. The concentration of lactic acid in the jejunum and ileum was 19.7 and 14.5 mmol/l in the group E, 11.42 and 12.26 mmol/l in the group L, 8.56 and 7.15 mmol/l in the group M, respectively. The concentration of acetic acid in the jejunum and ileum reached 34.45 and 47.33 mmol/l in the group E, 17.7 and 29.22 mmol/l in the group L, 9.77 and 26.04 mmol/l in the group M, respectively.

Of the conventional piglets, the highest numbers of leukocytes, lymphocytes and neutrophils were detected in the group of piglets preventively inoculated with lactobacilli with an addition of maltodextrin (group M). The comparison with the control (group E) showed significantly ($p < 0.05$) higher phagocytic activity (FA) and index of

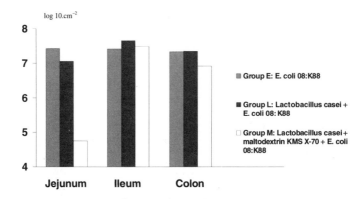

Figure 2. The numbers of *E. coli* 08: K88 adhered to the intestinal mucosa in 7 day old conventional pigs after administration of *Lactobacillus casei* and maltodextrin KMS X-70.

phagocytic activity (IFA) in piglets inoculated with lactobacilli (group L), while the addition of maltodextrin (group M) caused increase only in phagocytic activity.

4. DISCUSSION

The experiments showed that the preventive administration of *L. casei* alone resulted in only slight inhibitory effect on the adhesion of *E. coli* to jejunal mucosa, while *L. casei* administered in combination with maltodextrin decreased the number of *E. coli* colonizing jejunal mucosa by 1 logarithm in gnotobiotic pigs and by more than two and a half logarithm in conventional pigs. No significant differences between the groups were detected in the ileum and colon. Probiotics as natural bio-regulators help to mantain the balance of intestinal microflora by means of several mechanisms, such as competition for intestinal mucosa receptors, competition for nutrients, production of antibacterial substances and stimulation of immunity (Ávila et al., 1995; Vandenbergh, 1993). Our previous studies (Bomba et al., 1996; Bomba et al., 1997) showed that the competition for adhesion receptors on the intestinal mucosa did not play an important role in the mechanism of inhibiting enterotoxigenic *E. coli* by lactobacilli. More likely, it appears to be a metabolite—mediated inhibition. In our experiments on gnotobiotic pigs inoculated with lactobacilli, the levels of organic acids in the mucosal film of the jejunum and ileum were found to be higher than in the content. The significantly increased levels of organic acids in the mucosal film may present an efficient barrier inhibiting the adherence of digestive tract pathogens to the intestinal mucosa. Rodtong et al. (1993) and Watkins et al. (1982) concluded that lactobacilli can increase the concentration of organic acids, decreased pH in the intestine and thus inhibit the growth of bacteria, particularly of those which are pathogenic. In our study, lower numbers of *E. coli* and at the same time lower values of pH and higher concentrations of lactic and acetic acid were observed only in gnotobiotic pigs.

Perdigon et al. (1988) stated that application of probiotics stimulates cellular and humoral immunity. An increase in phagocytic activity and production of serum antibodies was observed (Lessard and Brisson, 1987). A stimulative effect of lactobacilli on the intestinal imunity in piglets was recorded (Tortuero et al., 1995). In our study, the phagocytic activity and the index of phagocytic activity reached significantly higher values in conventional piglets inoculated with *L. casei* in comparison with those in the control group. The administration of *L. casei* with maltodextrin increased only phagocytic activity. The results obtained indicated that the inhibitory effect of *Lactobacillus casei* and maltodextrin KMS X-70 on the adhesion of *E. coli* to the jejunal mucosa of gnotobiotic and conventional pigs was probably mediated by production of antibacterial substances and stimulation of immunity.

5. CONCLUSIONS

In conclusion, the continuous preventive administration of *L. casei* had only slight inhibitory effect on the adhesion of *E. coli* to the intestinal mucosa of gnotobiotic and conventional piglets. Maltodextrin KMS X-70 stimulated the inhibitory effect of *L. casei* on the adhesion of *E. coli* to the jejunal mucosa of gnotobiotic and conventional piglets. The inhibitory effect of *L. casei* and maltodextrin on the adhesion of *E. coli* to the jejunal mucosa of piglets was probably mediated by production of antibacterial substances and stimulation of imunity.

ACKNOWLEDGMENTS

The authors gratefully acknowledge the assistance of Kristína Ondrejová, Jana Karaffová and Ol'ga Hanzelová in the care of the animals. This work was financed by the Ministry of Agriculture of Slovak Republic.

REFERENCES

Ávila, F.A., Paulillo, A.C., Schocken-Iturrino, R.P., Lucas, F.A., Orgaz, A., and Quintana, J.L., 1995, A comparative study of the efficiency of a probiotic and the anti-A 14 vaccines in the control of diarrhea in calves in Brazil, Revue Élev. Méd. Vét. Pays trop. 48:239–243.

Bertschinger, H.U., Moon, H.W., and Whipp, S.C., 1972, Asociation of *Escherichia coli* with the small intestinal epithelium. I. Comparison of enteropathogenic and nonenteropathogenic porcine strains in pigs, Infect. Immun. 5:595–605.

Bomba, A., Kaštel', R., Gancarčíková, S., Nemcová, R., Herich, R., and Čížek, M., 1996, The effect of *Lactobacilli* inoculation on organic acid levels in the mucosal film and the small intestine contents in gnotobiotic pigs, Berl. Munch. Tierärztl. Wschr. 109:428–430.

Bomba, A., Kravjanský, I., Kaštel', R., Herich, R., Juhásová, Z., Čížek, M., and Kapitančík, B., 1997, Inhibitory effects of *Lactobacillus casei* upon the adhesion of enterotoxigenic *Escherichia coli* K 99 to the intestinal mucosa in gnotobiotic lambs, Small Rum. Res. 23:199–206.

Fairbrother, J.M., 1993, Les colibaciloses du porc, Ann. Méd. Vét. 137:369–375.

Fuller, R., 1989, Probiotics in man and animals, J. Appl. Bacteriol. 66:365–378.

Jones, G.W. and Rutter, J.M., 1972, Role of the K 88 antigen in the pathogenesis of neonatal diarrhea caused by *Escherichia coli* in piglets, Infect. Immun. 6:918–927.

Jonsson, E. and Conway, P., 1992, Probiotics for pigs, In: Probiotics the scientific basis, Editor: Fuller, R., Chapman and Hall, London, UK, P. 260–316.

Lessard, M. and Brisson, G.J., 1987, Effect of a *Lactobacillus* fermentation producton growth, imune response and fecal enzyme activity in weaned pigs, Can. J. Anim. Sci. 67:509–516.

Perdigon, G., Nader De Macias, M.E., Alvarez, S., Oliver, G., and Pesce De Ruiz Holgado, A., 1988, Systemic augmentation of immune response in mice by feeding fermented milks with *Lactobacillus casei* and *Lactobacillus acidophilus*, Immunology 63:17–23.

Rodtong, S., Dobbinson, S., Thode-Andersen, S., Mc Connell, M., and Tannock, G., 1993, Derivation of DNA probes for enumeration of a specific strain of *Lactobacillus acidophilus* in piglet digestive tract samples, Appl. Environ. Microbiol. 59:3871–3877.

Smith, H.W. and Gyles, C.L., 1970, The relationship between two apparently different enterotoxins produced by enteropathogenic strains of *Escherichia coli* of porcine origin, J., Med. Microbiol. 3:387–401.

Toman, M. and Pšikal, J., 1985, Test of phagocytic activity of leukocytes in blood of calves, Vet. Med. (Prague) 30:393–400.

Tortuero, F., Rioperez, J., Fernandez, E., and Rodriguez, M.L., 1995, Response of piglets to oral administration of Lactic acid bacteria, J. Food Protect. 58:1369–1374.

Vanderbergh, P.A., 1993, Lactic acid bacteria, their metabolic products and interference with microbial growth, FEMS Microbiol. Rev. 12:221–238.

Watkins, B.A., Muler, B.F., and Neil, D.H., 1982, In vivo inhibitory effect of *Lactobacillus acidophilus* against pathogenic *Escherichia coli* in gnotobiotic chicks, Poult. Sci. 61:1298–1308.

19

RECOVERY FROM COLONIC INFECTION ELICITS SERUM IgG ANTIBODIES TO SPECIFIC *SERPULINA PILOSICOLI* OUTER MEMBRANE ANTIGENS (SPOMA)

Peng Zhang, Nancy A. Witters, and Gerald E. Duhamel

Department of Veterinary and Biomedical Sciences
University of Nebraska-Lincoln
Lincoln, Nebraska 68583-0905

1. SUMMARY

Colonic spirochetosis caused by *S. pilosicoli* is a disease of human and animals characterized by intimate attachment of the spirochete to colonic epithelial cells and colitis. To identify antigens that are potentially involved in recovery from the disease, whole-cell lysate (WC) and various detergent extracts including Sarkosyl-soluble (SS) and insoluble (SI), and Triton X-114 detergent phase (TXD) and aqueous phase (TXA) of the human isolate SP16 were examined by Western blotting with *Serpulina* spp. periplasmic flagellar protein FlaB-specific monoclonal antibody 7G2 as well as pooled pre-immune serum (PS), hyperimmune serum (HS), and convalescent serum (CS) from swine. The HS reacted with several antigens that were not identified by the CS, including the periplasmic flagellar proteins and some lower molecular weight bands. The CS identified three major immunoreactive double (D) or single (S) bands of approximately: (i) 64-kDa in the WC(S), SS(D), and TXD/A(S), (ii) 54-kDa in the WC(S), SS/I(S), and TXD(S), and (iii) 47-kDa in the SS(S) fraction. The data indicate recovery from colonic infection elicits serum IgG antibodies to specific *S. pilosicoli* outer membrane antigens (SPOMA).

2. INTRODUCTION

In the early 1980's, investigations into the cause of a disease of growing pigs characterized by diarrhea and colitis identified certain spirochetes as the etiological agent

Mechanisms in the Pathogenesis of Enteric Diseases 2, edited by Paul and Francis.
Kluwer Academic / Plenum Publishers, New York, 1999.

(Taylor et al., 1980). The spirochete responsible for the disease of pigs designated intestinal or colonic spirochetosis (CS) has been recently classified as *Serpulina pilosicoli* (Duhamel et al., 1995; Trott et al., 1996). Since then, *S. pilosicoli* has been found in a broad range of hosts including human beings (Duhamel et al., 1995; Trivett-Moore et al., 1998), non-human primates (Duhamel, 1997; Duhamel et al., 1997), dogs (Duhamel et al., 1995; Duhamel, 1997; Duhamel et al., 1998), and several species of birds (Swayne and McLaren, 1997; Webb et al., 1997). A characteristic lesion of *S. pilosicoli* infection is intimate attachment of the spirochetes by one of their ends to the apical membrane of colonic enterocytes and invasion of the colonic mucosa (Duhamel, 1997; Trivett-Moore et al., 1998). Spirochetemia has been documented in critically ill human patients, some of whom had a history of intestinal disease (Trott et al., 1997).

The outer-membrane of pathogenic bacteria contains antigens that are involved in the generation of a protective immune response against infection (Rapp et al., 1986; Udhayakumar et al., 1987). Therefore, vaccination may be an effective intervention strategy for control of CS, but development of an efficacious vaccine for this disease is hindered by the lack of information on the immunogenic moieties involved in protection. The purpose of this study was to identify antigens of *S. pilosicoli* that are potentially involved in recovery from CS. Comparative analysis of hyperimmune and convalescent swine sera with whole-cell and various detergent extracts by Western blot revealed three major *S. pilosicoli* outer membrane antigens (SPOMA) that may be relevant to recovery from the disease.

3. MATERIALS AND METHODS

3.1. Bacterial Strains and Growth Conditions

Serpulina pilosicoli isolate SP16 (American Type Culture Collection [ATCC] 49776; Duhamel et al., 1995), obtained from an HIV-positive homosexual male with CS, was provided by R. M. Smibert (Virginia Polytechnic Institute, Blacksburg, VA). Porcine *S. pilosicoli* isolates B359 and B1555a were obtained from J. M. Kinyon, Iowa State University, Ames (Ramanathan et al., 1993; Muniappa et al., 1997). *Serpulina pilosicoli* isolate UNL-8 was isolated from a pig with CS and characterized in our laboratory (Muniappa et al., 1997; Duhamel, 1998). The spirochetes were propagated in prereduced anaerobically-sterilized Trypticase soy broth supplemented with 2% (vol/vol) fetal bovine serum as previously described (Ramanathan et al., 1993).

3.2. Convalescent and Hyperimmune Swine Sera

Convalescent serum (CS) was produced by oral inoculation of 5-week old conventional pigs with *S. pilosicoli* isolate UNL-8 as previously described (Duhamel, 1998). Equal volumes of sera collected prior to inoculation (pre-immune serum; PS) and at necropsy on day 49 post-inoculation of two pigs that developed diarrhea and shed *S. pilosicoli* in their feces, but became culture negative and had no colonic lesions at necropsy were pooled together. Hyperimmune sera (HS) were produced by oral inoculation of Specific Pathogen Free pigs with broth cultures containing approximately 5×10^{10} *S. pilosicoli* isolate B359 or isolate B1555a for three consecutive days. Seven weeks later, and for the next four weeks, each pig received weekly booster injections containing increasing protein concentrations, from 1, 2, 4, and 8 mg of the corresponding sonicated whole-cell antigen, respectively. The first and second boosters were mixed with an equal volume of Freund's incomplete adjuvant and administered by intramuscular and subcutaneous injections. Subsequent boosters were without adjuvant and administered intravenously. The pigs were euthanized three weeks after the last booster and equal volumes of each serum were pooled. The experimental protocols for animal experimentations were approved by the University's Institutional Animal Care and Use Committee. The presence of *S. pilosicoli*-specific immunoglobulin (Ig) G antibodies in the PS, CS, and HS was determined using a whole-cell enzyme-linked immunosobent assay (ELISA) as previously described (Fisher et al., 1990). Briefly, 5×10^5 late logarithmic phase *S. pilosicoli* isolate SP16 in phosphate-buffered saline (PBS) pH 7.4 were fixed to each well of 96-well polystyrene microtiter plates (Corning Costar Co., Cambridge, MA) with glutaraldehyde. After blocking with 1% polyvinyl alcohol in PBS (PVA/PBS), each serum pool was serially diluted 2-fold in PVA/PBS and applied to duplicate wells. After incubation and washing with PBS with 0.05% (vol/vol) Tween 20 (Sigma, St. Louis, MO), the antigen-specific antibody complexes were detected by adding peroxidase labeled goat anti-swine IgG (heavy and light chains) antibodies and substrate (Kirkegaard and Perry Laboratories Inc., Gaithersburg, MD). The end point titer was calculated as the last dilution which gave an optical density value at 405/490 nm greater than or equal to the optical density of the PS using an automated plate reader (Dynatech Laboratories Inc. Chantilly, VA). To remove non-specific reactivity, the pooled swine sera were absorbed with *Escherichia coli* DH5α before Western blotting.

3.3. Whole-Cell and Detergent Extracts

After washing with 0.05 M Tris-HCl pH 7.0, whole-cell (WC) lysate of *S. pilosicoli* isolate SP16 was prepared by solubilizing cells in distilled water with an equal volume of 2X sodium dodecyl sulfate (SDS) buffer (125 mM Tris-HCl [pH 6.8], 4% SDS, 5% β-mercaptoethanol, 20% glycerol, 0.005% bromophenol blue) and heating at 100°C for 5 min. Detergent extracts of isolate SP16 were prepared using the ionic detergent sodium *N*-lauroyl sarcosinate (Sarkosyl, Sigma) and designated Sarkosyl-soluble (SS) and Sarkosyl-insoluble (SI), as previously described (Carlone et al., 1986). Phase partitioning with the nonionic detergent Triton X-114 was done by the method of Bordier (1981), and the fraction containing amphiphilic integral membrane proteins was designated Triton X-114 detergent phase (TXD) and the fraction containing hydrophilic proteins was designated Triton X-114 aqueous phase (TXA).

3.4. SDS Polyacrylamide Gel Electrophoresis (SDS-PAGE)

Each bacterial preparation (10–15 μg) was mixed with an equal volume of $2 \times$ SDS buffer and heated at 100°C for 5 min, loaded in each lane of 10% SDS-polyacrylamide gels and electrophoresed in 25 mM Tris-192 mM glycine-0.1% SDS, pH 8.5 at 30 mA constant current until the dye maker was within 3–4 mm of the bottom of the gel. After separation, the proteins were electrotransferred to a nitrocellulose membrane (0.2-μm pore size; Midwest Scientific, Valley Park, MI) in 25 mM glycine-192 mM Tris-HCl-20% methanol with a TRANS-BLOT Cell (Bio-Rad, Hercules, CA) at a constant current of 0.8 mA/cm^2 for 1 h (Ausubel et al., 1990).

3.5. Western Blotting (Immunoblotting)

The immunoblots were completed as previously described (Fisher et al., 1997). Briefly, the membranes were blocked with wash buffer (50mM Tris-base [pH 7.5], 150 mM NaCl, 5mM $MgCl_2$, 5% nonfat dry milk, 0.05% Nonidet P-40) for 2h and incubated with either the *Serpulina* spp. periplasmic flagellar protein FlaB-specific monoclonal antibody 7G2 (Fisher et al., 1997), or the pre-absorbed PS (1:100), HS (1:400), or CS (1:100) for 2h at room temperature with rocking, followed by biotin-labeled goat anti-swine IgG (heavy and light chains) or anti-mouse IgM and IgG (heavy and light chains) antibodies, peroxidase labeled streptavidin, and 4-chloro-1-naphthol (Kirkegaard and Perry Laboratories Inc.). Three 5-min washes with wash buffer were performed between each incubation step.

4. RESULTS AND DISCUSSION

The HS and CS before absorbtion with *E. coli* had end point titers of 2,400 and 400, respectively. Immunoreactive bands of approximately 37-, 34-, and 32-kDa that

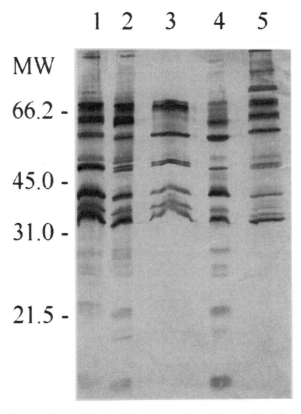

Figure 1. SDS-PAGE and immunoblotting of various preparations of human *Serpulina pilosicoli* isolate SP16 with pooled hyperimmune swine serum pre-absobed with *Escherichia coli* DH5α followed by biotin-labeled goat anti-swine IgG (H + L), peroxidase labeled streptavidin, and 4-chloro-1-naphthol substrate. Lane 1, whole-cell lysate; lane 2, sodium N-lauroylsarcosine-soluble; lane 3, sodium N-lauroylsarcosine-insoluble; lane 4, Triton X-114 detergent phase; lane 5, Triton X-114 aqueous phase. MW, molecular weight (in thousands).

presumably corresponded to the periplasmic flagellar proteins FlaB1, FlaB2, and FlaB3 respectively, were present in the WC, SS, SI, and TXA by immunoblotting with the monoclonal antibody 7G2 (data not shown). Immunoblotting with the absorbed PS revealed a single immunoreactive 68-kDa band with WC and each of the detergent extracts except the SI fraction (data not shown). The immunoreactivity of pre-absorbed HS was similar with WC, SS, and TXD and revealed 4 major immunoreactive double bands of approximately 72-, 64-, 54-, and 47-kDa in addition to the FlaB antigens (Fig. 1). Approximately 12 additional immunoreactive bands of lower intensity and less than 32-kDa also were present in these fractions. The SI and TXA fractions had fewer immunoreactive bands; the 64-kDa band was absent from the SI fraction, and a single 54-kDa band was present in the SI and TXA.

The CS identified three major immunoreactive double (D) or single (S) bands of approximately: (i) 64-kDa in the WC(S), SS(D), and TXD/A(S), (ii) 54-kDa in the WC(S), SS/I(S), and TXD(S), and (iii) 47-kDa in the SS(S) fraction.

The data indicate that recovery from colonic infection elicits serum IgG antibodies to specific *S. pilosicoli* outer membrane antigens (SPOMA). The HS reacted with several antigens that were not identified by the CS, including the periplasmic flagellar proteins and some lower molecular weight bands. At least four major antigens different from the flagellar proteins were identified using the HS. However, only 3 of the 4 immunoreactive bands also were identified with CS suggesting that these antigens are potentially involved in recovery from infection. The exact nature and relationship of each immunoreactive band present in different detergent extracts remain to be determined.

Laboratory mice experimentally infected with *S. pilosicoli* display a serum IgG response to *S. pilosicoli* 16- to 24-kDa antigens, presumably lipooligosaccharides, as well

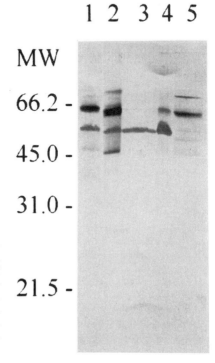

Figure 2. SDS-PAGE and immunoblotting of various preparations of human *Serpulina pilosicoli* isolate SP16 with pooled convalescent swine serum pre-absobed with *Escherichia coli* DH5α followed by biotin-labeled goat anti-swine IgG (H + L), peroxidase labeled streptavidin, and 4-chloro-1-naphthol substrate. Lane 1, whole-cell lysate; lane 2, sodium N-lauroylsarcosine-soluble; lane 3, sodium N-lauroylsarcosine-insoluble; lane 4, Triton X-114 detergent phase; lane 5, Triton X-114 aqueous phase. MW, molecular weight (in thousands).

as several antigens between 33- and 47-kDa, 30 to 45 days post-infection (Sacco et al., 1997). An earlier report suggested a lack of demonstrable serum antibody response in pigs three weeks after challenge-inoculation with *S. pilosicoli* (La et al., 1998). However, these results are easily reconciled when considering the incubation period for CS which can take up to three weeks post-inoculation. Thus in light of the present results and those of Sacco and coworkers (1997), we concluded that specific antibodies to *S. pilosicoli* antigens are elicited during colonic infection with *S. pilosicoli*. The present report further indicate recovery from infection elicits a serum IgG antibody response to a limited number of SPOMA.

ACKNOWLEDGMENTS

The authors thank M. R. Mathiesen for her technical assistance. The research was supported in part by funds provided by the U.S. Department of Agriculture, Regional Research Project NC-62, Enteric Diseases of Swine and Cattle: Prevention, Control, and Food Safety.

REFERENCES

Ausubel F.M., Brent R., Kingston R.E., Moore D.D., Seidman J.G., Smith J.A., and Struhl K., 1990, Current protocols in molecular biology. Vol. 1. New York: Wiley Interscience.

Bordier, C., 1981, Phase separation of integral membrane proteins in Triton X-114 solution. J. Biol. Chem. 256:1604–1607.

Carlone, G.M., Thomas, M.L., Rumschlag, H.S., and Sottnek, F.O., 1986, Rapidmicroprocedure for isolating detergent-insoluble outer membrane proteins from *Heamophilus* species. J. Clin. Microbiol. 24:330–332.

Duhamel, G.E., Muniappa, N., Mathiesen, M.R., Johnson, J.L., Toth, J., Elder, R.O., and Doster, A.R., 1995, Certain canine weakly beta-hemolytic intestinal spirochetes are phenotypically and genotypically related to spirochetes associated with human and porcine intestinal spirochetosis. J. Clin. Microbiol. 33:2211–2215.

Duhamel, G.E., 1997, Intestinal spirochaetes in non-production animals, In: Intestinalspirochaetosis in domestic animals and humans. Editors: Hampson, D.J. and Stanton, T.B., CAB International, Wallingford, UK, pp. 301–320.

Duhamel, G.E., Elder, R.O., Muniappa, N., Mathiesen, M.R., Wong, V.J., and Tarara, R.P., 1997, Colonic spirochetal infections in nonhuman primates that were associated with *Brachyspira aalborgi, Serpulina pilosicoli*, and unclassified flagellated bacteria. Clin. Infect. Dis. 25(Suppl. 2):S186–S188.

Duhamel, G.E., 1998, Colonic spirochetosis caused by *Serpulina pilosicoli*. Large Animal Pract. 19:14–22.

Duhamel, G.E., Trott, D.J., Muniappa, N., Mathiesen, M.R., Tarasiuk, K., Lee, J.I., and Hampson, D.J., 1998, Canine intestinal spirochetes consist of *Serpulina pilosicoli* and a newly identified group provisionally designated "*Serpulina canis*" sp. nov. J. Clin. Microbiol. 36:2264–2270.

Fisher, L.N., Duhamel, G.E., Mathiesen, M.R., and Bernard, R.J., 1990, Developmentand evaluation of a whole-cell ELISA for detection of serum antibodies to *Treponema hyodysenteriae* in swine. 71st Ann. Mtg. Conf. Res. Wkrs Anim. Dis., Chicago, Ill., p. 13.

Fisher, L.N., Duhamel, G.E., Westerman, R.B., and Mathiesen, M.R., 1997, Immunoblotreactivity of polyclonal and monoclonal antibodies with periplasmic flagellar proteins FlaA1 and FlaB of porcine *Serpulina* species. Clin. Diagn. Lab. Immun. 4:400–404.

La, T., Penhale, W.J., and Hampson, D.J., 1998, Lack of a significant systemic immuneresponse in pigs experimentally infected with *Serpulina pilosicoli*. Proc. 15th Int. Pig Vet. Soc. Conf. 3:131.

Muniappa, N., Mathiesen, M.R., and Duhamel, G.E., 1997, Laboratory identification and enteropathogenicity testing of *Serpulina pilosicoli* associated with porcine colonic spirochetosis. J. Vet. Diagn. Invest. 9:165–171.

Ramanathan M., Duhamel G.E., Mathiesen M.R., and Messier S., 1993, Identification and partial character-ization of a group of weakly β-hemolytic intestinal spirochetes of swine distinct from *Serpulina innocens,* isolate B256. Vet. Microbiol. 37:53–64.

Rapp, V.J. and Ross, R.F., 1986, Antibody response of swine to outer membrane components of *Haemophilus pleuropneumoniae* during infection. Infect. Immun. 54:751–760.

Sacco, R.E., Trampel, D.W., and Wannemuehler, M.J., 1997, Experimental infection of C3H mice with avian, porcine, or human isolates of *Serpulina pilosicoli.* Infect. Immun. 65:5349–5353.

Swayne, D.E. and McLaren, A.J., 1997, Avian intestinal spirochaetes and avian intestinal spirochaetosis, In: Intestinal spirochaetosis in domestic animals and humans, Editors: Hampson, D.J. and Stanton, T.B., CAB International, Wallingford, UK, pp. 267–300.

Taylor, D.J., Simmons, J.R., and Laird, H.M., 1980, Production of diarrhoea and dysentery in pigs by feeding pure cultures of a spirochaete differing from *Treponema hyodysenteriae.* Vet. Rec. 106:326–332.

Trivett-Moore, N.L., Gilbert, G.L., Law, C.L.H., Trott, D.J., and Hampson, D.J., 1998, Isolation of *Serpulina pilosicoli* from rectal biopsy specimens showing evidence of intestinal spirochetosis. J. Clin. Microbiol. 36:261–265.

Trott, D.J., Stanton, T.B., Jensen, N.S., Duhamel, G.E., Johnson, J.L., and Hampson, D.J., 1996, *Serpulina pilosi-coli* sp. nov., the agent of porcine intestinal spirochetosis. Int. J. Syst. Bacteriol. 46:206–215.

Trott, D.J., Jensen, N.S., Saint Girons, I., Oxberry, S.L., Stanton, T.B., Lindquist, D., and Hampson, D.J., 1997, Identification and characterization of *Serpulina pilosicoli* isolates recovered from the blood of criti-cally ill patients. J. Clin. Microbiol. 35:482–485.

Udhayakumar, V. and Muthukkaruppan, R., 1987, Protective immunity induced by outer membrane proteins of *Salmonella typhimurium* in mice. Infect. Immun. 55:816–821.

Webb, D.M., Duhamel, G.E., Mathiesen, M.R., Muniappa, N., and White, A.K., 1997, Cecal spirochetosis associated with *Serpulina pilosicoli* in captive juvenile ring-necked pheasants. Avian Dis. 41:997–1002.

20

MOTILITY-REGULATED MUCIN ASSOCIATION OF *SERPULINA PILOSICOLI*, THE AGENT OF COLONIC SPIROCHETOSIS OF HUMANS AND ANIMALS

Nancy A. Witters and Gerald E. Duhamel

Department of Veterinary and Biomedical Sciences
University of Nebraska-Lincoln
Lincoln, Nebraska 68583-0905

1. SUMMARY

Colonic spirochetosis is a disease of humans and animals characterized by colonization of the colonic mucus gel and intimate attachment of *Serpulina pilosicoli* to the apical membrane of enterocytes. Motility-regulated mucin association plays a key role in colonic infection by the related spirochete *Serpulina hyodysenteriae*, the cause of swine dysentery. In this study the chemotaxis of *Serpulina pilosicoli* porcine isolate P43/6/78, human isolate SP16, and canine isolate 16242-94 was examined by anaerobic incubation of each spirochete in control medium or medium containing increasing concentrations of D-L serine or porcine gastric mucin (PGM). The porcine isolate had a chemotactic response towards 10 mM D-L serine, but not towards PGM. By contrast, the human and canine isolates were attracted towards 0.1% PGM, but not towards DL-serine. The composition of the growth medium appeared to modulate the chemotactic response of *S. pilosicoli* towards PGM; the loss of a chemotactic response of spirochetes grown in medium without pig fecal extract was restored by growing the spirochetes in medium containing 0.1% PGM. *Serpulina pilosicoli* displays a chemotactic response towards PGM which is modulated by the presence of certain substrate during the growth phase of the spirochete.

2. INTRODUCTION

Serpulina pilosicoli is a Gram negative, anaerobic, but oxygen tolerant spirochete found in the colon of a broad range of hosts, including human beings, non-human

Mechanisms in the Pathogenesis of Enteric Diseases 2, edited by Paul and Francis.
Kluwer Academic / Plenum Publishers, New York, 1999.

199

primates, swine, dogs, and several species of birds (Duhamel et al., 1995; Trott et al., 1996a; Duhamel, 1997; Swayne and McLaren, 1997; Trott et al., 1997; Duhamel, 1998; Duhamel et al., 1998; Trivett-Moore et al., 1998; Johnston et al., 1998). Isolates from different hosts are genetically closely related and cause colonic spirochetosis (CS) a disease characterized by colonization of the colonic mucus gel and intimate attachment of the spirochetes by one of their ends to the apical membrane of enterocytes. Reproduction of CS lesions in chicks, laboratory mice and swine with isolates obtained from humans, non-human primates, dogs, swine, and birds suggest the potential for transmission between different hosts (Trott et al., 1995; Muniappa et al., 1996; Trott et al., 1996b; Muniappa et al., 1997; Sacco et al., 1997; Muniappa et al., 1998).

Colonization of the mucosal surface of the intestine by pathogenic bacteria involves the interplay between motility and chemotaxis (Allweiss et al., 1977; Hugdahl et al., 1988; Milner and Sellwood, 1994). Mucin chemotaxis plays a critical role in mucosal localization of *Campylobacter jejuni*, a major cause of enteric disease of humans and animals (Hugdahl et al., 1988). Similarly, motility-regulated mucin association is the predominant mechanism of mucosal association for *Serpulina hyodysenteriae*, a spirochete that causes swine dysentery (Milner and Sellwood, 1994; Kennedy and Yancey, 1996). Virulent strains of *S. hyodysenteriae* are attracted towards mucin, and major components of mucin, including the polypeptide backbone amino acid serine, and the terminal sugar of the O-linked oligosaccharide side chain fucose (Milner and Sellwood, 1994; Kennedy and Yancey, 1996). Because *S. pilosicoli* is different from *S. hyodysenteriae*, *S. pilosicoli* might respond differentially to mucin and mucin components. The purpose of this study was to assess the chemotactic response of *S. pilosicoli* towards mucin and serine. A potential relationship between the composition of the growth medium and the chemotactic response of *S. pilosicoli* also was examined. A better understanding of *S. pilosicoli* chemotaxis will help define the pathogenesis of CS and lead to possible early intervention strategies for prevention of the disease.

3. MATERIALS AND METHODS

3.1. Bacterial Strains

The reference porcine *S. pilosicoli* isolate P43/6/78[T] (American Type Culture Collection [ATCC] 51139; Trott et al., 1996a) was provided by T.B. Stanton, National Animal Disease Center, Ames, Iowa. *Serpulina pilosicoli* isolate SP16 (ATCC 49776; Duhamel et al., 1995), obtained from an HIV-positive homosexual male with CS, was provided by R.M. Smibert (Virginia Polytechnic Institute, Blacksburg, VA). The canine *S. pilosicoli* isolate 16242-94 was isolated in our laboratory from a puppy with CS and giardiasis (Duhamel et al., 1995; Muniappa et al., 1996; Duhamel et al., 1996; Duhamel et al., 1998).

3.2. Growth Conditions

The spirochetes were propagated in pre-reduced anaerobically-sterilized (PRAS) medium containing 5.0% (v/v) pig fecal extract (PFE) as previously described (Ramanathan et al., 1993). To determine whether the composition of the growth medium had an effect on the chemotactic response of *S. pilosicoli* towards porcine gastric mucin (PGM), the responses of the porcine and the human spirochete isolates harvested after three passages in PRAS medium without PFE were compared with that of the fifth passage without PFE but supplemented with 0.1% (w/v) PGM (Sigma, St. Louis, MO).

3.3. Chemotaxis Assays

The chemotaxis assays were done using a modification of previously described methods (Kennedy and Yancey, 1996; Milner and Sellwood, 1994). Solutions of attractants consisting of either 100.0 mM, 10.0 mM, 1.0 mM, or 0.1 mM DL-serine (Sigma), and either 1.0%, 0.1%, or 0.01% PGM were prepared in normal saline (NS; 0.9% [w/v] NaCl) under an atmosphere of 10% hydrogen, 10% carbon dioxide, and 80% nitrogen, and autoclaved. Mid- to late-logarithmic phase cultures of *S. pilosicoli* (approx. 10^9 cells/ml) were harvested by centrifugation at $1800 \times g$ for 15 min, washed twice in NS, and adjusted to approximately 1×10^9 per ml under anaerobic conditions. After incubating the spirochetes for 15 min at 37°C under constant stirring, 250 µl volumes were placed in each well of a chemotaxis chamber (Palleroni, 1976; Kelly-Wintenberg and Montie, 1994). In each assay, duplicate capillary tubes (5×23 mm, Scientific Manufacturing Industries, Emeryville, CA) containing 5 µl volumes of either attractant or NS control were incubated anaerobically for 1 h at 37°C. At the end of the incubation period, the contents of each capillary tube was expelled into 50 µl of NS, mixed, and the chemotaxis index (R_{che}) was calculated as the ratio of the mean number of spirochetes in the attractant capillaries over the mean number in the control capillaries as determined by direct microscope counts (Petroff-Hausser counting chamber; Hausser Scientific Partnership, Horsham, PA). Each isolate was examined for chemotaxis towards each concentration of attractant in at least three separate experiments. An R_{che} value >2 was considered significant (Moulton and Montie, 1979).

4. RESULTS AND DISCUSSION

The close association of *S. pilosicoli* with the cecal and colonic mucus gel suggests a role for chemotaxis or motility-regulated mucin association as a key early event in CS (Trott et al., 1995; Muniappa et al., 1996; Trott et al., 1996b; Muniappa et al., 1997; Sacco et al., 1997; Swayne and Mc Laren, 1997; Duhamel, 1998; Muniappa et al., 1998; Johnston et al., 1998; Trivett-Moore et al., 1998). The lack of chemotactic response of porcine isolate P43/6/78 towards PGM was consistent with previous observations with the same isolate (Milner and Sellwood, 1994). Conversely, the presence of a chemotactic response towards 10 mM DL-serine suggested that isolate P43/6/78 has functional sensory transduction mechanisms for motility and chemotaxis. By contrast, the human and the canine isolates had R_{che} values >2 with 0.1% PGM, but not with any concentration of DL-serine. The magnitude of the chemotactic responses of these isolates towards PGM was similar to previous observations with *S. hyodysenteriae* (Kennedy and Yancey, 1996). On the basis of these observations, a role for mucin chemotaxis in the pathogenesis of CS appears likely. As suggested from studies with other mucosal pathogens, a relationship between chemotaxis and virulence may exist among *S. pilosicoli* isolates (Allweiss et al., 1977; Hugdahl et al., 1988; Milner and Sellwood, 1994).

Passage of the human *S. pilosicoli* in medium without PFE resulted in a loss of the chemotactic response towards PGM. However, supplementation of the growth

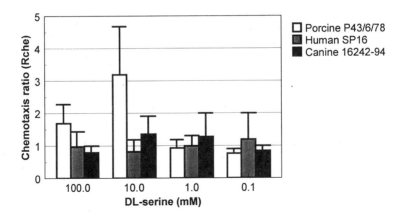

Figure 1. Chemotaxis of *Serpulina pilosicoli* isolates towards various concentrations of DL-serine. Each bar represents the mean and standard deviation of the R_{che} for at least three separate experiments.

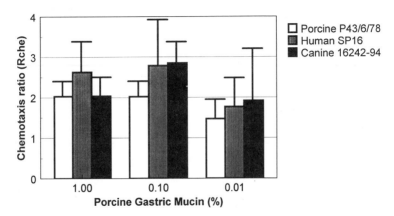

Figure 2. Chemotaxis of *Serpulina pilosicoli* isolates towards various concentrations of porcine gastric mucin. Each bar represents the mean and standard deviation of the R_{che} for at least three separate experiments.

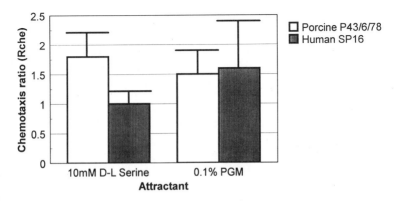

Figure 3. *Serpulina pilosicoli* isolates passaged three times in medium without pig fecal extract and examined for chemotaxis towards optimal concentrations of either DL-serine or porcine gastric mucin (PGM). Each bar represents the mean and standard deviation of the R_{che} for at least three separate experiments.

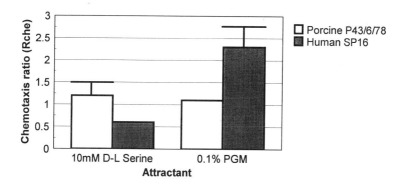

Figure 4. *Serpulina pilosicoli* isolates passaged in medium without pig fecal extract, but supplemented with 0.1% (w/v) porcine gastric mucin (PGM) on the fifth passage and examined for chemotaxis towards optimal concentrations of either DL-serine or PGM. Each bar represents the mean and standard deviation of the R_{che} for at least three separate experiments.

medium with PGM restored the chemotactic response of the human but not the porcine *S. pilosicoli* isolates towards PGM, suggesting that sensory transduction mechanisms associated with the chemotactic response of *S. pilosicoli* may be modulated by components present the gut environment.

Although susceptibility and resistance to bacterial enteric diseases is multifactorial, chemotaxis towards mucin appears to play a role in the pathogenesis of certain enteric bacterial infections (Allweiss et al., 1977; Hugdahl et al., 1988; Milner and Sellwood, 1994; Kennedy and Yancey, 1996). Mucin is the principal constituent of the colonic mucus-gel and consists of complex glycoproteins synthesized and secreted by goblet cells (Smith and Podolsky, 1986; Strous and Dekker, 1992). The primary function of mucin is to provide a selective diffusion barrier against penetration of the mucosa by bacteria, toxins, and dietary components. Variation in the physicochemical properties of mucin may account for differences in chemotactic responses to different mucin preparations, and perhaps susceptibility to disease among different hosts (Smith and Podolsky, 1986; Specian and Oliver, 1991; Strous and Dekker, 1992).

By analogy with *S. hyodysenteriae*, it appears that initial colonization of the colon by *S. pilosicoli* may be mediated by motility-regulated mucin association. As suggested from comparative studies with cultured cells and a chick infection model, attachment of *S. pilosicoli* involves a specific interaction between a spirochete ligand and a host cell membrane receptor (Muniappa et al., 1996; Muniappa et al., 1998). Movement of *S. pilosicoli* in close proximity to the mucosal epithelium may be required for establishment of intimate contacts between the spirochetes and the apical membrane of colonic enterocytes (Trott et al., 1995; Muniappa et al., 1996; Trott et al., 1996b; Duhamel, 1998; Johnston et al., 1998; Muniappa et al., 1998). Identification and molecular characterization of mediators and underlying mechanisms of motility-regulated chemotaxis in *S. pilosicoli* and contribution to disease require further investigation.

ACKNOWLEDGMENTS

The authors thank Kenneth W. Nickerson of the School of Biological Sciences for excellent technical assistance. This work was supported by funds from the University of Nebraska-Lincoln Agricultural Experiment Station, United States Department of Agriculture, Regional Research Project NC-62, Enteric Diseases of Swine and Cattle: Prevention, Control, and Food Safety.

REFERENCES

Allweiss, B., Dostal, J., Carey, K.E., Edwards, T.F., and Freter, R., 1977, The role of chemotaxis in the ecology of bacterial pathogens of mucosal surfaces. Nature, London 266:448–450.

Duhamel, G.E., Muniappa, N., Mathiesen, M.R., Johnson, J.L., Toth, J., Elder, R.O., and Doster, A.R., 1995, Certain canine weakly beta-hemolytic intestinal spirochetes are phenotypically and genotypically related to spirochetes associated with human and porcine intestinal spirochetosis. J. Clin. Microbiol. 33:2211–2215.

Duhamel, G.E., 1997, Intestinal spirochaetes in non-production animals, In: Intestinal spirochaetosis in domestic animals and humans. Editors: Hampson, D.J. and Stanton, T.B., CAB International, Wallingford, UK, pp. 301–320.

Duhamel, G.E., 1998, Colonic spirochetosis caused by *Serpulina pilosicoli*. Large Animal Pract. 19:14–22.

Duhamel, G.E., Trott, D.J., Muniappa, N., Mathiesen, M.R., Tarasiuk, K., Lee, J.I., and Hampson, D.J., 1998, Canine intestinal spirochetes consist of *Serpulina pilosicoli* and a newley identified group provisionally designated "*Serpulina canis*" sp. nov. J. Clin. Microbiol. 36:2264–2270.

Hugdahl, M.B., Beery, J.T., and Doyle, M.P., 1988, Chemotactic behavior of *Campylobacter jejuni*. Infect. Immun. 56:1560–1566.

Johnston, T., Duhamel, G.E., Mathiesen, M.R., Walter, D., Smart, N., and Dewey, C., 1998, Recent advances in diagnosis and control of porcine colonic spirochetosis caused by *Serpulina pilosicoli*. Comp. Cont. Educ., in press.

Kelly-Wintenberg, K. and Montie, T.C., 1994, Chemotaxis to oligopeptides by *Pseudomonas aeruginosa*. Appl. Env. Microbiol. 60:363–357.

Kennedy, M.J. and Yancey, R.J., 1996, Motility and chemotaxis in *Serpulina hyodysenteriae*. Vet. Microbiol. 49:21–30.

Milner, J.A. and Sellwood, R., 1994, Chemotactic response to mucin by *Serpulina hyodysenteriae* and other porcine spirochetes: Potential role in intestinal colonization. Infect. Immun. 62:4095–4099.

Moulton, R.C. and Montie, T.C., 1979, Chemotaxis by *Pseudomonas aeruginosa*. J. Bacteriol. 137:274–280.

Muniappa, N., Duhamel, G.E., Mathiesen, M.R., and Bargar, T.W., 1996, Light microscopic and ultrastructural changes in the ceca of chicks inoculated with human and canine *Serpulina pilosicoli*. Vet. Pathol. 33:542–550.

Muniappa, N., Mathiesen, M.R., and Duhamel, G.E., 1997, Laboratory identification and enteropathogenicity testing of *Serpulina pilosicoli* associated with porcine colonic spirochetosis. J. Vet. Diagn. Invest. 9:165–171.

Muniappa, N., Ramanathan, M.R., Tarara, R.P., Westernman, R.B., Mathiesen, M.R., and Duhamel, G.E., 1998, Attachment of human and rhesus *Serpulina pilosicoli* to cultured cells and comparison with a chick infection model. J Spiro. Tick-borne Dis., in press.

Palleroni, N.J., 1976, Chamber for bacterial chemotaxis experiments. Appl. Environ. Microbiol. 32: 729–730.

Ramanathan M., Duhamel G.E., Mathiesen M.R., and Messier S., 1993, Identification and partial characterization of a group of weakly β-hemolytic intestinal spirochetes of swine distinct from *Serpulina innocens*, isolate B256. Vet. Microbiol. 37:53–64.

Sacco, R.E., Trampel, D.W., and Wannemuehler, M.J., 1997, Experimental infection of C3H mice with avian, porcine, or human isolates of *Serpulina pilosicoli*. Infect. Immun. 65:5349–5353.

Smith, A.C. and Podolsky, D.K., 1986, Colonic mucin glycoproteins in health and disease, In: Clinics in Gastroenterology, Editor: Mendeloff, A.I., W.B. Saunders Company, Philadelphia, PA, pp. 815–837.

Specian, R.D. and Oliver, M.G., 1991, Functional biology of intestinal goblet cells. Am. Physiol. Soc. 260:C183–C192.

Strous G.J. and Dekker, J., 1992, Mucin-type glycoproteins. Critical Rev. Biochem. Mol. Biol. 27:57–92.

Swayne, D.E. and McLaren, A.J., 1997, Avian intestinal spirochaetes and avian intestinal spirochaetosis, In: Intestinal spirochaetosis in domestic animals and humans, Editors: Hampson, D.J. and Stanton, T.B. CAB International, Wallingford, UK, pp. 267–300.

Trivett-Moore, N.L., Gilbert, G.L., Law, C.L.H., Trott, D.J., and Hampson, D.J., 1998, Isolation of *Serpulina pilosicoli* from rectal biopsy specimens showing evidence of intestinal spirochetosis. J. Clin. Microbiol. 36:261–265.

Trott, D.J., McLaren, A.J., and Hampson, D.J., 1995, Pathogenicity of human and porcine intestinal spirochetes in one day old specific pathogen free chicks: an animal model of intestinal spirochetosis. Infect. Immunol. 63:3705–3710.

Trott, D.J., Stanton, T.B., Jensen, N.S., Duhamel, G.E., Johnson, J.L., and Hampson, D.J., 1996a, *Serpulina pilosicoli* sp. nov., the agent of porcine intestinal spirochetosis. Int. J. Syst. Bacteriol. 46:206–215.

Trott, D.J., Huxtable, C.R., and Hampson, D.J., 1996b, Experimental infection of newly weaned pigs with human and porcine strains of *Serpulina pilosicoli*. Infect. Immun. 64:4648–4654.

Trott, D.J., Jensen, N.S., Saint Girons, I., Oxberry, S.L., Stanton, T.B., Lindquist, D., and Hampson, D.J., 1997a, Identification and characterization of *Serpulina pilosicoli* isolates recovered from the blood of critically ill patients. J. Clin. Microbiol. 35:482–485.

Trott, D.J., Combs, B.G., Mikosza, A.S.J., Oxberry, S.L., Robertson, I.D., Passey, M., Taime, J., Sehuko, R., Alpers, M.P., and Hampson, D.J., 1997b, The prevalence of *Serpulina pilosicoli* in humans and domestic animals in the Eastern Highlands of Papua New Guinea. Epidemiol. Infect. 119:369–379.

21

COILING PHAGOCYTOSIS IS THE PREDOMINANT MECHANISM FOR UPTAKE OF THE COLONIC SPIROCHETOSIS BACTERIUM SERPULINA PILOSICOLI BY HUMAN MONOCYTES

Xiaoxing Cheng, Jeffrey D. Cirillo, and Gerald E. Duhamel

Department of Veterinary and Biomedical Sciences
University of Nebraska-Lincoln
Lincoln, Nebraska 68583-0905

1. SUMMARY

Serpulina pilosicoli is a newly identified pathogenic spirochete that establishes persistent colonic infections in human beings and animals. Macrophages are one of the key defenses against invasion of mucosal surfaces by bacterial pathogens. Macrophages engulf many bacteria by conventional phagocytosis; however recent studies indicate coiling phagocytosis as a new and important mechanism for internalization of *Legionella pneumophila* and spirochetes of the genus *Borrelia*, *Leptospira*, and *Treponema*. In this study, THP-1 human monocytic cells were incubated with the human *S. pilosicoli* strain SP16 and the contribution of coiling and conventional phagocytosis to the total number of phagocytic events were determined by sequential ultrastructural examination between 5 and 45 minutes. The frequency of phagocytosis increased over time from 5.1% after 5 minutes up to 21.9% after 45 minutes with greater than 70% of the events involving coiling phagocytosis. The data indicate that coiling phagocytosis may be a universal mechanism for uptake of pathogenic spirochetes.

2. INTRODUCTION

Serpulina pilosicoli is the etiologic agent of colonic spirochetosis (CS), a disease characterized by colonization of the large intestine with intimate attachment of

Mechanisms in the Pathogenesis of Enteric Diseases 2, edited by Paul and Francis.
Kluwer Academic / Plenum Publishers, New York, 1999.

spirochetes by one of their ends to the apical membrane of enterocytes in a picket-fence fashion (Trott et al., 1996; Duhamel, 1997; Trivett-Moore et al., 1998; Johnston et al., 1998). *Serpulina pilosicoli* has been identified in a broad range of hosts, including human beings, non-human primates, swine, dogs, and several species of birds (Duhamel et al., 1995; Trott et al., 1996; Duhamel, 1997; Duhamel et al., 1997; Swayne and McLaren, 1997; Trott et al., 1997a; Trott et al., 1997b; Duhamel et al., 1998; Trivett-Moore et al., 1998; Johnston et al., 1998). Invasion of the colonic mucosa by spirochetes has been documented in human beings, pigs, and dogs with CS (Takeuchi et al., 1974; Duhamel, 1997; Johnston et al., 1998). Epithelial erosions with local invasion of spirochetes also are present in the chick infection model and in pigs with CS (Muniappa et al., 1996; Muniappa et al., 1997; Johnston et al., 1998). Ultrastructurally, the spirochetes penetrate the mucosal barrier and invade the subepithelial connective tissue of the lamina propria. In this location spirochetes are found extracellularly, inside capillary vessels, and within macrophages.

Phagocytosis by macrophages is an important mechanism of defense against invasion of mucosal surfaces by microbial pathogens. Many bacteria are engulfed by conventional phagocytosis where the microorganism is surrounded by two symmetrical pseudopods that form a phagocytic vacuole by depression of the cell membrane in contact with the bacterial ligand. However, phagocytic uptake of certain pathogens, most notably *Legionella pneumophila* and spirochetes of the genus *Borrelia*, *Leptospira*, and *Treponema* involves a phenotypically different mechanism of internalization designated coiling phagocytosis (Horwitz, 1984; Rittig et al., 1992; Rittig et al., 1998). During coiling phagocytosis a single pseudopod rotates around the microorganism and internalization occurs through the formation of a self-apposed membranous whorl. The mechanism of coiling phagocytosis has been studied extensively using *L. pneumophia* for which it is the preferential mechanism of entry leading to inhibition of phagosome-lysosome fusion and intracellular replication (Horwitz, 1983; Cirillo et al., 1994). Although the outcome of this unusual uptake mechanism may have important implications in the pathogenesis of colonic spirochetal infections, no information is available about coiling phagocytosis of intestinal spirochetes. In this study, the morphology and kinetics of phagocytosis of human *Serpulina pilosicoli* by human THP-1 monocytic cells were characterized. These data indicate that coiling phagocytosis accounts for at least 70 percent of the phagocytic events, and may be a universal mechanism for uptake of pathogenic spirochetes.

3. MATERIALS AND METHODS

3.1. Bacterial Strain and Growth Conditions

Serpulina pilosicoli isolate SP16 (American Type Culture Collection [ATCC] 49776; Duhamel et al., 1995), obtained from an HIV-positive homosexual male with CS, was provided by R.M. Smibert (Virginia Polytechnic Institute, Blacksburg, VA). The spirochetes were propagated in prereduced anaerobically-sterilized Trypticase soy broth supplemented with 2% (vol/vol) fetal bovine serum (FBS; Sigma, St. Louis, MO) as previously described (Duhamel et al., 1995). Cultures were grown to late logarithmic phase (approximately 10^8 cells per ml) in 5-ml volumes by using Hungate tubes and were stirred constantly at 37°C under an atmosphere of 10% hydrogen, 10% carbon dioxide and 80% nitrogen.

3.2. Cell Line and Culture Conditions

The human THP-1 monocytic cell line (ATCC TIB 202) was grown in RPMI Medium 1640 (Gibco BRL, Life Technologies, Gaithersburg, MD) supplemented with 10% heat inactivated (HI, 30 minutes at 56°C) FBS at 37°C in a humidified atmosphere of 5% carbon dioxide in air.

3.3. Phagocytosis Assays

THP-1 cells were centrifuged and resuspended in RPMI supplemented with 1% HI-FBS and incubated for 24 h at 37°C and 5% carbon dioxide in air. On the day of the assay, the THP-1 cells were washed once, and the concentration was adjusted to 2.0 $\times 10^6$ cells/ml in cold RPMI supplemented with 10% HI-FBS. Then 500 μl volumes of THP-1 cell suspension were mixed with 50 μl volumes of medium containing 5×10^7 spirochetes (spirochete THP-1 cell ratio of 50:1) and rotated in a sterile tube for 1 h at 4°C. At the end of the incubation, each tube was centrifuged at $220 \times g$ for 10 min at 4°C followed by $500 \times g$ for 10 min at 4°C, and transferred to a 37°C water bath and incubated for either 5, 10, 20, 30 or 45 min. At the end of the incubation period, the supernatant was removed and the cells were fixed by adding Karnovsky's fixative (2% paraformaldehyde, 2.5% glutaraldehyde in 0.1 M Sorenson's buffer pH 7.2) and stored at 4°C.

3.4. Transmission Electron Microscopy

The cell pellets were washed in propylene oxide and incubated in a 1:1 propylene oxide araldite embedding resin overnight. The next day, the specimens were soaked in fresh araldite for 6 h and heated in molds at 65°C overnight to allow polymerization. Ultrathin sections were mounted onto 150-mesh copper grids, stained with 2% (wt/vol) uranyl acetate and lead citrate, and examined with a transmission electron microscope (Philips 201, Eindhoven, The Netherlands).

3.5. Collection and Reporting of the Data

Individual grid square of ultrathin sections were examined at a magnification of 1500× and the total number of THP-1 cells with a complete outline and a visible nucleus was determined. Then, the number and type of phagocytic events were recorded for each cell at a magnification of 7000×. For each time point, a total of between 137 and 310 cells were counted using serial ultrathin sections cut at 25 μm intervals. Conventional and coiling phagocytic events were classified as a single or a group of spirochetes either partially or completely surrounded by one or more pseudopods with morphologic features indicative of each mechanism (Horwitz, 1984).

4. RESULT AND DISCUSSION

Sequential ultrastructural examination of THP-1 cells incubated with *S. pilosicoli* revealed coiling phagocytosis as the predominant mechanism for uptake of the spirochetes by the phagocytic cells. This is consistent with previous observations indicating coiling phagocytosis as the preferential mechanism for uptake of other

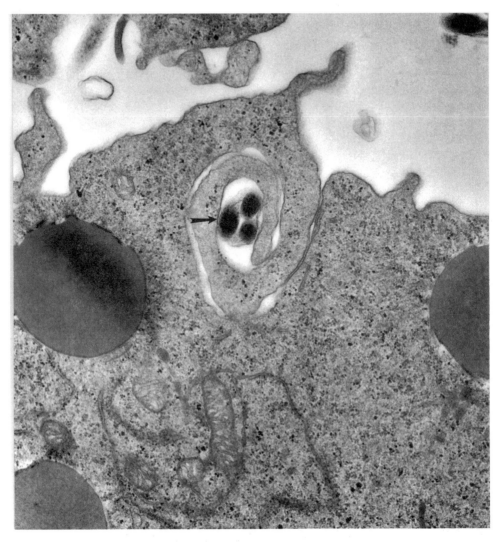

Figure 1. Transmission electron micrograph of a THP-1 human monocyte incubated with the human *Serpulina pilosicoli* isolate SP16 for 30 minutes. Cross-section through a monocyte shows a single pseudopod rotating around a spirochete (arrow) and internalization of the bacterium by a self apposed membranous whorl typical of coiling phagocytosis. Uranyl acetate and lead citrate. ×3500.

spirochetes in the genus *Borrelia*, *Leptospira* and *Treponema* (Rittig et al., 1992; Rittig et al., 1998).

The morphology of the coiling phagocytosis was identical to other spirochetes and to *L. pneumophila* (Horwitz, 1984; Rittig et al., 1992; Rittig et al., 1998). The THP-1 cells formed a single pseudopod that became tightly coiled around one or more spirochetes (Fig. 1). In more advanced stages of this process, spirochetes were internalized by a self apposed membranous whorl with localized rarefaction of cytoplasmic ribosomes and multifocal condensation of microfilaments (Fig. 2).

Although the morphology of individual coiling phagocytosis events was not markedly different between 5 min and 45 min of incubation, the frequency of such

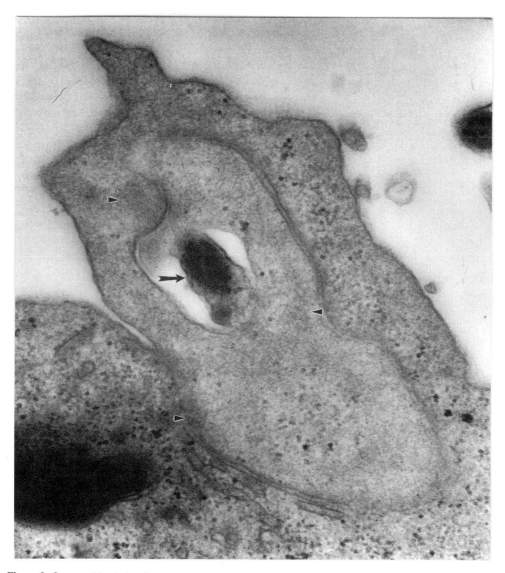

Figure 2. Same as Fig. 1 showing localized rarefaction of monocyte cytoplasmic ribosomes and condensation of microfilaments (arrow heads) in a membranous whorl surrounding a spirochete (arrow). Uranyl acetate and lead citrate. ×8400.

events increased dramatically from 5.1% to 21.9% over the same time period (Fig. 3). Additionally, coiling phagocytosis accounted for greater than 70% of the phagocytic events after 5, 30, or 45 min of incubation (Fig. 4).

    Coiling phagocytosis has been reported with a variety of microorganisms, but much of the experimental data has been generated with *L. pneumophila*. Although kinetic experiments have not been reported with spirochetes previously, it appears that 45 min is required for uptake of spirochetes by coiling phagocytosis (Rittig et al., 1992; Rattig et al., 1998). By contrast, internalization of *L. pneumophila* by this mechanism is completed within 5 min (Horwitz, 1984; Cirillo et al., 1994). The possibility that the differences in the timing of phagocytosis are caused by the origin of the phagocytic cells

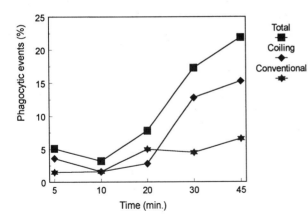

Figure 3. Relative contribution of coiling and conventional phagocytic events to total percentage of phagocytosis by THP-1 human monocytes incubated with the *Serpulina pilosicoli* isolate SP16 over time.

is unlikely since rapid uptake of *L. pneumophila* by THP-1 cells is similar to alveolar macrophages, blood monocytes and polymorphonuclear leukocytes (Horwitz, 1984; Cirillo et al., 1994).

It has been suggested that *S. pilosicoli* outer membrane subtilisin-like serine protease participates in invasion of the gut wall by dissociating junctional complexes between enterocytes (Muniappa et al., 1996; Muniappa and Duhamel, 1997). Translocation of *S. pilosicoli* to extraintestinal sites including the blood stream of terminally ill human patients, and the mesenteric lymph nodes of experimentally inoculated pigs has been documented (Trott et al., 1997a; Hampson et al., 1998). On the basis of these observations, the possibility exists that extraintestinal spread of *S. pilosicoli* involves evasion of the bactericidal mechanisms of mononuclear phagocytic cells.

Serpulina pilosicoli infections are commonly found in immunocompetent children with diarrhea in developing countries, and among human immunodeficiency virus-positive immunocompromised adults in developed countries (Trivett-Moore et al., 1998; Trott et al., 1997a; Trott et al., 1997b). The increased prevalence of this infection in developing countries is suggestive of poor hygienic environment, however, the

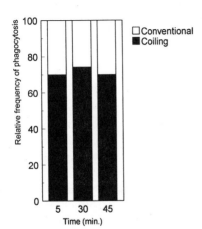

Figure 4. Relative frequency of coiling and conventional phagocytosis by THP-1 human monocytes at different time points after incubation with *Serpulina pilosicoli* isolate SP16.

situation in individuals with HIV infection is less clear. Increased risk of *S. pilosicoli* infection in individuals with HIV infection suggests a possible relationship between a direct spirochete-induced alteration of monocyte function or an indirect immunological alteration of T-cell function. Further investigation into the role of coiling phagocytosis in the pathogenesis of *S. pilosicoli* infection is warranted.

ACKNOWLEDGMENTS

The authors thank M.R. Mathiesen of for her technical assistance. The research was supported in part by funds provided by the U.S. Department of Agriculture, Regional Research Project NC-62, Enteric Diseases of Swine and Cattle: Prevention, Control, and Food Safety, and a grant from the Center for Indoor Air Research to J.D. Cirillo.

REFERENCES

Cirillo, J.D., Falkow, S., and Tompkins, L.S., 1994, Growth of *Legionella pneumophila* in *Acanthamoeba castellanii* enhances invasion. Infect. Immun. 62:3254–3261.

Duhamel, G.E., Muniappa, N., Mathiesen, M.R., Johnson, J.L., Toth, J., Elder, R.O., and Doster, A.R., 1995, Certain canine weakly beta-hemolytic intestinal spirochetes are phenotypically and genotypically related to spirochetes associated with human and porcine intestinal spirochetosis. J. Clin. Microbiol. 33:2211–2215.

Duhamel, G.E., 1997, Intestinal spirochaetes in non-production animals, In: Intestinal spirochaetosis in domestic animals and humans. Editors: Hampson, D.J. and Stanton, T.B., CAB International, Wallingford, UK, pp. 301–320.

Duhamel, G.E., Elder, R.O., Muniappa, N., Mathiesen, M.R., Wong, V.J., and Tarara, R.P., 1997, Colonic spirochetal infections in nonhuman primates that were associated with *Brachyspira aalborgi*, *Serpulina pilosicoli*, and unclassified flagellated bacteria. Clin. Infect. Dis. 25(Suppl. 2):S186–S188.

Duhamel, G.E., Trott, D.J., Muniappa, N., Mathiesen, M.R., Tarasiuk, K., Lee, J.I., and Hampson, D.J., 1998, Canine intestinal spirochetes consist of *Serpulina pilosicoli* and a newly identified group provisionally designated "*Serpulina canis*" sp. nov. J. Clin. Microbiol. 36:2264–2270.

Hampson, D.J., Robertson, I.D., Oxberry, S.L., and Pethick, D.W., 1998, Evaluation of vaccination and diet for the control of *Serpulina pilosicoli* infection (porcine intestinal spirochaetosis). Proc 15th International Pig Veterinary Society Conference 2:56.

Horwitz, M.A., 1983, The Legionnaires' disease bacterium (*Legionella pneumophila*) inhibits phagosome-lysosome fusion in human monocytes. J. Exp. Med. 158:2108–2126.

Horwitz, M.A., 1984, Phagocytosis of the Legionnaires' disease bacterium (*Legionella pneumophila*) occurs by a novel mechanism: Engulfment within a pseudopod coil. Cell 36:27–33.

Johnston, T., Duhamel, G.E., Mathiesen, M.R., Walter, D., Smart, N., and Dewey, C., 1998, Recent advances in diagnosis and control of porcine colonic spirochetosis caused by *Serpulina pilosicoli*. Comp. Cont. Educ., in press.

Muniappa, N., Duhamel, G.E., Mathiesen, M.R., and Bargar, T.W., 1996, Light microscopic and ultrastructural changes in the ceca of chicks inoculated with human and canine *Serpulina pilosicoli*. Vet. Pathol. 33:542–550.

Muniappa, N. and Duhamel, G.E., 1997, Outer membrane-associated serine protease of intestinal spirochetes. FEMS Microbiol. Lett. 154:159–164.

Muniappa, N., Mathiesen, M.R., and Duhamel, G.E., 1997, Laboratory identification and enteropathogenicity testing of *Serpulina pilosicoli* associated with porcine colonic spirochetosis. J. Vet. Diagn. Invest. 9:165–171.

Rittig, M.G., Krause, A., Haupl, T., Schaible, U.E., Modolell, M., Kramer, M.D., Lutjen-Drecoll, E., Simon, M.M., and Burmester, G.R., 1992, Coiling phagocytosis is the preferential phagocytic mechanism for *Borrelia burgdorferi*. Infect. Immun. 60:4205–4212.

Rittig, M.G., Jagoda, J.C., Wilske, B., Murgia, R., Cinco, M., Repp, R., Burmester, G.R., and Krause, A., 1998, Coiling phagocytosis discriminates between different spirochetes and is enhanced by phorbol myristate acetate and granulocyte-macrophage colony-stimulating factor. Infect. Immun. 66:627–635.

Swayne, D.E. and McLaren, A.J., 1997, Avian intestinal spirochaetes and avian intestinal spirochaetosis, In: Intestinal spirochaetosis in domestic animals and humans, Editors: Hampson, D.J. and Stanton, T.B., CAB International, Wallingford, UK, p. 267–300.

Takeuchi, A., Jervis, H.R., Nakazawa, H., and Robinson, D.M., 1974, Spiral-shaped organisms on the surface colonic epithelium of the monkey and man. Am. J. Clin. Nutr. 27:1287–1296.

Trivett-Moore, N.L., Gilbert, G.L., Law, C.L.H., Trott, D.J., and Hampson, D.J., 1998, Isolation of *Serpulina pilosicoli* from rectal biopsy specimens showing evidence of intestinal spirochetosis. J. Clin. Microbiol. 36:261–265.

Trott, D.J., Stanton, T.B., Jensen, N.S., Duhamel, G.E., Johnson, J.L., and Hampson, D.J., 1996, *Serpulina pilosicoli* sp. nov., the agent of porcine intestinal spirochetosis. Int. J. Syst. Bacteriol. 46:206–215.

Trott, D.J., Jensen, N.S., Saint Girons, I., Oxberry, S.L., Stanton, T.B., Lindquist, D., and Hampson, D.J., 1997a, Identification and characterization of *Serpulina pilosicoli* isolates recovered from the blood of critically ill patients. J. Clin. Microbiol. 35:482–485.

Trott, D.J., Combs, B.G., Mikosza, A.S.J., Oxberry, S.L., Robertson, I.D., Passey, M., Taime, J., Sehuko, R., Alpers, M.P., and Hampson, D.J., 1997b, The prevalence of *Serpulina pilosicoli* in humans and domestic animals in the Eastern Highlands of Papua New Guinea. Epidemiol. Infect. 119:369–379.

22

IDENTIFICATION OF PROTEINS REQUIRED FOR THE INTERNALIZATION OF *CAMPYLOBACTER JEJUNI* INTO CULTURED MAMMALIAN CELLS

Michael E. Konkel, Bong J. Kim, Vanessa Rivera-Amill, and Steven G. Garvis

Department of Microbiology
Washington State University
Pullman, Washington 99164

1. SUMMARY

Clinical and *in vitro* experimental data suggest that invasion of intestinal epithelial cells is an essential step in the pathogenesis of *Campylobacter jejuni*-mediated enteritis. However, the molecular mechanism of *C. jejuni* internalization remains poorly defined. The goal of this study was to identify a gene that encodes a protein required for the internalization of *C. jejuni* into host cells. A *C. jejuni* gene, designated *ciaB*, was identified upon immunoscreening *C. jejuni* genomic DNA-phage libraries with an antiserum generated against *C. jejuni* co-cultivated with INT 407 cells. The *C. jejuni ciaB* gene encodes a protein of 610 amino acids with a calculated molecular mass of 73,154 Da. The deduced amino acid sequence of the CiaB protein shares similarity with type III secreted proteins, associated with invasion of host cells, from other more extensively characterized bacterial pathogens. *In vitro* binding and internalization assays revealed that the binding of *C. jejuni ciaB* null mutants was indistinguishable from that of the parental isolate, whereas a significant reduction was noted in internalization. Immunoblot analysis using an anti-CiaB specific antibody revealed that CiaB is secreted into the supernatant fluids upon co-cultivation of *C. jejuni* with INT 407 cell conditioned medium. Metabolic labeling experiments revealed that at least eight *C. jejuni* proteins, ranging in size from 12.8 to 108 kDa, are secreted into the culture medium. *C. jejuni ciaB* null mutants were deficient in the secretion of all proteins, indicating that CiaB is required for the secretion process. Identification of the *C. jejuni ciaB* gene represents a significant advance in understanding the molecular mechanism of *C. jejuni* internalization.

Mechanisms in the Pathogenesis of Enteric Diseases 2, edited by Paul and Francis.
Kluwer Academic / Plenum Publishers, New York, 1999.

2. INTRODUCTION

Elucidation of the molecular mechanisms of pathogenic bacteria has revealed common themes. One common pathogenic mechanism is a specialized protein secretion system termed type III (reviewed in Hueck, 1998). This secretion system enables a variety of distantly related gram-negative bacteria to secrete and translocate virulence proteins into the cytoplasm of eukaryotic cells. These secreted proteins often trigger signal transduction events that result in reorganization of the host cell cytoskeletal components or in incapacitating host immune responses. While the type III secretion apparatus is conserved among distantly related pathogens, the proteins secreted via this pathway vary greatly in size, structure, and function. Not all of the secreted proteins have anti-host functions, but instead serve as accessory proteins in the secretion and translocation of the actual virulence determinants (Collazo and Galán, 1997). Interestingly, secretion of proteins via the type III secretion system is enhanced upon contact of bacteria to host cells (Ménard et al., 1994).

Campylobacter jejuni is a frequent cause of gastrointestinal disease worldwide (Blaser et al., 1983). Despite the prevalence of *C. jejuni* infections, the pathogenic mechanisms associated with *C. jejuni*-mediated enteritis are ill-defined. The dominating presentation of *Campylobacter* enteritis is acute enterocolitis. More specifically, the infection is characterized by severe abdominal pain, fever, and grossly bloody diarrhea containing leukocytes (Black et al., 1988; Blaser et al., 1979). Potential *C. jejuni* virulence factors include the proteins that facilitate the organism's binding and entry into the cells lining the gastrointestinal tract and the production of toxins (reviewed in Ketley, 1997).

The ability of *C. jejuni* to bind to the cells lining the intestinal tract is a prerequisite for *C. jejuni*-mediated enteritis, as binding prevents the colonizing bacteria from being swept away by mechanical cleansing forces such as peristalsis and fluid flow. The ability of *C. jejuni* to invade the cells lining the gastrointestinal tract is hypothesized to be required for disease production. This hypothesis is based on the clinical presentation of epithelial cell damage and inflammation in *C. jejuni*-infected individuals. In support of this hypothesis, intracellular organisms have been observed upon electron microscopic examination of biopsy specimens from *C. jejuni*-infected individuals with colitis (Van Spreeuwel et al., 1985). Intracellular bacteria have also been observed in infected infant macaque monkeys (Russell et al., 1993) and newborn piglets (Babakhani et al., 1993). These models closely mimic human *C. jejuni*-infections with the development of self-limiting diarrheal disease with acute colitis. Finally, the gentamicin-protection assay has been used extensively to demonstrate the invasive potential of *C. jejuni*.

A number of studies have been performed to gain a better understanding of the molecular mechanism of *C. jejuni* entry into host cells. Heat-inactivated or gentamicin-killed *C. jejuni* adhere efficiently to INT 407 cells but are not internalized, indicating that the internalization of *C. jejuni* into host cells is an energy-requiring process (Konkel and Cieplak, 1992). Previous studies have also revealed that *de novo* protein synthesis is required for the maximal internalization of *C. jejuni* into host cells, as chloramphenicol significantly reduces the number of *C. jejuni* internalized (Konkel and Cieplak, 1992; Oelschlaeger et al., 1993). Metabolic labeling experiments have revealed that *C. jejuni* synthesize at least fourteen new proteins upon cocultivation with mammalian cells (Konkel and Cieplak, 1992; Konkel et al., 1993). Interestingly, the internalization of *C. jejuni* was found to be significantly reduced in the presence of an antiserum that reacts with a subset of the newly synthesized proteins (Konkel et al., 1993). Collectively, these data suggest that distinct bacterial proteins promote the binding and entry of *C. jejuni* to host cells. The purpose of this investigation was to identify a *C. jejuni* gene that encodes an entry-promoting protein.

3. RESULTS

3.1. Cloning of a *C. jejuni* Entry-Promoting Protein

To clone a gene coding for a *C. jejuni*-entry promoting protein, *C. jejuni* genomic DNA-expression libraries were screened with an antiserum generated by immunization of a rabbit with whole-cell *C. jejuni* cultured in the presence of INT 407 cells (Cj + INT or 1588) (Konkel et al., 1993). The Cj + INT immunoreactive plaques were then screened with a second antiserum generated against *C. jejuni* cultured in tissue culture medium alone (Cj − INT or 1622) as the proteins that promote the entry of *C. jejuni* into cultured cells are synthesized only upon co-cultivation of *C. jejuni* with tissue culture cells (Konkel and Cieplak, 1992; Konkel et al., 1993). One differentially immunoreactive phage, designated PL3-4, was identified (Fig. 1). The PL3-4 phage reacted with the Cj + INT antiserum and not with the Cj − INT antiserum.

Two additional *C. jejuni*-genomic phage clones were isolated by screening the libraries with oligonucleotide primers that were designed based on the insert contained within the PL3-4 clone. The physical map of PL3-4 and overlapping PL3412 and PL3415 phage clones are shown in Fig. 2. Sequencing of overlapping gene inserts revealed an open reading frame (orf) of 1833 nucleotides, capable of encoding a protein of 610 amino acids with a calculated molecular mass of 73,154 Da. This *C. jejuni* gene was designated *ciaB*, for *Campylobacter* *invasion* *antigen* *B*. The deduced amino acid sequence of CiaB exhibited the greatest identity with the P50 adhesin protein from *Mycoplasma hominis* (Table 1). Direct sequence comparisons revealed that the CiaB deduced amino acid sequence also shared some similarity with type III secreted proteins from other Gram-negative pathogenic bacteria (Table 1).

3.2. CiaB Is Required for *C. jejuni* Invasiveness

To determine whether CiaB was required for the entry of *C. jejuni* into INT 407 cells, three *C. jejuni ciaB* mutants were isolated. The *ciaB* gene in *C. jejuni* F38011 was disrupted by homologous recombination via a single crossover event between the *ciaB* gene on the chromosome and an internal fragment of the *ciaB* gene on a suicide vector. Disruption of the *ciaB* gene in each of the three *C. jejuni ciaB* mutants was confirmed

Table 1. Similarity of *C. jejuni* CiaB with other proteins

Protein	Organism	No. of amino acid residues	mass (Da)	% similarity (% identity)
CiaB	*Campylobacter jejuni*	610	73,154	—
SipB	*Salmonella typhimurium*	593	62,450	45.0 (16.8)
IpaB	*Shigella flexneri*	580	62,185	40.6 (18.1)
YopB	*Yersinia pseudotuberculosis*	401	41,795	45.4 (20.1)
P50	*Mycoplasma hominis*	467	53,395	45.3 (21.1)

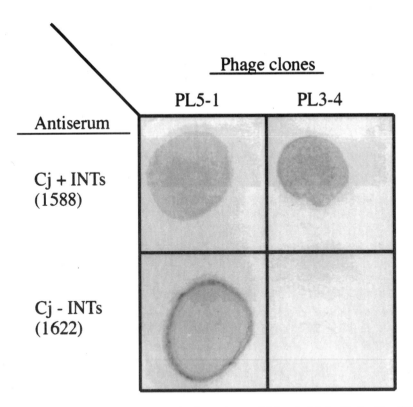

Figure 1. Immunoreactivity of *C. jejuni* genomic phage clones pL5-1 and pL3-4 with the Cj + INT (1588) and Cj – INT (1622) antisera. Bacteriophage infections were performed as described elsewhere (Stratagene, La Jolla, CA). Briefly, phage stocks (20 μl) were spotted onto the surface of solidified NYZ top agar [10 g of NZ amine (casein hydrolysate), 5 g of yeast extract, 5 g of sodium chloride, 2 g of $MgSO_4$-$7H_2O$, and 7.5 g agar per liter] containing *Escherichia coli*, and plates incubated at 37°C for 24 hours. The plaques were transferred to Duralose-U.V. membranes (Stratagene) and incubated with a 1:250 dilution of the Cj + INT and Cj – INT antisera in PBS/Tween-20 with 20% bovine serum. Bound antibodies were detected using peroxidase-conjugated goat anti-rabbit IgG (Organon Teknika Corp., West Chester, PA) and 4-chloro-1-naphthol (Sigma) as the chromogenic substrate. pL5-1 contains an insert of approximately 3.0 kb and pL3-4 an insert of approximately 3.3 kb. The orientation of the *C. jejuni* chromosomal DNA contained within each clone is such that the *C. jejuni* genes are transcribed from the *lac* promoter. pL5-1 harbors part of the *C. jejuni flbA* gene encoding a protein involved in flagellar biogenesis that is reactive with both the Cj + INT and Cj – INT antisera. pL3-4 harbors a gene encoding a protein that is only reactive with the Cj + INT antiserum.

by Southern hybridization (Fig. 3) and immunoblot analyses with an anti-CiaB antibody (not shown). The three *C. jejuni ciaB* mutants were then tested for their ability to bind to and enter INT 407 cells (Fig. 4). The binding efficiency of each of the *C. jejuni ciaB* isogenic mutants was indistinguishable from that of the F38011 parental isolate. However, a significant reduction was noted in the internalization of all three mutants when compared to the parental isolate, indicating that the synthesis of CiaB is required for the internalization of *C. jejuni* into host cells.

3.3. Identification of *C. jejuni* Secreted Proteins

Labeling experiments with [^{35}S]-methionine revealed at least eight bacterial proteins, tentatively designated CiaA through CiaH (in order of the highest to the lowest

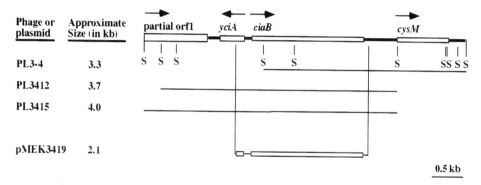

Figure 2. Physical map of the inserts of PL3-4 and overlapping PL3412 and PL3415 phage clones depicting approximately 5350-bp of *C. jejuni* chromosomal DNA containing three complete orfs and one partial orf. Also shown is the pMEK3419 recombinant plasmid, which contains the entire *ciaB* gene. The arrows show the direction in which the genes are transcribed. Restriction endonuclease sites, S = *Sau*3A I, are indicated. Identified orfs: Partial orf, 435 bases, 145 amino acid residues, shares 59.7% similarity with the CstA protein from *E. coli*; *yciA*, 414 bases, 137 amino acid residues, shares 58% similarity to YciA from *E. coli*; *ciaB*, 1833 bp, 610 amino acid residues, gene encoding *C. jejuni* invasion-antigen B; *cysM*, 900 bp, 299 amino acid residues, gene encoding *O*-acetylserine sulfhydrylase B.

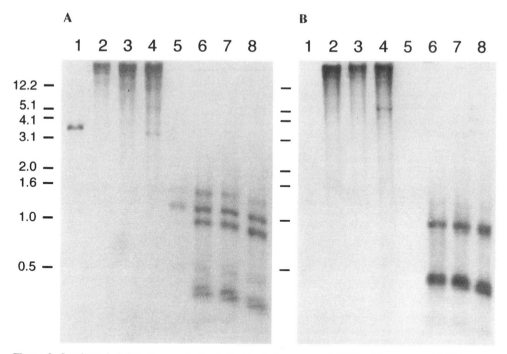

Figure 3. Southern hybridization analysis of *C. jejuni* chromosomal DNAs. Chromosomal DNAs were digested with *Bgl* II (lanes 1–4) and *Sau*3A I (lanes 5–8) restriction endonucleases, separated by agarose gel electrophoresis, transferred to a membrane, and probed with the nick-translated pMEK3419 recombinant plasmid containing the *C. jejuni ciaB* gene (panel A) or the *Campylobacter* kanamycin resistance gene (panel B). Lanes: 1 and 5, F38011; 2 and 6, mut*ciaB*1; 3 and 7, mut*ciaB*4; 4 and 8, mut*ciaB*5. Size standards, in kilobases, are indicated to the right of each panel.

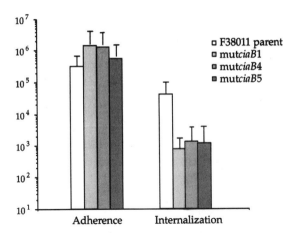

Figure 4. Binding and internalization of the *C. jejuni* parental isolate and *ciaB* isogenic mutants to INT 407 cells. The assays were performed as described previously (Konkel et al., 1993). Briefly, semi-confluent mono-layers (1.0×10^5 cells per well) were rinsed once with Eagle's Minimal Essential Medium supplemented with 1% fetal bovine serum (EMEM-1% FBS) and inoculated with 5×10^7 cfu of a bacterial suspension. The tissue culture trays were then centrifuged at 600 g for 5 min, and incubated at 37°C in a humidified, 5% CO_2 incubator. For binding, the infected monolayers were incubated for 30 min, rinsed three times with PBS, and the epithelial cells lysed with a solution of 0.5% (wt/vol) sodium deoxycholate. The suspensions were serially diluted and number of viable, adherent bacteria determined by counting the resultant colonies on Mueller-Hinton plates supplemented with 5% citrated bovine blood (MH/blood). To measure bacterial internalization, the infected monolayers were incubated for 3 hours, rinsed three times with EMEM-1% FBS, and incubated for an additional 3 hours in EMEM-1% FBS containing 250 µg per ml of gentamicin. The monolayers were then rinsed three times with PBS, epithelial cells lysed with a solution of sodium deoxycholate, and suspensions serially diluted and plated onto MH/blood plates. The number of internalized bacteria was determined by counting the resultant colonies on the MH/blood plates. The values represent the mean counts (± std. deviations) derived from triplicate wells.

molecular mass), in the supernatant fluids of *C. jejuni* co-cultured in INT 407 conditioned medium (Fig. 5). Secreted proteins were not observed in the supernatant fluids of the mut*ciaB*5 isolate, indicating that CiaB is required for the secretion process (Fig. 5, panel A). The 73 kDa secreted protein was identified as CiaB as judged by immunoblot analysis with the anti-CiaB antibody (Fig. 5, panel B).

4. DISCUSSION

Although significant progress has been made in defining both the bacterial and host cell requirements for *C. jejuni* internalization, the molecular mechanism of *C. jejuni* entry has remained elusive due to the lack of identification of genes encoding *C. jejuni*-entry promoting proteins. Here, a *C. jejuni* gene termed *ciaB* was implicated in invasion by demonstrating that a null mutation in this gene results in a non-invasive phenotype without altering adherence. Direct sequence comparisons revealed that the deduced amino acid sequence of CiaB exhibited from 40.6 to 45.4% similarity with the *Salmonella* SipB, *Shigella* IpaB, and *Yersinia* YopB proteins (Kaniga et al., 1995). Also similar to SipB, IpaB, and YopB, no typical signal sequence was identified at the amino terminus of the CiaB protein using the algorithm of Von Heijne (1985). Based on the data presented here, we hypothesize that *C. jejuni* possess a type III secretion system and that CiaB is a target of the secretion apparatus.

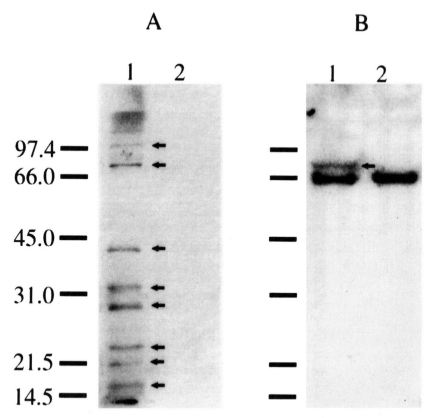

Figure 5. Analyses of the proteins secreted by *C. jejuni* F38011 parental and isogenic mut*ciaB*5 isolates. The isolates were incubated for 3 hours in INT 407 cell-conditioned media, after which the media were collected and bacteria pelleted by centrifugation at 6000 rpm for 10 min. The supernatant fluids were collected, concentrated fourfold, and subjected to SDS-PAGE. Panel A shows an autoradiograph of the [³⁵S]-methionine labeled proteins secreted by the *C. jejuni* parental (lane 1) and *ciaB* isogenic mutant (lane 2). The eight secreted Cia proteins are indicated (arrows). Panel B shows an immunoblot of the secreted proteins that were reactive with the rabbit anti-CiaB serum. The CiaB protein is indicated (arrow). Immunoblot detection of secreted CiaB was performed using a 1:250 dilution of the anti-CiaB antibody and a 1:2000 dilution of a peroxidase-conjugated goat-anti-rabbit IgG by enhanced chemiluminesence (SuperSignal; Pierce, Rockford, IL). Molecular mass standards, in kilodaltons, are indicated on the left.

Culturing *C. jejuni* in INT 407-conditioned medium resulted in the secretion of eight proteins, one of which is CiaB, into the culture medium. The apparent molecular masses of the eight bacterial proteins ranged in size from 12.8 to 108 kDa. CiaB is also required for the secretion of other proteins as *C. jejuni ciaB* null mutants are deficient in the secretion of all proteins as judged by metabolic labeling experiments. Mutations in two *Salmonella* genes, *invJ* (*spaN*) and *spaO*, completely abolish the secretion of all targets of the type III secretion apparatus, whereas mutations in other genes, *sipD* and to a lesser extent *sipB*, lead to an increase in secretion of a subset of secreted proteins. Both InvJ and SpaO are secreted proteins. These data, in part, have led Collazo and Galán (1997) to propose that there is a hierarchy in the secretion process in *Salmonella* spp., such that a subset of the exported proteins facilitates the translocation of other secreted proteins. The specific functions of InvJ and SpaO in the secretion process are unknown. CiaB apparently shares one feature with InvJ and SpaO (i.e., a null mutation abolishes secretion of all targets of the secretion system), but is more similar to SipB with respect to its relative molecular mass and deduced amino acid sequence.

Pathogenic bacteria often harbor one or more pathogenicity islands. Pathogenicity islands are commonly defined as blocks of foreign genes, differing in their mol% (G + C) content from the remainder of the chromosome, which confer a variety of virulence traits upon host bacteria (Galán, 1996; Lee, 1996). It is presently unclear whether the *C. jejuni ciaB* gene resides within a pathogenicity island. The *C. jejuni ciaB* gene has a mol% (G + C) of 25.9%, which is only slightly more AT rich than that of the rest of the *C. jejuni* chromosome (Owen and Leaper, 1981). It is interesting to note that the G + C content of the type III secretion genes thus far identified in *Chlamydia psittaci*

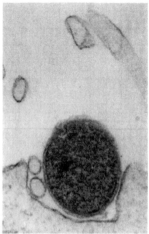

Requirements:
- metabolically active bacteria
- *de novo* protein synthesis
- bacterial protein secretion
- signal-dependent secretion (contact-mediated)
- active host cell participation

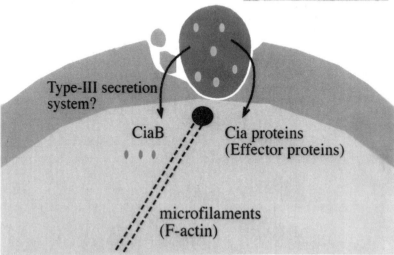

Figure 6. Model of *C. jejuni* internalization. Previous work has shown that *C. jejuni* synthesize a minimum of fourteen new proteins upon cultivation with host cells (Konkel et al., 1993). Here, at least eight bacterial proteins were found secreted in the culture medium upon culturing *C. jejuni* with host cells. We propose that a subset of this group of eight proteins is translocated into the cytoplasm of the target cell, triggering cell signalling events that lead to *C. jejuni* uptake. Interestingly, inhibitors of tyrosine kinases, heterotrimeric G-proteins, and phosphatidylinositol 3-kinase (PI 3-kinase) reduce *C. jejuni* internalization (Ketley, 1997).

are similar to the G + C content of the chlamydial genome. Regions upstream and downstream of *ciaB* are currently being sequenced to identify additional genes that may encode proteins associated with the entry process. Also noteworthy is the genetic organization of the *C. jejuni ciaB* gene. In nearly all pathogenic organisms, genes encoding type III secreted proteins are organized in blocks with many being located in operons. In contrast, the *C. jejuni ciaB* gene appears to be monocistronic based on the sequence data and physical map of the surrounding chromosomal region (see Fig. 1).

The ability of *C. jejuni* to cause disease is clearly a complex, multifactorial process requiring the contact-dependent expression of many genes. Previous work has shown that *C. jejuni* can sense and respond to co-cultivation with host cells by synthesizing at least fourteen new proteins. A subset of these fourteen newly synthesized proteins mediate the organism entry into host cells. Here, we present data that show that some of the newly synthesized proteins are secreted. These data suggest that there is global regulation governing the expression of *C. jejuni* virulence genes. The non-invasive phenotype of the *C. jejuni ciaB* mutant also suggests that one or more of the secreted proteins alters host cell signalling to stimulate bacterial uptake. Based on the literature and the data presented here, a model of the mechanism of *C. jejuni* entry into host cells is presented in Fig. 6. Although this model is simplified, mainly due to the lack of knowledge regarding the function of the *Campylobacter* secreted proteins and host cell signalling events, it represents a foundation from which further work can be done.

Future work will focus on the molecular and functional characterization of the *C. jejuni* Cia proteins. More specifically, studies will be done to determine whether a *C. jejuni ciaB* mutant is virulent *in vivo* using the piglet model. Our working hypothesis is that an adherent but non-invasive strain of *C. jejuni* would be avirulent, making it potentially useful as a vaccine candidate. One vaccine strategy currently being employed for dysentery is the use of a non-invasive *Shigella* strain administered orally (Lindberg and Pál, 1993). This vaccine strategy has the advantages of being safe and producing a long-lasting protective response. A similar, inexpensive and easily administered vaccine for *C. jejuni*-mediated enteritis would benefit developing countries where *Campylobacter* infections are hyperendemic.

ACKNOWLEDGMENTS

This work was supported by grants from the NIH (1R01 DK50567-01A1) and the USDA National Research Initiative Competitive Grants Program (USDA/NRICGP, No. 9601496) awarded to MEK.

REFERENCES

Babakhani, F.K., Bradley, G.A., and Joens, L.A. (1993) Newborn piglet model for *Campylobacteriosis*. *Infect. Immun.* 61:3466–3475.

Black, R.E., Levine, M.M., Clements, M.L., Hughes, T.P., and Blaser, M.J. (1988) Experimental *Campylobacter jejuni* infection in humans. *J. Infect. Dis.* 157:472–479.

Blaser, M.J., Berkowitz, I.D., LaForce, F.M., Cravens, J., Reller, L.B., and Wang, W.L. (1979) *Campylobacter enteritis*: clinical and epidemiological features. *Ann. Intern. Med.* 91:179–185.

Blaser, M.J., Wells, J.G., Feldman, R.A., Pollard, R.A., and Allen, J.R. (1983) The collaborative disease study group. *Campylobacter* enteritis in the USA. *Ann. Intern. Med.* 98:360–365.

Collazo, C.M. and Galán, J.E. (1997) The invasion-associated type-III protein secretion system in *Salmonella*—a review. *Gene* 192:51–59.

Galán, J.E. (1996) Molecular genetic bases of *Salmonella* entry into host cells. *Mol. Microbiol.* 20:263–271.

Hueck, C.J. (1998) Type III secretion systems in bacterial pathogens of animals and plants. *Microbiol. Mol. Biol. Rev.* 62:379–433.

Kaniga, K., Tucker, S., Trollinger, D., and Galán, J.E. (1995) Homologs of the *Shigella* IpaB and IpaC invasins are required for *Salmonella typhimurium* entry into cultured epithelial cells. *J. Bacteriol.* 177:3965–3971.

Ketley, J.M. (1997) Pathogenesis of enteric infection by *Campylobacter*. *Microbiology* 143:5–21.

Konkel, M.E. and Cieplak, W., Jr. (1992) Altered synthetic response of *Campylobacter jejuni* to co-cultivation with human epithelial cells is associated with enhanced internalization. *Infect. Immun.* 60:4945–4949.

Konkel, M.E., Mead, D.J., and Cieplak, W., Jr. (1993) Kinetic and antigenic characterization of altered protein synthesis by *Campylobacter jejuni* during cultivation with human epithelial cells. *J. Infect. Dis.* 168:-948–954.

Lee, C.A. (1996) Pathogenicity islands and the evolution of bacterial pathogens. *Infectious Agents and Disease* 5:1–7.

Lindberg, A.A. and Pál, T. (1993) Strategies for development of potential candidate *Shigella* vaccines. *Vaccine* 11:168–179.

Ménard, R., Sansonetti, P., and Parsot, C. (1994) The secretion of the *Shigella flexneri* Ipa invasins is activated by epithelial cells and controlled by IpaB and IpaD. *EMBO J.* 13:5293–5302.

Oelschlaeger, T.A., Guerry, P., and Kopecko, D.J. (1993) Unusual microtubule-dependent endocytosis mechanisms triggered by *Campylobacter jejuni* and *Citrobacter freundii*. *Proc. Natl. Acad. Sci. USA* 90:6884–6888.

Owen, R.J. and Leaper, S. (1981) Base composition, size and nucleotide sequence similarities of genome deoxyribonucleic acids from species of the genus *Campylobacter*. *FEMS Microbiol. Lett.* 12:395–400.

Russell, R.G., O'Donnoghue, M., Blake, D.C., Jr., Zulty, J., and DeTolla, L.J. (1993) Early colonic damage and invasion of *Campylobacter jejuni* in experimentally challenged infant *Macaca mulatta*. *J. Infect. Dis.* 168:210–215.

Van Spreeuwel, J.P., Duursma, G.C., Meijer, C.J.L.M., Bax, R., Rosekrans, P.C.M., and Lindeman, J. (1985) *Campylobacter* colitis: Histological immunohistochemical and ultrastructural findings. *Gut* 26:945–951.

Von Heijne, G. (1985) Signal sequences. The limits of variation. *J. Mol. Biol.* 184:99–105.

23

SECRETION OF *CAMPYLOBACTER JEJUNI* CIA PROTEINS IS CONTACT DEPENDENT

Vanessa Rivera-Amill and Michael E. Konkel

Washington State University
Department of Microbiology
Pullman, Washington 99164-4233

SUMMARY

Campylobacter jejuni is a common cause of human gastrointestinal disease world-wide. Despite the prevalence of *C. jejuni* infections, the mechanisms of *C. jejuni* pathogenesis remain ill-defined. Invasion of the cells lining the intestinal tract is hypothesized to be essential for the development of *C. jejuni*-mediated enteritis. Recent studies in our laboratory have revealed that *C. jejuni* secrete proteins, termed Cia for Campylobacter invasion antigens, upon incubation with human intestinal cells. A mutation in one of the genes encoding a secreted protein resulted in an invasion-deficient phenotype. The purpose of this study was to identify a component capable of stimulating the synthesis and secretion of the Cia proteins from *C. jejuni*. Here, we report that these processes can be induced upon incubating *C. jejuni* in medium supplemented with fetal bovine serum. The synthesis and secretion of the Cia proteins were not affected by heat-treatment of the fetal bovine serum, indicating that the stimulating molecule in serum is heat stable. The stimulatory molecule was not unique to fetal bovine serum as sera from other sources including human, pig, sheep, goat, rabbit, mouse, and chicken also induced the synthesis and release of the Cia proteins. These findings indicate that the synthesis and secretion of the Cia proteins can be induced in a cell-free system by incubating *C. jejuni* in serum-supplemented tissue culture medium.

1. INTRODUCTION

Although *Campylobacter jejuni* is now recognized as a leading cause of gastrointestinal disease in industrialized countries, the mechanism of *C. jejuni*-mediated enteritis remains unclear. Several studies support a role for invasion in the disease process

Mechanisms in the Pathogenesis of Enteric Diseases 2, edited by Paul and Francis.
Kluwer Academic / Plenum Publishers, New York, 1999.

of *C. jejuni*-mediated enteritis (Reviewed in Walker et al., 1986; Konkel et al., 1989; Russell et al., 1993; Wooldridge et al., 1997). *C. jejuni* has been detected inside intestinal epithelial cells of experimentally infected infant monkeys and new born piglets (Russell et al., 1993; Babakhani et al., 1993). *C. jejuni* has also been shown to be capable of translocating across polarized Caco-2 cell monolayers (Konkel et al., 1992). Given these observations, cell invasion has been proposed to be the primary mechanism of colon damage and diarrheal disease (Russell et al., 1993).

Studies have revealed that the binding of *C. jejuni* to intestinal cells in vitro is independent of protein synthesis, whereas internalization requires newly synthesized bacterial proteins. *C. jejuni* engage in an adaptive response upon co-cultivation with intestinal cells or upon incubation in media exposed to intestinal cells. Inhibition of the synthesis of these proteins blocks invasion of *C. jejuni* to host cells in vitro (Konkel and Cieplak, 1992). These results indicate that *C. jejuni* is able to respond upon contact with intestinal cells by synthesizing the proteins that mediate internalization. Additionally, studies in our laboratory have also demonstrated that *C. jejuni* secrete proteins upon co-cultivation with INT407 cells or INT407 cell-conditioned medium. These bacterial secreted proteins, termed Cia for <u>C</u>ampylobacter <u>i</u>nvasion <u>a</u>ntigens, are required for *C. jejuni* internalization into cultured mammalian cells. One of the secreted proteins, termed CiaB (<u>C</u>ampylobacter <u>i</u>nvasion <u>a</u>ntigen <u>B</u>), shares similarity with type III secreted proteins from *Salmonella*, *Shigella*, and *Yersinia* (Konkel et al., submitted for publication). Like other type III secreted proteins, CiaB lacks a typical cleavable signal sequence. Taken together, these results suggest that *C. jejuni* possess a type III secretion system.

The type III secretion system is an essential virulence determinant utilized by a wide variety of Gram-negative bacteria for the secretion of virulence factors (Salmon and Reeves, 1993). This system has been extensively studied in pathogens such as *Salmonella*, *Shigella*, and *Yersinia* (Reviewed in: Hueck, 1998). Most of the proteins secreted via a type III secretion machinery have effector functions inside the host cell, resulting in alteration of the signal transduction pathways of the target cell.

2. METHODS AND RESULTS

Secretion of *Salmonella typhimurium* InvJ protein, a target of the *inv*-encoded type III secretion system has been shown to be stimulated by contact with cultured epithelial cells or by incubation with medium supplemented with calf serum (Zierler and Galán, 1995). Similar results have been observed for *Shigella flexneri* and the secretion of the Ipa proteins (Ménard et al., 1994). To determine whether incubation of *C. jejuni* in the presence of serum would stimulate the secretion of the Cia proteins, *C. jejuni* was incubated in Eagle's Minimal Essential Medium (EMEM) supplemented with different concentrations of fetal bovine serum (FBS). FBS triggered the synthesis and secretion of the *C. jejuni* Cia proteins as judged by autoradiography (Fig. 1). Although no differences were observed in the amount of secreted proteins when *C. jejuni* were cultured in media supplemented with 1% to 10% FBS, incubation of *C. jejuni* in media containing 1% to 0.01% FBS resulted in a dose-dependent reduction in the secretion of the Cia proteins. In addition, heat treatment of EMEM containing 1% FBS did not affect the secretion of the Cia proteins. These results indicate that there is a molecule in serum responsible for stimulating the synthesis and secretion of

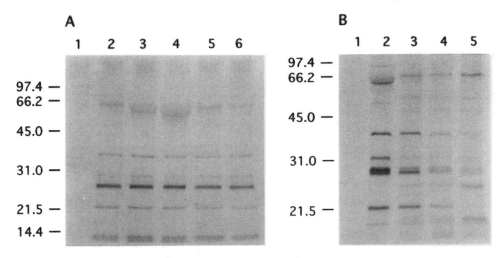

Figure 1. Fetal bovine serum stimulates the synthesis and secretion of the Cia proteins. *C. jejuni* F38011 were incubated in Eagle's Minimal Essential Medium (EMEM) without methionine and with or without fetal bovine serum (FBS). After an 1 hour pre-incubation period, [^{35}S]-methionine was added and incubation continued for 2 additional hours. Following the labeling of the newly synthesized proteins, the bacterial cells were pelleted by centrifugation and the supernatant fluids collected. Secreted proteins were concentrated fourfold with four volumes of 1 mM HCL-acetone and then resuspended in water. Secreted proteins were analyzed by SDS-PAGE and autoradiography. (A) Effect of 1 to 10% FBS on the secretion of the Cia proteins. Lanes: 1, no FBS; 2, 1% FBS; 3, 5% FBS; 4, 10% FBS; 5, 1% heat-treated 60°C for 30 min; 6, 1% FBS heat-treated 100°C for 15 min. (B) Effect of 1 to 0.01% FBS on the secretion of the Cia proteins. Lanes: 1, no FBS; 2, 1% FBS; 3, 0.1% FBS; 4, 0.05% FBS; 5, 0.01% FBS. Molecular mass standards are indicated, in kDa, on the left.

the Cia proteins and this molecule is not heat-labile. Sera from different sources were also used to test their ability for stimulating the synthesis and secretion of *C. jejuni* target proteins (Fig. 2). Incubation of *C. jejuni* in EMEM supplemented with different sera resulted in the synthesis and secretion of the Cia proteins. These data indicate that the stimulating molecule is conserved between the sera tested.

3. CONCLUSION

In summary, the Cia proteins are essential for the internalization of *C. jejuni* into host cells. These proteins are synthesized and released upon contact of *C. jejuni* with a soluble factor present in serum. We are in the process of identifying the serum component that stimulates the synthesis and secretion of the Cia proteins. Continued molecular and functional analyses of the Cia proteins will provide more insight into the molecular mechanisms utilized by *C. jejuni* to gain access into host cells.

ACKNOWLEDGMENTS

This work was supported by a grant from the NIH (1RO1 DK50567-01A1) awarded to MEK.

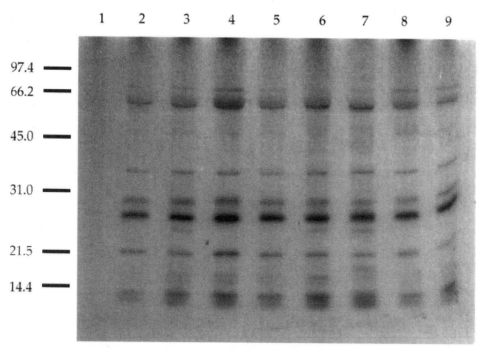

Figure 2. Stimulation of synthesis and secretion of Cia proteins by serum from different sources. *C. jejuni* was incubated in EMEM without methionine and without (lane 1) or with serum (lanes 2–9). Metabolic labeling and preparation of secreted proteins were carried out as described in Fig. 1. Lanes: 1, no serum; 2, 1% bovine serum; 3, 1% human serum; 4, 1% pig serum; 5, 1% goat serum; 6, 1% sheep serum; 7, 1% rabbit serum; 8, 1% mouse serum; 9, 1% chicken serum. Molecular mass standards are indicated, in kDa, on the left.

REFERENCES

Babakhani, F.K. and Joens, L.A. (1993) Primary swine intestinal cells as a model for studying *Campylobacter jejuni* invasiveness. *Infec Immun* **61**:2723–2726.

Fauchere, J.L., Rosenau, A., Veron, M., Moyen, E.N., Richard, S., and Pfister, A. (1986) Association with HeLa cells of *Campyloabacter jejuni* and *Campylobacter coli* isolated from human feces. *Infec and Immun* **54**:283–287.

Hueck, C.J. (1998) Type III protein secretion system in bacterial pathogens of animals and plants. *Micro and Mo Bio Revs* **62**:379–433.

Kleipstein, F.A. and Engert, R.F. (1984) Purification of *Campylobacter jejuni* enterotoxin. *Lancet* **1**:1123–1124.

Konkel, M.E. and Joens, L.A. (1989) Adhesion to and invasion of Hep-2 cells by *Campylobacter* ssp. *Infec and Immun* **57**:2984–2990.

Konkel, M.E. and Cieplak, W., Jr. (1992) Altered synthetic response of *Campylobacter jejuni* to cocultivation with human epithelial cells is associated with enhanced internalization. *Infec and Immun* **60**:-4945–4949.

Konkel, M.E., Mead, D.J., Hayes, F., and Cieplak, W., Jr. (1992) Translocation of *Campylobacter jejuni* across human polarized epithelial cells. *J Infec Dis* **166**:308–315.

Konkel, M.E., Mead, D.J., and Ciplak, W., Jr. (1993) Kinetic and antigenic characterization of altered protein synthesis by *Campylobacter jejuni* during cultivation with human epithelial cells. *J Infec Dis* **168**:-948–954.

Konkel, M.E. and Cieplak, W., Jr. (1996) Molecular pathogenesis of *Campylobacter jejuni* pathogenesis. *In:* Enteric Infections and Immunity. Plenum Press, New York. pp. 133–147.

Konkel, M.E., Kim, B.J., Rivera-Amill, V., and Garvis, G.S. (1998) Bacterial secreted proteins are required for the internalization of *C. jejuni* into cultured mammalian cells. Submitted for publication.

Ménard, R., Sansonetti, P., and Parsot, C. (1994) The secretion of the *Shigella flexneri* Ipa invasins is activated by epithelial cells and controlled by IpaB and IpaD. *EMBO J* **13**:5293–5302.

Ruiz-Palacios, G.M., Torres, J., Torres, N.I., Escamilla, E., Ruiz-Palacios, B.R., and Tamayo, J. (1983) Cholera-like enterotoxin produced by *Campylobacter jejuni*. Characterization and clinical significance. *Lancet* **2**:250–253.

Russell, R.G., O'Donnoghue, M., Blake, D.C., Jr., Zulty, J., and De Tolla, L.J. (1993) Early colonic damage and invasion of *Campylobacter jejuni* in experimentally challenged infant *Macaca mulatta*. *J of Infec Dis* **168**:210–215.

Salmon, G.P.C. and Reeves, P.J. (1993) Membrane traffic wardens and protein secretion in Gram-negative bacteria. *Trends Biochem Sci* **18**:7–12.

Walker, R.I., Caldwell, M.B., Lee, E.C., Guerry, P., Trust, T.J., and Ruiz-Palacios, G.M. (1986) Pathophysiology of *Campylobacter* enteritis. *Micro Rev* **50**:81–94.

Wooldridge, K.G. and Ketley, J.M. (1997) *Campylobacter*-host cell interactions. *Trends in Microbiol* **5**:96–102.

Zierler, M.K. and Galán, J.E. (1995) Contact with cultured epithelial cells stimulates the secretion of *Salmonella typhimurium* invasion protein InvJ. *Infec Immun* **63**:4024–4028.

24

CODON USAGE IN THE A/T-RICH BACTERIUM *CAMPYLOBACTER JEJUNI*

Sean A. Gray and Michael E. Konkel

Department of Microbiology
Washington State University
Pullman, Washington 99164-4233

1. SUMMARY

Campylobacter jejuni is a Gram negative, microaerophilic pathogen that causes gastroenteritis in humans. The genome of *C. jejuni* is AT-rich, with a mol% G + C of 30.4. This high AT content was hypothesized to result in unique codon usage. In the present study, we analyzed the codon usage of sixty-seven C. jejuni genes and generated a codon frequency table. As predicted, the codon usage of C. jejuni revealed a strong bias towards codons ending in A or U. In addition to determining codon usage frequencies, the relative synonymous codon usage values were calculated to identify rare and optimal codons. Seventeen codons were identified as optimal and twelve codons as rare. Thirty-two codons exhibited little or no bias. A plot of the effective number of codons versus the third position %G + C values for the sixty-seven genes revealed that *C. jejuni* uses an average of 39 of the 61 codons to encode proteins. These data will be useful for various molecular analyses including selection of degenerate primers to screen C. jejuni-genomic DNA libraries.

2. INTRODUCTION

Campylobacter jejuni is one of the most common causes of diarrhea, and is acquired by eating undercooked chicken or drinking unpasteurized milk or contaminated water (Blaser et al., 1979). *C. jejuni* is a Gram-negative, microaerophilic, spiral-shaped bacterium that frequently causes an acute gastroenteritis in humans, similar to that caused by *Salmonella typhimurium* (Blaser et al., 1979). Infections with *C. jejuni* are characterized by malaise, fever, abdominal cramps, and bloody diarrhea often containing leukocytes. Although the mechanism of pathogenesis of *C. jejuni* has been the

Mechanisms in the Pathogenesis of Enteric Diseases 2, edited by Paul and Francis.
Kluwer Academic / Plenum Publishers, New York, 1999.

focus of many studies in recent years, few genes have been shown conclusively to play a role in virulence. To date, only about seventy genes have been characterized from *C. jejuni*. Recently, the genome of *C. jejuni* was sequenced (The Sanger Group, data not published), yet the limiting factor in working with this organism is that there are relatively few tools for performing molecular analyses. Few heterologous genes have been shown to be expressed in *C. jejuni*. Some of the problems with expression of heterologous genes might be explained by the fact that the genomic mol% G + C content of *C. jejuni* is 30.4. The purpose of this study was to analyze genes from *C. jejuni* for codon usage and generate a codon frequency table (Andersson and Sharp, 1996).

3. RESULTS AND DISCUSSION

Sixty-seven genes, containing 18,888 codons, were used for codon analyses. Ribosomal RNA sequences, noncoding sequences, and incomplete sequences were eliminated from the analyses. Codon usage and relative synonymous codon usage (RSCU) analyses were performed using the program CodonFrequency found in the GCG-Wisconsin package (Edelman et al., 1996). Third position percent G + C (GC3$_s$) and effective number of codons (N$_c$) calculations were performed using the FORTRAN program CODONS described by Lloyd and Sharp (1992).

The codon usage for the sixty-seven genes is shown in Table 1. Overall, *C. jejuni* genes showed a bias for codons ending in adenine (A) or uracil (U) over codons ending in cytosine (C) or guanine (G). This bias was most pronounced at the third position "wobble" base of codons as the position-specific mol% G + C was 46.89 at the first position, 34.99 at the second position, and 19.55 at the third position. Furthermore, there was also bias for the use of U over A in every case examined where an amino acid could be encoded by a synonym ending in either A or U. When a C or G occurred in the third position, no bias was observed for either base. Examination of codon usages allowed for selection of seventeen optimal codons and twelve rare codons based on the RSCU values. The selection of optimal codons was arbitrary and based on the method used for *E. coli* except that a higher RSCU value was used for *C. jejuni* given the greater bias in *C. jejuni* (Guoy and Gautier, 1982; Ikemura, 1985; Medigue et al., 1991). The selection of optimal codons reflects the U over A bias in that twelve of the seventeen optimal codons end in U while five end in A. The underlined codons are the ones identified as optimal codons by having a RSCU value greater to or equal to 1.60. The codons followed by an asterisk indicate rare codons by having a RSCU value less than or equal to 0.20.

Figure 1 shows the N$_c$ versus GC3$_s$ plot for each of the sixty-seven genes analyzed. Each point represents a single *C. jejuni* gene. The GC3$_s$ versus N$_c$ plot is a commonly used plot which correlates the effective number of codons that an organism uses to encode the standard 20 amino acids as a function of its genomic G + C content (Wright, 1990). The %G + C at the third position of all *C. jejuni* codons was 19.8, ranging between 12 and 25, in contrast to its overall genomic mol% G + C of 30.4. *C. jejuni* most frequently uses 39 of the 61 codons, with a range of 32 to 48 codons, to encode the 20 amino acids, probably due to its bias for A or U ending codons.

There are many reasons why a heterologous gene may not be expressed in *C. jejuni*. Wosten et al. (1998) recently showed that promoter compatibility is one important factor in expression of heterologous genes. Several researchers have also demonstrated that transcriptional or translational initiation may also play important roles in

Table 1. *C. jejuni* codon preferences

AA	Codon	Freq[a]	RSCU[b]	AA	Codon	Freq[a]	RSCU[b]	AA	Codon	Freq[a]	RSCU[b]
F	UUU	4.29	1.86	S	UCU	1.88	1.56	Y	UAU	2.39	1.74	C	UGU	0.59	1.36
F	UUC*	0.34	0.14	S	UCC*	0.16	0.12	Y	UAC	0.35	0.26	C	UGC	0.28	0.64
L	UUA	4.18	2.75	S	UCA	1.48	1.26	Z	UAA	0.24	2.07	Z	UGA	0.05	0.42
L	UUG	1.30	0.84	S	UCG*	0.20	0.18	Z	UAG	0.06	0.51	W	UGG	0.61	1.00
L	CUU	2.79	1.86	P	CCU	1.45	2.32	H	CAU	1.08	1.66	R	CGU	0.73	1.37
L	CUC*	0.21	0.12	P	CCC*	0.07	0.12	H	CAC	0.22	0.34	R	CGC	0.31	0.59
L	CUA	0.51	0.36	P	CCA	0.89	1.40	Q	CAA	3.24	1.80	R	CGA*	0.05	0.11
L	CUG*	0.08	0.06	P	CCG*	0.09	0.16	Q	CAG*	0.37	0.20	R	CGG*	0.02	0.05
I	AUU	4.04	1.54	T	ACU	2.54	2.40	N	AAU	5.35	1.66	S	AGU	2.30	1.92
I	AUC	1.61	0.61	T	ACC	0.80	0.76	N	AAC	1.11	0.34	S	AGC	1.14	0.95
I	AUA	2.23	0.85	T	ACA	0.65	0.60	K	AAA	7.23	1.74	R	AGA	1.80	3.34
M	AUG	2.27	1.00	T	ACG	0.27	0.24	K	AAG	1.09	0.26	R	AGG	0.28	0.54
V	GUU	2.71	1.88	A	GCU	4.29	2.04	D	GAU	5.69	1.86	G	GGU	3.00	1.76
V	GUC*	0.17	0.12	A	GCC*	0.56	0.28	D	GAC*	0.44	0.14	G	GGC	0.95	0.56
V	GUA	2.03	1.40	A	GCA	3.02	1.40	E	GAA	5.22	1.62	G	GGA	2.48	1.44
V	GUG	0.90	0.60	A	GCG	0.55	0.28	E	GAG	1.26	0.38	G	GGG	0.44	0.24

aThe overall percentage of use of each codon in the 67 genes.
bThe RSCU value for each codon.
*rare codons.
_optimal codons.

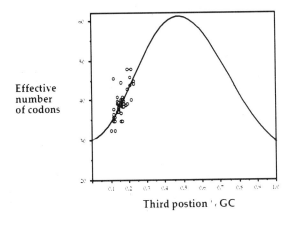

Figure 1. *Campylobacter jejuni* uses a small subset of the 61 codons to encode the 20 amino acids as a result of its low third position %G + C content.

Effective number of codons

Third position % GC

gene expression (Guoy and Gautier, 1982; Ikemura et al., 1985). This study focuses on codon usage, an aspect that we consider fundamental, as yet another important factor of gene expression. We have identified the codon usage for *C. jejuni* based on sixty-seven genes and identified optimal and rare codons based on relative synonymous codon usages. These data indicate that codon usage in *C. jejuni* is extremely biased towards codons ending in A or U due to the AT-richness of the genome. The results of this study will be useful in molecular analyses of *C. jejuni* by facilitating degenerate primer selection, construction of cloning vectors, and revealing potential problems with codon usage when attempting to express heterologous genes.

ACKNOWLEDGMENTS

The authors wish to thank Steven M. Thompson and Susan Jean-Johns for their assistance with the computer analyses, Gwyn Glaser for her assistance in compiling the gene sequences, and Dr. Mike Kahn for critically reviewing the article. This work was supported by grants from the NIH (1R01 DK50567-01A1) and the USDA National Research Initiative Competitive Grants Program (USDA/NRICGP, No. 9601496) awarded to MEK.

REFERENCES

Andersson, S.G.E. and P.M. Sharp. 1996. Codon usage in the *Mycobacterium tuberculosis* complex. *Microbiol.* 142:915–925.

Blaser, M.J., I.D. Berkowitz, F.M. LaForce, J. Cravens, L.B. Reller, and W.L. Wang. 1979. *Campylobacter* enteritis: clinical and epidemiological features. *Ann. Intern. Med.* 91:179–185.

Dong, H., L. Nilsson, and C.G. Kurland. 1996. Co-variation of tRNA abundance and codon usage in *Escherichia coli* at different growth rates. *J. Mol. Biol.* 260:645–663.

Edelman, I., S. Olsen, and J. Devereux. 1996. *Program manual for the Wisconsin Package*, Version 9.1. Genetics Computer Group (GCG), Madison, Wisconsin, U.S.A. 53711.

Gouy, M. and C. Gautier. 1982. Codon usage in bacteria: correlation with gene expressivity. *Nucleic Acids Res.* 10:7055–7074.

Ikemura, T. 1985. Codon usage and tRNA content in unicellular and multicellular organisms. *Mol. Biol. Evol.* 2:13–34.

Lloyd, A.T. and P.M. Sharp. 1992. CODONS: A microcomputer program for codon usage analysis. *J. Hered.* 83:239–240.

Medigue, C., T. Rouxel, P. Vigier, A. Henaut, and A. Danchin. 1991. Evidence for horizontal gene transfer in *Escherichia coli* speciation. *J. Mol. Biol.* 222:851–856.

Wosten, M.M.S.M., M. Boeve, M.G.A. Koot, A.C. van Nuenen, and B.A.M. van der Zeijst. 1998. Identification of *Campylobacter jejuni* promoter sequences. *J. Bacteriol.* 180:594–599.

Wright, F. 1990. The 'effective number of codons' used in a gene. *Gene.* 87:23–29.

25

PREVALENCE OF *CAMPYLOBACTER*, *SALMONELLA*, AND *ARCOBACTER* SPECIES AT SLAUGHTER IN MARKET AGE PIGS

Roger B. Harvey,*[1] Robin C. Anderson,[1] Colin R. Young,[1]
Michael E. Hume,[1] Kenneth J. Genovese,[2] Richard L. Ziprin,[1]
Leigh A. Farrington,[2] Larry H. Stanker,[1] and David J. Nisbet[1]

[1] Food Animal Protection Research Laboratory
USDA, ARS, College Station
Texas 77845 USA
[2] College of Veterinary Medicine
Texas A&M University
College Station
Texas 77843 USA

1. SUMMARY

A survey was conducted to determine the prevalence of *Campylobacter*, *Salmonella*, and *Arcobacter* species in market age pigs from an integrated swine operation in Texas. Our findings indicate that farms from this commercial operation were heavily contaminated with *Campylobacter* and *Salmonella*, that the isolation rates of *C. jejuni* were higher than predicted, and that there was a low prevalence of *Arcobacter*.

2. INTRODUCTION

Losses to the U.S. swine industry from *Salmonella* species are estimated at >$100 million annually. *Salmonella*-contaminated meat, including pork, is an important source of infection for human salmonellosis. Due to public health concerns, there has been an increased effort to survey the incidence of on-farm salmonellae in swine production (Centers for Disease Control and Prevention, 1998). Although not as strictly monitored or controlled as salmonellae, the presence of *Campylobacter spp.* in food items has generated a great deal of attention in the past few years. *Campylobacter* has emerged as one of the most common causes of human enteric disease in developed countries. In the

Mechanisms in the Pathogenesis of Enteric Diseases 2, edited by Paul and Francis.
Kluwer Academic / Plenum Publishers, New York, 1999.

U.S., *Campylobacter* is considered by many to be the chief cause of enteric illness (Wesley and Bryner, 1989). *Campylobacter* has been isolated from raw beef, pork, lamb, chicken, cooked meats, and seafood (Nielsen et al., 1997; Fricker and Park, 1989; Zanetti et al., 1996). Pigs are probably one of the natural reservoirs of *Campylobacter spp. Arcobacter*, found in some domestic and wild animals, can cause enteric disease in humans and animals (Zanetti et al., 1996). This organism has been reported infrequently in pigs; however, very few studies have focused on recovery of the bacteria from domestic swine. Because of the public health concerns surrounding these enteropathogens, the purpose of the present study was to survey the prevalence of *Salmonella, Campylobacter*, and *Arcobacter* in market age pigs from an integrated swine operation in Texas.

3. ISOLATION PROCEDURES

The experimental design called for 4 representative farms (farrow-to-finish) to be sampled 3 times each over a nine-month period. Samples of ileocolic lymph nodes and cecal contents were collected at slaughter from 50 pigs per sampling period (for a total of 595 pigs sampled). Enteric bacteria were cultured and identified by utilization of enrichment broth, restrictive media, biochemical analyses, antibody agglutination, differential stains, microscopic examination, and ELISA techniques.

4. RESULTS AND DISCUSSION

The mean prevalence rate for salmonellae was 61% (range of 11–88%) with 30+ serovars of *Salmonella* identified. A total of 362 *Salmonella* isolates were typed. Ten serovars accounted for 87% of isolates and 5 serovars (*S. schwartzengrund, S. montevideo, S. livingstone, S. anatum*, and *S. typhimurium*) accounted for 68% of all isolates. Fifty-one pigs (14%) had more than one serovar isolated. Of the salmonellae isolates, 271 came from lymph nodes, whereas 216 originated from cecal contents. When evaluating two pre-enrichments used for salmonellae isolations, we noted that tetrathionate broth was considerably more efficient than GN Hajna for isolations from cecal contents (65% vs. 34%), whereas GN Hajna was slightly better than tetrathionate for recovery from lymph nodes (56% vs. 44%). Antibiotic sensitivity profiles were performed on all of the typed *Salmonella* isolates. The results of that study are presented elsewhere at this conference (Farrington et al., 1998).

Approximately one-half the farms were sampled for *Arcobacter* and the mean prevalence rate was 5% (range of 0–20%). Our isolation rate is similar to that reported for *Arcobacter* prevalence (2.4%) in pork sausage in Italy (Zanetti et al., 1996).

The prevalence rate for *Campylobacter* was 92% (range of 70–100%) with 60% *C. coli* and 31% *C. jejuni. C. lari* was isolated from 2 pigs. Our results are similar to an epidemiological study in the Netherlands in which young pigs had a *Campylobacter* prevalence of 85% (Weijtens et al., 1997). We sampled replacement gilts and 9–14 day old piglets for *Campylobacter* and *Salmonella*, and our results show that colonization by both organisms occurs at an early age and suggest that the source of transmission is from dam to offspring. This is in agreement with that of Weijtens et al. (1997) in which piglets became colonized by 14 days of age and obtained *Campylobacter* infection from their sows.

5. CONCLUSIONS

Our findings indicate that farms from this commercial operation were heavily contaminated with *Campylobacter* and *Salmonella*, that the isolation rates of *C. jejuni* in pigs were higher than predicted, and that there was a low prevalence of *Arcobacter*. It is unknown if carcass contamination rates mirror the prevalence of *Salmonella* and *Campylobacter* seen in the slaughter pigs. These food safety issues will be addressed in the next phase of our survey. We will also attempt to reduce the on-farm prevalence of *Salmonella* and *Campylobacter* through some promising intervention strategies we have developed.

REFERENCES

Centers for Disease Control and Prevention, April 1998, In: FoodNet, 1997 Surveillance Results: CDC/USDA/FDA Foodborne Diseases Active Surveillence Network, CDC's Emerging Infections Program. U.S. Department of Human Services, Washington DC.

Farrington, L.A., Harvey, R.B., Buckley, S.A., et al., 1998, A survey of antibiotic resistance of *Salmonella* in market-age swine, In: Proceedings, 2nd Int. Rushmore Conference on Mechanisms in the Pathogenesis of Enteric Disease.

Fricker, C.R. and Park, R.W.A., 1989, A two-year study of the distribution of "thermophilic" campylobacters in human, environmental and food samples from the Reading area with particular reference to toxin production and heat-stable serotype, J. Appl. Bacteriol. 66:477–490.

Nielsen, E.M., Enberg, J., and Madsen, M., 1997, Distribution of serotypes of *Campylobacter jejuni* and *C. coli* from Danish patients, poultry, cattle, and swine, FEMS Immunol. Med. Microbiol. 19:47–56.

Weijtens, M.J.B.M., van der Plas, J., Bijker, P.G.H., et al., 1997, The transmission of campylobacter in piggeries; an epidemiological study, J. Appl. Microbiol. 83:693–698.

Wesley, R.D. and Bryner, J., 1989, Re-examination of *Campylobacter hyointestinalis* and *C fetus*, In: Proceedings, International Workshop on *Campylobacter* Infections, p. 122.

Zanetti, F., Varoli, O., Stampi, S., et al., 1996, Prevalence of thermophilic *Campylobacter* and *Arcobacter butzleri* in food of animal origin, Int. J. Food Microbiol., 33:315–321.

26

CRYPTOSPORIDIUM PARVUM GENE DISCOVERY

Mitchell S. Abrahamsen

Department of Veterinary PathoBiology
University of Minnesota

SUMMARY

Cryptosporidium parvum is a well-recognized cause of diarrhea in humans and animals throughout the world, and is associated with a substantial degree of morbidity and mortality in patients with acquired immunodeficiency syndrome (AIDS). At the present time, there is no effective therapy for treating or preventing infection with *C. parvum*. This is primarily due to a lack of understanding of the basic cellular and molecular biology of this pathogen in terms of virulence factors, genome structure, gene expression, and regulation. Over the past few years, large-scale sequencing of randomly selected cDNAs or fragments of genomic DNA has proven to be an efficient approach for obtaining large amount of genomic information. Recently, large-scale sporozoite expressed sequence tag (EST) and genomic sequence tag (GST) projects have been initiated for *C. parvum*. These projects have greatly increased the number of *C. parvum* genes identified and demonstrate the usefulness of large-scale sequencing for expanding our understanding of *C. parvum* biology. Continued characterization of the *C. parvum* genome will increase our basic understanding of the cellular and molecular biology of *C. parvum* in terms of gene and genome structure, and will identify key metabolic and pathophysiologic features of the organism for future development of safe and effective strategies for prevention and treatment of disease.

Correspondence Address: Department of Veterinary PathoBiology, University of Minnesota, 1988 Fitch Ave., St. Paul, MN 55108, USA, Phone: (612) 624-1244, Fax: (612) 625-0204, Electronic mail address: abrah025@tc.umn.edu.

Mechanisms in the Pathogenesis of Enteric Diseases 2, edited by Paul and Francis.
Kluwer Academic / Plenum Publishers, New York, 1999.

1. INTRODUCTION

Cryptosporidium belongs to the phylum Apicomplexa and is one of several genera that are referred to as coccidia. The life cycle and morphological stages of *Cryptosporidium parvum* resemble that of other coccidia. The parasite primarily infects the microvillous border of the intestinal epithelium, and to a lesser extent extraintestinal epithelia, causing acute gastrointestinal disease in a wide range of mammalian hosts (Dubey et al., 1990). The first case of human *Cryptosporidium* infection was reported in 1976 (Navin and Harden, 1987), and only seven additional cases were documented before 1982 (Tzipori, 1988). Since then, the number of cases identified has increased dramatically, largely due to the recognition of a life-threatening form of infection in patients with AIDS. In addition, seroprevalence rates of 25–35% in the U.S. indicate that infection with *Cryptosporidium* is very common among healthy persons (Campbell and Current, 1983). *C. parvum* infection is now a well-recognized cause of diarrhea in immunocompetent and immunocompromised humans and animals of veterinary and agricultural interest throughout the world. Typically, the duration of infection and ultimate outcome of intestinal cryptosporidiosis is dependent on the immune status of the patient. In the most severely immunocompromised host, such as persons with AIDS, diarrhea caused by *C. parvum* infection of the gastrointestinal tract becomes progressively worse with time and may be a major factor leading to death. While immunologically healthy patients usually recover spontaneously within 30 days, their clinical signs can be severe and their potential for transmission can be persistent for as long as 60 days after symptoms cease (Smith et al., 1988; Connolly et al., 1988; Dias et al., 1988). Currently, there are no effective therapies for treating or preventing infection by *C. parvum*. Of the more than 150 antimicrobial drugs tested in animals and humans infected with *Cryptosporidium*, none have been found to be consistently effective against this parasite (Dubey et al., 1990; Fayer and Ungar, 1986; Tzipori, 1988; Petersen, 1993).

Transmission is by fecal-oral spread of the oocyst stage. When oocysts in food, water, or the general environment are ingested by a suitable host, sporozoites excyst, and parasitize epithelial cells of the gastrointestinal tract. Experimental infections in mammals have established that *C. parvum* has little or no host specificity. It is therefore not surprising that calves, and perhaps companion animals such as dogs, cats or rodents, have served as sources of human infection. Thus, cryptosporidiosis is included in the list of more than 150 diseases caused by agents that are naturally transmitted between other vertebrate animals and man. In addition, human to human transmission of *Cryptosporidium* has been established between household and family members, sexual partners, children in day care centers and their caretakers, and healthcare workers and their patients (Dubey et al., 1990).

2. CHARACTERIZATION OF *C. PARVUM* GENES

Despite the medical and veterinary importance of *C. parvum*, studies of this organism at the genetic level have only begun in recent years and are still in their infancy. Limited genetic studies have identified *C. parvum* genes encoding a relatively small number of basic metabolic and structural genes, as well as several genes encoding immunogenic antigens (Bonafonte et al., 1997; Jenkins and Petersen, 1997; Khramtsov et al., 1997; Spano et al., 1997). Currently, less than 70 non-EST/GST derived (discussed below) *C. parvum* sequences are available in the GenBank database, 11 of which are reports for ribosomal RNA. The limited number of gene sequences is representative of the lack of understanding of *Cryptosporidium* biology.

A common feature of coccidian parasites is that all development, sexual or asexual, occurs within cells of the host. This requires a complex association between two distinct eukaryotic organisms and is likely to represent some of the most unique aspects of coccidian biology. Until recently, the majority of research on coccidian parasites has focused on the identification and characterization of genes and antigens expressed by the invasive forms, (i.e., sporozoites and merozoites), with little consideration being given to understanding the biology of the parasite-infected cell. Although electron microscopy has been performed to study the association of *C. parvum* and other coccidians with their host cells (Dubey et al., 1990), little is known of the basic developmental biology of *C. parvum* or the molecular mechanisms involved in host-parasite interaction. Considering the absolute dependence of coccidian development on the host cell, it is crucial that we develop a better understanding of the molecular mechanisms involved in the unique intracellular developmental pathways of these parasites. Experiments to identify these biochemical pathways have been hindered by the lack of purification methods for the intracellular developmental stages, and the relatively small mass of parasite mRNA and proteins relative to the host cell. Previously, Jones et al. (1994) successfully used a PCR-based cDNA subtraction procedure to identify mRNAs specifically expressed in *C. parvum*-infected MDCK cells. These included *C. parvum* genes and host genes upregulated during infection. The development of differential mRNA display (Liang and Pardee, 1992) provides another powerful approach for use in examining genes whose expression is regulated during intracellular *C. parvum* development. These genes will represent some of the biochemical mechanisms that are crucial for *C. parvum* development and involved in the unique biochemistry of host-parasite interaction. To begin to understand these complex biochemical pathways, we have used differential mRNA display PCR to identify *C. parvum* genes, which are expressed during intracellular development (Abrahamsen et al., 1996; Schroeder et al., 1998, 1999). Although this approach has been successful, it is relatively time consuming and inefficient at identifying large-numbers of expressed *C. parvum* genes within the background of the ~15,000 genes estimated to be normally expressed in a mammalian cell.

3. EXPRESSED SEQUENCE TAGS

One approach for rapidly identifying large numbers of unknown genes is by the partial sequencing of gene transcripts, known as expressed sequence tags (ESTs). This approach has proven to be a very rapid and effective means of identifying and characterizing genes expressed in a variety of organisms and has become a standard method for the identification of tissue-specific and developmentally-regulated genes in a variety of higher and lower eukaryotic organisms. EST projects for several pathogenic protozoa including *Plasmodium falciparum*, *Toxoplasma gondii*, *Trypanosoma brucei*, and *Schistosoma mansoni*, have been conducted (Franco, 1995; Chakrabarti, 1994; El-Sayed, 1995). Recently, a large-scale EST project was initiated for *C. parvum* sporozoites (www.ebi.ac.uk/parasites/cparvEST.html). In a relatively short period of time, this project has identified 384 unique ESTs, greatly expanding the number of genes known to be expressed by *C. parvum* sporozoites. In addition to the identification of large numbers of *C. parvum* genes unique to any currently in the sequence databases, this project has identified numerous expressed sequences with similarities to known genes of other organisms.

Although the ongoing *C. parvum* sporozoite EST project will continue to provide valuable information concerning the parasite's biology, there are several technical issues associated with an EST approach which greatly limits the amount of information that can be obtained with regard to *C. parvum* genes. The first and major limitation of an EST approach for *C. parvum* gene discovery is the inability to obtain purified samples of the various asexual, sexual, and intracellular developmental stages of the parasite. Therefore, an EST approach for this parasite can only identify those genes which are expressed during the sporozoite stage of the life cycle. Genes whose expression is limited to merozoites, macrogametes, microgametes, or genes which are only expressed during intracellular development will not be identified. Considering the absolute dependence of *C. parvum* development on the host cell, many unique and novel biochemical pathways and molecular mechanisms involved in host-parasite interaction are unlikely to be identified by the ongoing sporozoite EST project. Indeed, during gene discovery projects of the related coccidian parasite *Eimeria bovis*, we have demonstrated that the merozoite developmental stage expresses numerous genes which are not expressed by the sporozoite stage (Abrahamsen et al., 1993, 1995).

A second limitation of an EST approach is that, in general, the frequency of identification of a particular gene is directly related the level of expression of the corresponding mRNA species in the cell. Therefore, the most abundantly expressed genes are characterized multiple times during the course of the project, and genes which are expressed at very low levels may not be identified. Of the 567 total ESTs generated from the *C. parvum* sporozoite cDNA libraries, 284 were redundant, resulting in the identification of 384 unique sequences (68%). In addition, the continued sequencing of random cDNA clones rapidly becomes less productive, as fewer new sequences will be identified. Although there are some technically difficult and time consuming manipulations of the cDNA library which can minimize the problems associated with abundant mRNAs, it is well-recognized that an EST approach is most efficient at identifying genes which are expressed at moderate to high levels.

4. LARGE-SCALE ANALYSIS OF THE *C. PARVUM* GENOME

4.1. GST Approach to *C. parvum* Genome Characterization

Over the past few years, large-scale sequencing of random fragments of genomic DNA has proven to be an efficient approach for obtaining large amount of genomic information. This type of an approach has the potential to rapidly identify a large amount of sequence distributed throughout the genome of an organism. In order to identify *C. parvum* genes independent of their developmental expression, we initiated a large-scale sequencing of random *C. parvum* genomic segments. A total of 654 genomic sequence tags (GSTs) were generated, representing >250 kb of unique sequence, or ~2.5% of the *C. parvum* genome. Comparison of the GSTs with sequences in the public DNA and protein databases revealed that 134 GSTs (20.1%) displayed similarity to previously identified proteins, ribosomal RNA and tRNA genes. These included putative genes involved in the glycolytic pathway, DNA, RNA, and protein metabolism, and signal transduction pathways. During the course of our GST project, we became aware of another effort to identify 5000 genome sequence tags of *C. parvum* (www.ebi.ac.uk/parasites/cparvGST.html). Information provided by the GST web site revealed that ~21% of the unique GSTs generated, display significant sequence homology with sequences present in GenBank. This is consistent with the results of our own pilot GST project.

These GST projects demonstrate the usefulness of a this approach to rapidly identify large numbers of *C. parvum* genes. However, a limitation of a GST approach is that only those tags which contain sequences which display homology to known genes in the database will be identified as genes. For those GSTs which do not display any sequence homology, it cannot be determined if they represent intragenic, intergenic, non-coding, or coding sequences. Therefore, unless the GST contains a complete open reading frame, previously uncharacterized gene homologues or genes unique to *C. parvum* will not be identified by this approach.

4.2. Genome Sequencing

Since the genomic DNA sequence encodes all of the heritable information responsible for development, disease pathogenesis, virulence, species permissiveness, and immune resistance, a comprehensive knowledge of the *C. parvum* genome will provide the necessary information required for cost-effective and targeted research into disease prevention and treatment. The complex life cycle of *C. parvum* and lack of access to purified populations of the different developmental stages, makes other gene discovery approaches difficult and very inefficient. A genomic sequencing approach for *C. parvum* gene discovery is not subject to the same limitations of an EST approach; all genes can be identified, irrespective of their developmental expression. In addition, all of the genes on a sequenced chromosome can be identified. By having the entire chromosomal sequence, the complete open reading frame (ORF) for each gene can be identified based on structure, not homology, as is the case for a GST approach.

An important issue to consider when proposing to obtain the genomic sequence of any organism, and in particular, eukaryotic organisms, is the organization and size of the genome. Recently, improved separation of *C. parvum* chromosomes using contour-clamped homogeneous electric fields combined with scanning densitometry has determined that the most likely number of chromosomes is eight (Blunt et al., 1997). The chromosomes range in size from 1.03 Mb to 1.54 Mb with a total genome size of ~10.4 Mb. This is relatively small for a eukaryotic organism, and the limited number and size of each chromosome allows for the genomic sequencing of *C. parvum* to be pursued in discrete steps for each chromosome or group of chromosomes. Even the largest chromosome is small enough to be completely sequenced using current technologies, without the need for expensive and time consuming genome mapping. Therefore, *C. parvum* appears to be an ideal candidate for a complete genome sequencing project.

5. CONCLUSIONS

The obligate intracellular nature of *C. parvum* presents many hurdles for identifying and characterizing the genes controlling the development of the multiple asexual and sexual life cycle stages, or the unique biochemistry and molecular mechanisms involved in host-parasite interaction. With the recent advances in high-throughput automated DNA sequencing capabilities, large-scale genomic sequencing has become a cost-effective and time-efficient approach to understanding the biology of an organism. In addition, the continued development and implementation of new software tools that can scan raw sequences for signs of genes and then identify clues as to potential functions, has provided the final realization of the potential rewards of genome sequencing. This is in stark contrast to the cost and time associated with single-gene studies where a substantial amount of effort can be directed at characterizing a known biochemical activity or searching for genes based on homology that may not be conserved between different organisms.

The ongoing *C. parvum* EST and GST projects demonstrate that large-scale sequencing efforts are an efficient and cost-effective method for identifying *C. parvum* genes which are expressed throughout the parasite's life cycle. Future efforts to sequence the entire *C. parvum* genome, or individual chromosomes, will provide a vast amount of information regarding the biology of *C. parvum* which will have many long-term benefits. In addition to identifying hundreds of *C. parvum* genes independent of their developmental expression or transcript level, these efforts will provide sequence information on the promoters of *C. parvum* genes, the structural organization of the genome, and the basis for future comparative genome analysis with other eukaryotic organisms. These efforts will identify novel biochemical pathways, antigens, and virulence mechanisms which are critical for parasite survival, disease pathogenesis and the development of immunity. These targets will provide the basis for future efforts to design new and effective drugs, vaccines, and diagnostics for *C. parvum* infection in normal and immunocompromised hosts.

REFERENCES

Abrahamsen, M.S., Clark, T.G., Mascolo, P., Speer, C.A., and White, M.W., 1993, Developmental gene expression in *Eimeria bovis*, Mol. Biochem. Parasitol. 57:1–14.

Abrahamsen, M.S., Johnson, R.R., Hathaway, M., and White, M.W., 1995, Identification of *Eimeria bovis* merozoite cDNAs using differential mRNA display, Mol. Biochem. Parasitol. 71:183–191.

Abrahamsen, M.S., Schroeder, A.A., and Lancto, C.A., 1996, Differential mRNA display analysis of gene expression in *Cryptosporidium parvum*-infected HCT-8 cells, J. Euk. Microbiol. 43:80–81S.

Blunt, D.S., Khramtsov, N.V., Upton, S.J., and Montelone, B.A., 1997, Molecular karyotype analysis of *Cryptosporidium parvum*: evidence for eight chromosomes and a low-molecular-size molecule, Clin. Diag. Lab. Immunol. 4:11–13.

Bonafonte, M.T., Priest, J.W., Garmon, D., Arrowood, M.J., and Mead, J.R., 1997, Isolation of the gene coding for elongation factor-1 alpha in *Cryptosporidium parvum*, Biochim. Biophys. Acta. 1351:256–260.

Campbell, P.N. and Current, W.L., 1983, Demonstration of serum antibodies to *Cryptosporidium* sp in normal and immunodeficient humans with confirmed infections, J. Clin. Micro. 18:165–169.

Chakrabarti, D., Reddy, G.R., Dame, J.B., Almira, E.C., Laipis, P.J., Ferl, R.J., Yang, T.P., Rowe, T.C., and Schuster, S.M., 1994, Analysis of expressed sequence tags from *Plasmodium falciparum*, Mol. Biochem. Parasitol. 66:97–104.

Connolly, G.M., Dryden, M.S., Shanson, D.C., and Gassard, B.G., 1988, Cryptosporidial diarrhea in Aids and its treatment, Gut 29:593–597.

Dias, R.M.D., Mangini, A.C.S., Torres, D.M.G.V., Correa, M.O.A., Lupetti, N., Correa, F.A., and Chieffe, P.P., 1988, Cryptosporidiosis among patients with acquired immunodeficiency syndrome (AIDS) in the county of Sao Paulo, Brazil, Rev. Inst. Med. Trop. Sao Paulo 30:310.

Dubey, J.P., Speer, C.A., and Fayer, R., 1990, Cryptosporidiosis of man and animals, CRC Press, Inc., Boca Raton. Fl.

El-Sayed, N.M.A., Alarcon, C.M., Beck, J.C., Sheffield, V.C., and Donelson, J.E., 1995, cDNA expressed tags of *Trypanosoma brucei rhodesiense* provide new insights into the biology of the parasite, Mol. Biochem. Parasitol. 73:75–90.

Fayer, R. and Ungar, B.L.P., 1986, *Cryptosporidium* spp. and cryptosporidiosis, Microbiol. Rev. 50:458–483.

Franco, G.R., Adams, M.D., Soares, M.B., Simpson, A.J., Venter, J.C., and Pena, S.D., 1995, Identification of new *Schistosoma mansoni* genes by the EST strategy using a directional cDNA library, Gene 152:141–147.

Jenkins, M.C. and C. Petersen, 1997, Molecular biology of *Cryptosporidium*, In: *Cryptosporidium* and cryptosporidiosis, Editor: Fayer, R., CRC Press, Boca Raton, Florida, p. 225–232.

Jones, D.E., Tu, T.D., Sweeney, R.W., and Clark, D.P., 1994, Isolation of *Cryptosporidium* and bovine cDNA clones from a *Cryptosporidium*-infected MDBK cell line subtraction library, J. Euk. Microbiol. 41:46–47S.

Khramtsov, N.V., Oppert, B., Montelone, B.A., and Upton, S.J., 1997, Sequencing, analysis and expression in *Escherichia coli* of a gene encoding a 15 kDa *Cryptosporidium parvum* protein, Biochem. Biophys. Res. Com. 230:164–166.

Liang, P. and Pardee, A.B., 1992, Differential display of eukaryotic messenger RNA by means of the polymerase chain reaction, Science 257:967–971.

Navin, T.R. and Harden, A.M., 1987, Cryptosporidiosis in patients with Aids, J. Infect. Dis. 155:150.

Petersen, C., 1993, Cellular biology of *Cryptosporidium parvum*, Parasitol. Today 9:87–91.

Schroeder, A.A., Lawrence, C.E., and Abrahamsen, M.S., 1999, Differential mRNA display cloning and characterization of a *Cryptospordium parvum* gene expressed during intracellular development, J. Parasitol. (in press).

Schroeder, A.A., Brown, A.M., and Abrahamsen, M.S., 1998, Identification of a developmentally-regulated *Cryptosporidium parvum* gene by differential mRNA display PCR, Gene 216:327–334.

Smith, P.D., Lane, H.C., Gill, V.J., Manischewitz, J.F., Quinnan, G.V., Fauci, A.S., and Masur, H., 1988, Intestinal infections in patients with the acquired immunodeficiency syndrome (AIDS): Etiology and response to therapy, Ann. Intern. Med. 108:328–333.

Spano, F., Puri, C., Ranucci, L., Putignani, L., and Crisanti, A., 1997, Cloning of the entire COWP gene of *Cryptosporidium parvum* and ultrastructural localization of the protein during sexual parasite development, Parasitol. 114:427–437.

Tzipori, S., 1988, Cryptosoporidiosis in perspective, Adv. Parasitol. 27:63–129.

27

NOREPINEPHRINE STIMULATES *IN VITRO* GROWTH BUT DOES NOT INCREASE PATHOGENICITY OF *SALMONELLA CHOLERAESUIS* IN AN *IN VIVO* MODEL

Jerome C. Nietfeld,[1] Teresa J. Yeary,[1] Randall J. Basaraba,[1] and Konrad Schauenstein[2]

[1] Department of Diagnostic Medicine/Pathobiology, College of Veterinary Medicine, 1800 Denison Ave, Kansas State University, Manhattan, Kansas 66506
[2] Department of General and Experimental Pathology, School of Medicine, University of Graz, Graz, Austria

1. SUMMARY

Norepinephrine stimulates growth of *Escherichia coli, Yersinia enterocolitica*, and *Pseudomonas aeruginosa* in serum-supplemented media, and *in vivo* increases in norepinephrine may be important in the pathogenesis of sepsis by gram-negative bacteria. Because salmonellosis often is associated with stress, the effects of norepinephrine on *in vitro* growth, and *in vivo* pathogenicity of the swine pathogen *Salmonella choleraesuis* were investigated. When RPMI 1640 with and without pig serum was inoculated with fewer than 100 *S. choleraesuis*/ml and incubated overnight, bacterial numbers were 10^4 to 10^6 lower in RPMI containing serum. Norepinephrine restored bacterial growth in RPMI with serum to normal levels, but it did not increase growth in serum-free RPMI. Similar results were obtained with SAPI, a nutrient-poor medium previously used to study the effect of norepinephrine on growth of gram-negative bacteria. Conditioned media were produced by growing *S. choleraesuis* in RPMI containing serum with and without norepinephrine and filter sterilizing. Conditioned medium produced with norepinephrine stimulated growth of *S. choleraesuis* but not *E. coli*, whereas conditioned medium produced without norepinephrine stimulated growth of both bacteria. To determine the *in vivo* effects of norepinephrine, rats were implanted with tablets that secrete norepinephrine for 20 to 24 hours or with identical tablets without norepinephrine and infected intraperitoneally with graded doses of *S. choleraesuis*. The

Mechanisms in the Pathogenesis of Enteric Diseases 2, edited by Paul and Francis.
Kluwer Academic / Plenum Publishers, New York, 1999.

LD-50 of *S. choleraesuis* was the same in both groups, and norepinephrine did not affect the carrier rate at 30 days after infection. We concluded that although norepinephrine stimulates *in vitro* growth of *S. choleraesuis* in serum-based media, the increase in norepinephrine levels in the present *in vivo* system was probably not sufficient to influence the pathogenesis of *S. choleraesuis* infection.

2. INTRODUCTION

Recent reports indicated that the neuroendocrine hormone norepinephrine stimulates *in vitro* growth of the gram-negative bacteria *Escherichia coli*, *Yersinia enterocolitica*, and *Pseudomonas aeruginosa* (Lyte and Ernst, 1992; Lyte and Ernst, 1993). Neither α- nor β-adrenergic receptor agonists or antagonists prevented or mimicked the growth enhancement by norepinephrine, and Lyte and Ernst concluded that growth enhancement was receptor mediated, but not by either α- or β-adrenergic receptors (Lyte and Ernst, 1993). The same group then demonstrated that norepinephrine increases *in vitro* expression of K99 pilus adhesion and production of Shiga-like toxins by *E. coli* (Lyte, Arulanandam, and Frank, 1996; Lyte et al., 1997). They then demonstrated that when grown in the presence of norepinephrine, *E. coli* produces and secretes into the growth medium an autoinducer that stimulates its growth by an amount comparable to the response to norepinephrine (Lyte, Frank, and Green, 1996). All experiments used a minimal medium (referred to by the authors as SAPI) that contained 30% normal bovine serum and was inoculated initially with low numbers of bacteria, typically fewer than 100/ml. The growth medium and low level of inoculation were designed to mimic *in vivo* growth conditions. A second group confirmed that norepinephrine stimulates growth of *E. coli* in serum-based medium, but they did not find the growth stimulation to be receptor mediated (Lenard and VanDeroef, 1995). Instead, they found that serum inhibits growth of *E. coli*, and norepinephrine prevents that growth inhibition.

Based on these findings, Lyte (1992, 1993) proposed that *in vivo* increases in serum and tissue norepinephrine probably stimulate growth of gram-negative bacteria and may be important in the pathogenesis of sepsis caused by those bacteria. Because the intestinal tract is richly supplied with norepinephrine-secreting nerves, factors that increased the release of norepinephrine into the intestines might encourage overgrowth of intestinal gram-negative bacteria, which are important causes of sepsis. In support of this theory is the finding that chemical destruction of norepinephrine-secreting neurons, which results in release of norepinephrine, caused a three to five log increase in gram-negative bacteria in the ceca of mice (Lyte and Bailey, 1997). Also, plasma norepinephrine is increased significantly in septic humans and rats, and prolonged elevation of plasma norepinephrine in humans suffering from shock due to sepsis, hemorrhage, or trauma is associated with increased mortality (Benedict and Grahame-Smith, 1978; Groves et al., 1973; Jones et al., 1988; Kovarik et al., 1987).

In humans and domestic animals, the incidence of salmonellosis is increased by stressors such as cold, crowding, transportation, and hospitalization (Peterson et al., 1991; Sheridan et al., 1994; Wilcock and Schwartz, 1992). *Salmonella choleraesuis* is the most common cause of salmonellosis in swine and causes both enteritis and septicemia (Wilcock and Schwartz, 1992). The purpose of this study was to determine the effects of norepinephrine on the *in vitro* growth of *S. choleraesuis* and on its *in vivo* pathogenicity for rats. Norepinephrine has a short *in vivo* half-life; therefore, to avoid the stress of repeated injections, rats were implanted subcutaneously with tablets that continuously secreted a controlled amount of norepinephrine for 20 to 24 hours (Felsner et al., 1992; Felsner et al., 1995; Korsatko et al., 1982).

3. MATERIALS AND METHODS

3.1. *In Vitro* Determination of the Effect of Norepinephrine on Growth of *S. choleraesuis*

The bacteria used were field isolates cultured from pigs and consisted of two isolates of *S. choleraesuis*, one isolate of *S. typhimurium*, and one isolate of *E. coli* that expressed the F18 (F107) pilus adhesion and produced heat-labile toxin and heat-stable toxin b. Pig sera were from three sources: two lots of commercial pooled pig sera (Sigma Chemical Co, St. Louis, MO); pigs that had been infected orally with *S. choleraesuis* as part of an unrelated experiment 3 weeks prior to collection of sera; and a Cesarean-derived, colostrum-deprived pig that was isolated in a stainless steel cage until the serum was collected at 6 weeks of age. Unless otherwise specified, the basic growth medium for all experiments was RPMI 1640 with HEPES buffer (Sigma Chemical Co.) pH 7.0 to 7.2, and incubation was at 37 C. When used, SAPI medium was prepared as previously described (Lyte and Ernst, 1992).

Norepinephrine bitartrate (Sigma Chemical Co.) was dissolved in RPMI 1640 at a concentration of 10^{-2} M, and the mixture was filter sterilized and stored at -80 C until use when it was thawed and added to the culture medium at the appropriate dilutions. Iron-poor, bovine transferrin (Sigma Chemical Co.) was dissolved in RPMI 1640 at 2 mg transferrin/ml, and the mixture was filter sterilized and stored at -80 C until used. The concentration of 2 mg transferrin/ml was chosen to approximate the average concentration (1.8 mg/ml) in normal pig plasma (Baldwin et al., 1990). Iron dextran (Injectable Iron, Phoenix Pharamaceutical Inc., St. Joseph, MO) was added to the culture medium at the time of use.

Conditioned media were prepared as follows: Conditioned medium 1 (CM1)— *S. choleraesuis* was added at less than 100 bacteria/ml to 10 ml of RPMI 1640 containing 30% pig serum and 10^{-4} M norepinephrine, and the mixture was incubated overnight; conditioned medium 2 (CM2)—*S. choleraesuis* was added at 10^{7}/ml to 10 ml RPMI 1640 containing 30% pig serum and 10^{-4} M norepinephrine, and the mixture was incubated 5 hours; conditioned medium 3 (CM3)—was prepared at the same time and in the same manner as CM2 except that the growth medium did not contain norepinephrine. After incubation, the bacteria were pelleted by centrifugation, and the supernatants were filter sterilized and used as conditioned media.

To prepare the bacterial inocula, the bacterial isolates were grown in RPMI 1640 until the medium became cloudy, and then two serial 1 : 1000 dilutions were made in phosphate buffered saline solution (PBSS), pH 7.0 to 7.2. Two milliliters of RPMI with and without supplements were added to wells of 12-well cell culture dishes. Twenty microliters of the second 1 : 1000 bacterial dilution was added to each well of culture medium to give an initial bacterial inoculum of less than 100 bacteria/ml, and the plates were incubated overnight. The actual number of bacteria added to each well and the bacterial numbers after incubation were determined by plate counts. In each *in vitro* experiment, each combination of media and additives was tested in triplicate and each experiment was performed a minimum of three times.

3.1.1. In Vivo *Determination of the Effect of Norepinephrine on the Pathogenicity of* S. choleraesuis. Forty eight Sprague-Dawley rats were purchased, housed in 19 cages with two rats/cage and in 10 cages with one rat/cage, maintained on commercial rat chow and water ad libitum, and allowed to acclimatize for 8 days. The rats were weighed, and based on their weights (197 to 269 grams) each cage of rats was assigned to one of six groups with eight rats/group. All rats were fasted overnight but allowed free access to water and anesthetized by intramuscular injection of ketamine (44 mg/kg) and xylazine (4 mg/kg). All rats in a group were injected intraperitoneally with 0.25 ml of PBSS containing 10^9, 10^7, 10^5, 10^3, 10^1, or 0 *S. choleraesuis*. At each bacterial dosage, four rats were implanted subcutaneously in the neck with a retard tablet containing a slow release base and 5 mg norepinephrine, and four rats were implanted with a placebo tablet containing only slow release base (Felsner et al., 1992; Felsner et al., 1995; Korsatko et al., 1982). The retard tablets were designed to continuously release a constant amount of norepinephrine over 20 to 24 hours. The rats were evaluated twice daily for 30 days for clinical signs of illness—anorexia, huddling, ruffled fur, diarrhea, and cyanosis of the extremities. All rats were weighed daily for 10 days and then twice weekly for an additional 20 days. Using criteria set forth in the Institutional Animal Use and Care Committee protocol for the project, rats with prolonged or excessive weight loss or with signs of severe illness were euthanized to prevent unnecessary suffering. Thirty days after infection, the remaining animals were euthanized and necropsied, and samples collected for culture for *S. choleraesuis*. Euthanasia was accomplished by CO_2 after anesthesia with ketamine and xylazine. Lung, liver, spleen, and colon contents were cultured from all rats. In addition, heart blood was cultured from all rats euthanized before 30 days after infection.

4. RESULTS

4.1. Effects of Norepinephrine and Serum on *In vitro* Growth of *Salmonella*

When RPMI 1640 containing 30% normal pig serum was inoculated with low numbers (100 or fewer/ml) of *S. choleraesuis* and incubated overnight, the addition of norepinephrine resulted in an increase of 10^4 to 10^6 *S. choleraesuis*/ml (Fig. 1). Although not calculated exactly, the minimum concentration of norepinephrine required to enhance bacterial growth was between 10^{-5} and 10^{-4} molar, which is the same concentration required to enhance growth of other gram-negative bacteria (Lyte and Ernst, 1992). Increasing the norepinephrine concentration to 10^{-3} M did not increase growth; therefore, subsequent experiments were performed using a concentration of 10^{-4} M.

Growth stimulation by norepinephrine occurred only when *S. choleraesuis* was grown in RPMI supplemented with serum. Pig serum inhibited *S. choleraesuis* growth, and norepinephrine restored bacterial growth to a level comparable to that in RPMI alone (Fig. 2). However, norepinephrine did not increase *S. choleraesuis* growth in RPMI not containing serum (Fig. 2). Most previous studies of the effects of norepinephrine on the growth of gram-negative bacteria used a nutrient poor-medium, referred to as SAPI, but RPMI is a nutrient-rich medium. Therefore, the effects of serum and norepinephrine on growth of *S. choleraesuis* in SAPI medium also were determined. Similar to the results with RPMI, norepinephrine stimulated *S. choleraesuis* growth in SAPI containing pig serum but not in SAPI alone (Fig. 3).

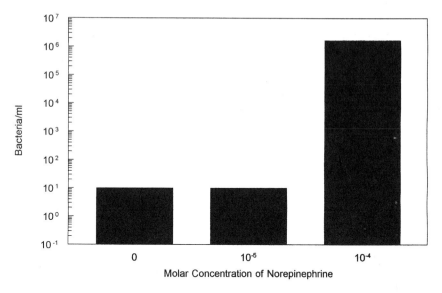

Figure 1. Effect of norepinephrine on the growth of *S. choleraesuis* in RPMI 1640 + 30% pig serum. Each bar represents the average number of *S. choleraesuis*/ml in eight wells each inoculated with approximately 5 to 20 *S. choleraesuis*/ml and incubated for 24 hours.

To determine if the inhibitory effect of pig serum was limited to a single strain of *S. choleraesuis* or lot of serum, the experiments were repeated using a second isolate of *S. choleraesuis*; an isolate of *S. typhimurium*; a second lot of commercial pig serum; sera from pigs orally inoculated with *S. choleraesuis* 3 weeks before collection of the sera; and serum from a 6 week-old, Cesarean-derived, colostrum-deprived pig raised in isolation. Each salmonella isolate was inhibited by pig serum, and all sera were

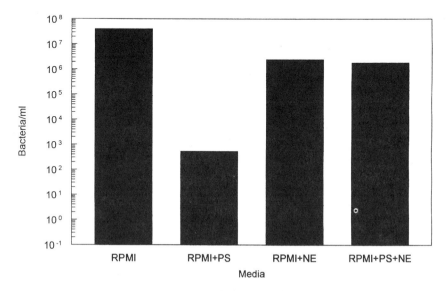

Figure 2. Effects of 30% pig serum (PS), 10^{-4} M norepinephrine (NE), and the combination of PS and NE on growth of *S. choleraesuis* in RPMI. Each bar represents the average numbers of *S. choleraesuis*/ml in three wells after overnight incubation.

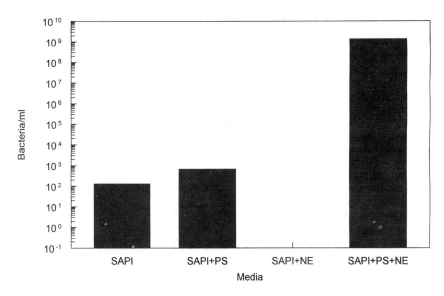

Figure 3. Effects of 30% pig serum (PS), 10^{-4} M norepinephrine (NE), and the combination of PS and NE on growth of *S. choleraesuis* in SAPI medium. Each bar represents the average numbers of *S. choleraesuis*/ml in three wells after overnight incubation. Bacterial growth was not detected by direct plating in any of the three wells supplemented only with NE, whereas each well supplemented with both NE and PS contained greater than 10^9 *S. choleraesuis*/ml.

inhibitory. Serum concentrations of 0.1% or greater inhibited bacterial growth, and heat inactivation (56 C for 30 minutes) did not decrease the inhibitory effect on *S. choleraesuis* growth (data not shown). To determine if the growth inhibition was partly due to serum antibodies specific for *S. choleraesuis*, sera were absorbed twice with either heat-killed or living *S. choleraesuis*. Absorption with heat-killed *S. choleraesuis* had no effect on the growth inhibition by serum. Similar to normal serum, serum absorbed with living *S. choleraesuis* inhibited bacterial growth at a concentration of 0.1% but had no effect at 0.01% or less (Fig. 4). Unlike normal serum, increasing the concentration of serum absorbed with living *S. choleraesuis* to 1% or greater stimulated *S. choleraesuis* growth, which indicated that the living bacteria were secreting something into the serum that enhanced growth.

4.1.1. Effects of Iron, Transferrin, and Conditioned Media on In Vitro Growth of S. choleraesuis. Because serum iron-binding proteins, such as transferrin, decrease free iron available for bacterial growth, the effects of iron and transferrin on growth of *S. choleraesuis* were investigated. Similar to norepinephrine, iron prevented inhibition of *S. choleraesuis* growth by serum (Fig. 5). Bovine transferrin solution (2 mg transferrin/ml) at concentrations of 5% and 40% did not affect growth of *S. choleraesuis* in RPMI without serum (Fig. 5). However, the combination of transferrin and norepinephrine inhibited growth of *S. choleraesuis* by an amount comparable to that in response to serum (Fig. 5).

Conditioned medium 1 (CM1), prepared by adding low numbers of *S. choleraesuis* to serum-based media with norepinephrine and incubating overnight, stimulated *S. choleraesuis* growth in serum-based medium at concentrations of 0.5% and 1.0% (data not shown). CM2, prepared by inoculating serum-based medium containing

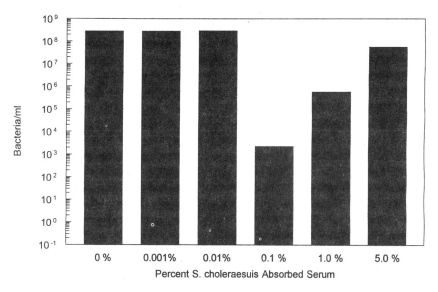

Figure 4. Effect of serum absorbed twice with living *S. choleraesuis* on growth of *S. choleraesuis*. Each bar is the average number of bacteria/ml in three wells.

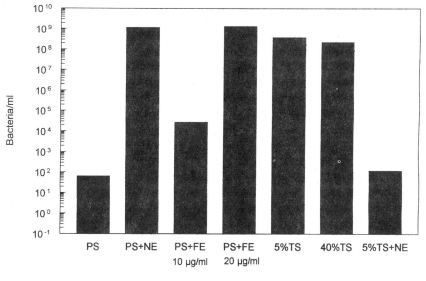

Figure 5. Effects of 5% pig serum (PS), 10^{-4} M norepinephrine (NE), iron (FE), transferrin solution (TS), and TS plus NE on growth of *S. choleraesuis* in RPMI 1640. Each bar represents the average numbers of *S. choleraesuis* in three wells after overnight incubation.

norepinephrine with high numbers of *S. choleraesuis* and incubating for only 5 hours, at concentrations of 0.5% and 1.0% stimulated growth of *S. choleraesuis*, but not *E. coli* (Fig. 6) CM3, prepared exactly like CM2 with the exception that the medium used for CM3 did not contain norepinephrine, stimulated both *S. choleraesuis* and *E. coli* when added at the same concentrations as CM1 and CM2 (Fig. 6).

4.1.1.1. Effect of Norepinephrine on *S. choleraesuis* Infection in Rats. The rats implanted with norepinephrine retard tablets and inoculated with PBSS had lost an average of 7% of their body weight 24 hours after implantation, whereas the PBSS inoculated rats implanted with placebo tablets did not lose weight. Over the next 24 hours, the body weights of rats in both the placebo- and norepinephrine-implanted groups that were inoculated with PBSS increased an average of 6 to 7%. Seventy two hours after infection, all rats in both the norepinephrine and placebo groups that were inoculated with 10^9 *S. choleraesuis* were euthanized because of anorexia and excessive weight loss. *S. choleraesuis* was isolated from the heart blood, lung, liver, and spleen of each rat. The rats given norepinephrine tablets and inoculated with 10^7 *S. choleraesuis* were approximately 1% lighter at 72 hours after infection than they were before infection, but they had gained weight between 48 and 72 hours after infection. The rats given the placebo tablets and infected with 10^7 *S. choleraesuis* were approximately 2% heavier at 72 hours after infection than they were prior to infection, and rats in the other groups also were gaining weight at that time. No additional deaths occurred and the rats continued to eat and gain weight during the remainder of the experiment. When the rats were euthanized 30 days after infection, *S. choleraesuis* was isolated from only four rats, two that received placebo tablets and two that received norepinephrine tablets.

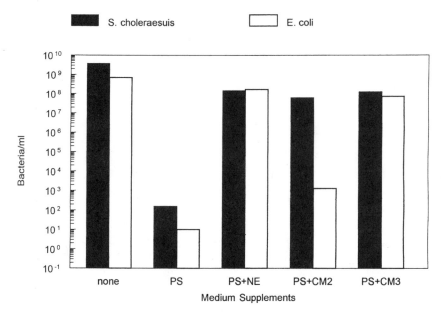

Figure 6. The effects of 30% pig serum (PS), PS plus 10^{-4} M norepinephrine (NE), PS plus 1% conditioned medium 2 (CM2), and PS plus 1% conditioned medium 3 (CM3) on growth of *S. choleraesuis* and *E. coli* in RPMI 1640. Each bar represents the average numbers of bacteria in four wells after overnight incubation.

5. DISCUSSION

Similar to its effects on other gram-negative bacteria, norepinephrine stimulated growth of *S. choleraesuis* and *S. typhimurium* when they were grown in serum-based media. Serum inhibited salmonella growth, and the addition of norepinephrine prevented the growth inhibition in both nutrient-rich and nutrient-poor media. However, norepinephrine did not stimulate bacterial growth in the absence of serum. This supports the earlier findings that serum is bacteriostatic for *E. coli* and that norepinephrine blocks the bacteriostatic effect (Lenard and VanDeroef, 1995) but does not support the report that norepinephrine stimulates growth of gram-negative bacteria by a receptor mediated process (Lyte and Ernst, 1993).

Heat inactivation and absorption with killed *S. choleraesuis* did not affect the bacteriostatic effect of serum, which indicates that complement activation and specific antibodies are not responsible for the growth inhibition. Added iron also reversed the bacteriostatic effect of serum on salmonella growth, which is similar to results previously reported for *E. coli* (Erickson and Crawford, 1996). That report suggested that norepinephrine stimulated growth and increased expression of K99 pilus adhesion by enterotoxigenic *E. coli* through an iron-based mechanism. The mechanisms for growth stimulation by norepinephrine and iron are unknown but most likely are different. When transferrin was added to growth medium to decrease the availability of free iron, suppression of *S. choleraesuis* was not observed, which suggests that the bacteriostatic effect of serum is due to a mechanism other than simple iron depletion of the media. Also, the combination of norepinephrine and transferrin decreased growth of *S. choleraesuis*, but the addition of iron overcame this bacteriostatic effect (data not shown). Inhibition of *S. choleraesuis* growth by norepinephrine in combination with transferrin was unexpected, and we do not know why norepinephrine enhances *S. choleraesuis* growth in combination with serum and inhibits growth in combination with transferrin.

The production of an autoinducer of growth by *S. choleraesuis* when grown overnight in the presence of serum and norepinephrine was similar to results published for *E. coli* (Lyte, Frank, and Green, 1996). The *S. choleraesuis* autoinducer reversed the bacteristatic effects of both serum and the combination of norepinephrine and transferrin. Preliminary experiments indicated that any medium used to grow *S. choleraesuis* would stimulate *S. choleraesuis* growth in serum-based media. Therefore, CM2 and CM3 were produced to determine if norepinephrine was necessary for *S. choleraesuis* to produce an autoinducer of growth. High numbers of *S. choleraesuis* were used to inoculate the initial cultures in order to get good bacterial growth in the sample not containing norepinephrine, because other experiments (data are not shown) had demonstrated that inoculation with high numbers of bacteria would quickly overcome the inhibitory effects of serum. The CM2 and CM3 were incubated only 5 hours because the audoinducer produced by *E. coli* was detectable after only 8 hours of incubation (Lyte, Frank, and Green, 1996). *S. choleraesuis* produced autoinducers after only 5 hours of incubation with and without norepinephrine; but they were different. The one produced without norepinephrine stimulated growth of both *S. choleraesuis* and *E. coli*, whereas the autoinducer produced in the presence of norepinephrine stimulated only *S. choleraesuis*. We can only guess at the nature of these autoinducers, because our efforts to identify them so far have failed.

Based on the *in vitro* results, it seemed reasonable that increased *in vivo* levels of norepinephrine would stimulate *in vivo* growth of *S. choleraesuis* and increase the virulence of the organism. However, persistent stimulation for 20 to 24 hours by nor-epinephrine did not affect the LD-50 or persistence of *S. choleraesuis* in intraperi-toneally infected rats. Norepinephrine levels were not measured, so we cannot be certain that the retard tablets secreted norepinephrine as designed. However, we feel that the tablets did work correctly because the norepinephrine retard tablets caused a 7% weight loss in the PBSS-inoculated controls. This is similar to the weight loss reported previously in Sprague-Dawley rats implanted with retard tablets similar to those used in this study (Felsner et al., 1992). In that study at 20 hours after implanta-tion, plasma norepinephrine levels in rats implanted with norepinephrine retard tablets were 13-fold higher than those in rats receiving placebo tablets (Felsner et al., 1992).

Clinical and experimental data in humans and laboratory animals show that persistent increases in norepinephrine levels are associated with increased mortality from sepsis (Benedict and Grahame-Smith, 1978; Groves et al., 1973; Jones et al., 1988; Kovarik et al., 1987). However, whether the increased norepinephrine is the cause or the result of sepsis is unknown. Rats administered a chemically defined, fat-free, carbohydrate-based, total, parenteral, nutrition formula exhibited increased transloca-tion of intestinal bacteria to the mesenteric lymph nodes and increased urinary excre-tion of norepinephrine (Helton et al., 1995). The addition of polymyxin B, an antibiotic that neutralizes the effects of lipopolysaccharide (LPS), decreased the translocation of bacteria to mesenteric lymph nodes and prevented the increase in urinary excretion of norepinephrine (Johnson et al., 1995). This indicates that the increased norepinephrine was the result of LPS absorption and bacterial translocation from the intestines. In another study, anesthetized rabbits were infused continuously with one of two dosages of norepinephrine, injected intravenously with *E. coli* 60 minutes after beginning the norepinephrine infusion, and the number of *E. coli*/ml of blood were determined every 30 minutes for 180 minutes (Koch et al., 1996). Norepinephrine infusion caused a dose-dependent increase in the time required for elimination of *E. coli* from the blood, but even in the high-dose norepinephrine group, the number of bacteria/ml of blood con-tinuously decreased during the 3 hour monitoring period. Norepinephrine at the high dosage caused a 20% decrease in oxygen uptake, and although direct stimulation of *E. coli* growth cannot be ruled out entirely, the decreased bacterial clearance more likely was the result of decreased phagocyte function due to hypoxia. Norepinephrine also has been shown to inhibit macrophage function at levels lower than those required to stimulate growth of gram-negative bacteria (Hu et al., 1991), and this could have contributed to prolonged bacterial clearance in norepinephrine-infused rabbits. Bacte-rial clearance also was increased in rats with endotoxin induced shock, but infusion of norepinephrine at a dosage that did not decrease oxygen uptake restored bacterial clearance back to a level only slightly less than normal (Koch et al., 1996). This seems to indicate that *in vivo* increases in norepinephrine do not normally increase the *in vivo* growth of gram negative bacteria.

The concentration of norepinephrine required to stimulate growth of gram-negative bacteria is relatively high. Previous studies (Lenard and VanDeroef, 1995; Lyte and Ernst, 1992; Lyte and Ernst, 1993) used 5×10^{-5} M or 8450 ng norepinephrine /ml, which is the minimum concentration that we found to stimulate growth of *S. cholerae-suis*. Results from a study in which Sprague-Dawley rats were implanted with retard tablets similar to those used in this study indicate that norepinephrine levels may not reach this level *in vivo* (Felsner et al., 1995). Twenty hours after implantation, the nor-epinephrine levels were 707 ± 58 ng/gm in the spleens of rats receiving the placebo tablets and 1971 ± 230 ng/gm in the spleens of rats receiving the norepinephrine tablets.

Norepinephrine levels in the heart and plasma were much lower. We have not found published results to indicate that tissue or plasma levels of norepinephrine naturally exceed the 707 ng/gm found in the spleens of the placebo-implanted controls. For example, norepinephrine levels were measured in the gastric wall, gastric mucosa, interstitial fluid of the gastric submucosa, lumbar cerebrospinal fluid, and plasma of rabbits (Meirieu et al., 1986). The norepinephrine levels ranged from 0.98 ng/ml in the plasma to 82.6 ng/gm in the gastric wall. Most likely, the norepinephrine in the rats in the current study did not reach levels high enough to directly stimulate growth of *S. choleraesuis*. Currently, studies are underway in one of the laboratories (K. Schauenstein) to further test the validity of the theory of neuroendocrine-bacterial interactions in the pathogenesis of infectious disease by utilizing norepinephrine pellets of higher concentration and shorter duration of release to more closely mimic actual trauma events which are known to result in massive release of catecholamines and increased infections.

ACKNOWLEDGMENTS

This project was supported by the Kansas Agricultural Experiment Station, NC-62 Technical Committee "Prevention and control of enteric diseases of swine." Published as contribution No. 99-197-A from the Kansas Agricultural Experiment Station, Kansas State University, Manhattan, KS 66506, USA.

REFERENCES

Baldwin, G.S., Bacic, T., Chandler, R., Grego, B., Pedersen, J., Simpson, R.J., Toh, B.H., and Weinstock, J., 1990, Isolation of transferrin from porcine gastric mucosa: comparison with porcine serum transferrin, Comp. Biochem. Physiol. 95B:261–268.

Benedict, C.R. and Grahame-Smith, D.G., 1978, Plasma noradrenaline and adrenaline concentrations and dopamine-β-hydroxylase activity in patients with shock due to septicaemia, trauma, and haemorrhage, Quart. J. Med. 185:1–20.

Erickson, A.K. and Crawford, M.A., 1996, Norepinephrine-induced increase in growth rate and fimbrial adhesion expression of K99+ *Escherichia coli* strain B44 occur through an iron-based mechanism, 77th Annual Meeting of Conference of Research Workers in Animal Diseases, Chicago, IL, abstract 109.

Felsner, P., Hofer, D., Rinner, I., Mangge, H., Gruber, M., Korsatko, W., and Schauenstein, K., 1992, Continuous in vivo treatment with catecholamines suppresses in vitro reactivity of rat peripheral blood T-lymphocytes via α-mediated mechanisms, J. Neuroimmunol. 37:47–57.

Felsner, P., Hofer, D., Rinner, I., Porta, S., Korsatko, W., and Schauenstein, K., 1995, Adrenergic suppression of peripheral blood T cell reactivity in the rat is due to activation of peripheral α_2-receptors, J Neruoimmunol. 57:27–34.

Groves, A.C., Griffiths, J., Leung, F., and Meek, R.N., 1973, Plasma catecholamines in patients with serious postoperative infection, Ann. Surg. 178:102–107.

Helton, W.S., Rockwell, M., Garcia, R.M., Maier, R.V., and Heitkemper, M., 1995, TPN-induced sympathetic activation is related to diet, bacterial translocation, and an intravenous line, Arch. Surg., 130:209–214.

Hu, X., Goldmuntz, E.A., and Brosnan, C.F., 1991, The effect of norepinephrine on endotoxin-mediated macrophage activation, J. Neuroimmunol. 31:35–42.

Johnson, K.M., Garcia, R.M., Heitkemper, M., and Helton, W.S., 1995, Polymyxin B prevents increased sympathetic activity and alveolar macrophage tumor necrosis factor release in parenterally fed rats, Arch. Surg. 130:1294–1299.

Jones, S.B., Westfall, J.V., and Sayeed, M.M., 1988, Plasma catecholamines during *E. coli* bacteremia in conscious rats, Am. J. Physiol 254:R470–R477.

Koch, T., Heller, S., van Ackern, K., Schiefer, H.G., and Neuhof, H., 1996, Impairment of bacterial clearance induced by norepinephrine infusion in rabbits, Intensive Care Med. 22:637–643.

Korsatko, W., Porta, S., Sadjak, A., and Supanz, S., 1982, Implantierbare adrenalin-retard-tabletten zur langzeituntersuchung in ratten, Pharmazie 37:565–567.

Kovarik, M.F., Jones, S.B., and Romano, F.D., 1987, Plasma catecholamines following cecal ligation and puncture in the rat, Circul Shock 22:281–290.

Lenard, J. and VanDeroef, R., 1995, A novel bacteristatic action of bovine and porcine serum that is reversed by norepinephrine, Life Sci. 57:443–447.

Lyte, M., 1992, The role of catecholamines in gram-negative sepsis, Med. Hypotheses, 37:255–258.

Lyte, M., 1993, The role of microbial endocrinology in infectious disease, J. Endocrinol. 137:343–345.

Lyte, M., Arulanandam, B.P., and Frank, C.D., 1996, Production of Shiga-like toxins by *Escherichia coli* O157:H7 can be influenced by the neuroendocrine hormone norepinephrine, J. Lab. Clin. Med. 128:392–398.

Lyte, M. and Bailey, M.T., 1997, Neuroendocrine—bacterial interactions in a neurotoxin-induced model of trauma, J. Surgical Res. 70:195–201.

Lyte, M., Erickson, A.K., Arulanandam, B.P., Frank, C.D., Crawford, M.A., and Francis, D.H., 1997, Norepinephrine-induced expression of the K99 pilus adhesin of enterotoxigenic *Escherichia coli*, Biochem. Biophys. Res. Commun. 232:682–686.

Lyte, M. and Ernst, S., 1992, Catecholamine induced growth of gram negative bacteria, Life Sci. 50:203–212.

Lyte, M. and Ernst, S., 1993, Alpha and beta adrenergic receptor involvement in catecholamine-induced growth of gram-negative bacteria, Biochem. Biophys. Res., Commun. 190:447–452.

Lyte, M., Frank, C.D., and Green, B.T., 1996, Production of an autoinducer of growth by norepinephrine cultured *Escherichia coli* O157:H7, FEMS Microbiol. Let. 139:155–159.

Meirieu, O., Pairet, M., Sutra, J.F., and Ruckebusch, M., 1986, Local release of monoamines in the gastrointestinal tract: an in vivo study in rabbits, Life Sci., 38:827–837.

Peterson, P.K., Chao, C.C., Molitor, T., Murtaugh, M., Strgar, F., and Sharp, B.M., 1991, Stress and pathogenesis of infectious disease, Rev. Infect. Dis. 13:710–720.

Sheridan, J.F., Dobbs, C., Brown, D., and Zwilling, B., 1994, Psychoneuroimmunology: Stress effects on pathogenesis and immunity during infection, Clin. Microbiol. Rev. 7:200–212.

Wilcock, B.P. and Schwartz, K.J., 1992, Salmonellosis, In: Diseases of swine, 7th edition, Editor: Leman, A.D., Straw, B.E., Mengeling, W.L., D'Allaire, S., and Taylor, D.J., Iowa State University Press, Ames, IA, pp. 570–583.

28

OF MICE, CALVES, AND MEN

Comparison of the Mouse Typhoid Model with Other *Salmonella* Infections

Renée M. Tsolis,[1] Robert A. Kingsley,[2] Stacy M. Townsend,[2] Thomas A. Ficht,[1] L. Garry Adams,[1] and Andreas J. Bäumler[2]*

[1] Department of Veterinary Pathobiology
College of Veterinary Medicine
Texas A&M University
College Station, Texas
77843-4467
[2] Department of Medical Microbiology and Immunology
College of Medicine
Texas A&M University Health Science Center
407 Reynolds Medical Building
College Station, Texas
77843-1114

1. SUMMARY

Numerous *Salmonella typhimurium* virulence factors have been identified and characterized using experimental infection of mice. While the murine typhoid model has been used successfully for *Salmonella typhi* vaccine development and to infer virulence mechanisms important during typhoid fever, information derived from infection of mice has been of limited value in elucidating the mechanism by which *S. typhimurium* causes enteritis in humans. Progress in our understanding of virulence mechanisms contributing to diarrheal disease comes from recent studies of bovine enteritis, a *S. typhimurium* infection, which manifests as acute gastroenteritis. This review compares virulence genes and mechanisms required during murine typhoid, typhoid fever, and bovine enteritis. Comparison of illnesses caused in different animal hosts identifies

* For correspondence: e-mail: abaumler@tamu.edu, Fax: 409-845-3479, Phone: 409-862-7756

Mechanisms in the Pathogenesis of Enteric Diseases 2, edited by Paul and Francis.
Kluwer Academic / Plenum Publishers, New York, 1999.

virulence mechanisms involved in species specific disease manifestations. The determination of the relative importance of virulence factors for disease manifestations in different host species provides an important link between the in vitro characterization of genes and their role during host pathogen interaction.

2. INTRODUCTION

Salmonella enterica serotype Typhimurium (*S. typhimurium*) was discovered in 1892 by Loeffler as the causative agent of an epidemic disease in mice. The signs of disease observed in mice as well as the course of infection closely resemble typhoid fever caused by *S. enterica* serotype Typhi (*S. typhi*) in humans (Ørskov and Moltke, 1929). For these reasons, murine typhoid is commonly used as an experimental model for the study of typhoid fever. The popularity of the murine typhoid model is in part due to the lack of animal models to study *S. typhi* virulence. Aside from humans, chimpanzees are the only natural hosts for *S. typhi*, and the scarcity and high cost of these animals limit their use. The widespread use of *S. typhimurium* and *S. enterica* serotype Enteritidis (*S. enteritidis*) infection in mice to model typhoid fever has greatly advanced our understanding of *Salmonella*-host interactions. However, the mouse typhoid model has some obvious shortcomings, which need to be considered when extrapolating the data back to interactions with other hosts, such as humans or livestock. First, *S. typhimurium* does not cause typhoid fever in humans, and therefore, lacks virulence factors present in *S. typhi*. Secondly, mice do not develop diarrhea, the prominent symptom in infections with non-typhoidal serotypes in humans, and therefore murine typhoid may not accurately model all aspects of disease caused by *Salmonella* serotypes. This chapter will review the murine typhoid model with an emphasis on its strengths and limitations for the study of *Salmonella* pathogenesis in other hosts. The focus of our article is to review preferentially those virulence factors or mechanisms, which have been studied in mice and, in addition, in a different animal host or in man. A more comprehensive overview of *Salmonella* virulence factors can be found in (Groisman and Ochman, 1997).

3. THE MOUSE TYPHOID MODEL

3.1. Course of Infection

S. typhimurium and *S. enteritidis* are natural pathogens of mice and can both be isolated frequently from their rodent animal reservoir (Edwards and Bruner, 1943). The course of infection in the mouse was described by Ørskov and Moltke using *S. typhimurium* (Ørskov and Moltke, 1929) and later by Carter and Collins using *S. enteritidis* (Carter and Collins, 1974). After oral infection, the lumen of the cecum contains most of non-tissue associated organisms. Bacteria invade the intestinal epithelium in the small intestine, preferentially M cells located in the follicle associated epithelium of Peyer's patches (Jones et al., 1994). In addition to invasion of intestinal epithelial cells, *S. typhimurium* is translocated across the mucosa by CD18 positive leucocytes, which phagocytose the organism in the intestinal lumen and then enter the circulation (Vazquez-Torres et al., 1999). Upon intestinal penetration by either pathway, *S.*

typhimurium causes a transient bacteremia and seeds the liver and spleen. Subsequent to bacterial spread, *S. typhimurium* multiplies in Peyer's patches of the terminal ileum and these organs therefore contain the bulk of organisms associated with the intestinal wall (Carter and Collins, 1974; Hohmann et al., 1978). During growth in Peyer's patches, *S. typhimurium* can be co-localised with dendritic cells in the dome of lymph follicles (Hopkins and Kraehenbuhl, 1997). In parallel to multiplication in Peyer's patches, *S. typhimurium* replicates in the mesenteric lymph node, the liver and the spleen at a net growth rate of 0.5–1.5 log/day (Maw and Meynell, 1968; Hormaeche, 1980). There is good evidence suggesting that growth in liver and spleen occurs intracellularly, most likely within macrophages (Fields, 1986; Dunlap et al., 1991; Gulig and Doyle, 1993; Richter-Dahlfors et al., 1997). Bacterial growth at these sites leads to granuloma formation and hepato- and splenomegaly. After bacterial numbers in liver and spleen reach between 10^8 and 10^9 CFU (colony forming units)/organ, bacteria re-enter the blood, causing a secondary bacteremia. Death in murine typhoid is caused by lipopolysccharide (LPS) induced damage of liver and spleen, which appears to be distinct from endotoxic shock (Khan et al., 1998).

3.2. Virulence Factors

Numerous virulence factors have been identified using the mouse typhoid model (Groisman and Ochman, 1997). One class consists of factors, which are specifically required to overcome host defense mechanisms and which may thus be considered bona fide virulence genes. Bona fide virulence genes have in common that they are not present in related avirulent organisms, such as *E. coli* K-12, thereby fulfilling the first molecular Koch's postulate (Falkow, 1988). Some bona fide virulence factors act at the initial stages of infection, i.e. in the intestine. A fimbrial adhesin encoded by the *lpf* operon mediates adherence of *S. typhimurium* to murine Peyer's patches (Bäumler et al., 1996). The major pathway for invasion of the intestinal epithelium is encoded by *Salmonella* pathogenicity island 1 (SPI-1), a 40 kb DNA region encoding a type III secretion apparatus (Mills et al., 1995). This secretion apparatus forms a needle complex, which injects type III secreted effector proteins into epithelial cells (Kubori et al., 1998). One of the proteins, which is injected into epithelial cells by this mechanism, SopE, induces signaling events by directly engaging Rho GTPases (Hardt et al., 1998). These signaling events result in bacterial uptake by macropinocytosis (Frances et al., 1993). Mutations, which inactivate the type III secretion apparatus encoded on SPI1 cause a marked reduction in bacterial colonization of murine Peyer's patches (Galán and Curtiss III, 1989). However, SPI1 mutants are only modestly attenuated in mice (15 to 50-fold), because *S. typhimurium* can reach the liver and spleen by alternate pathways, including transepithelial migration of CD18 positive leukocytes (Galán and Curtiss III, 1989; Bäumler et al., 1997; Vazquez-Torres et al., 1999).

Other bona fide virulence factors facilitate growth of *Salmonella* within phagocytic cells. The *spv* (*Salmonella* plasmid virulence) genes increase the intracellular growth rate of *S. typhimurium* within macrophages by an unknown mechanism (Gulig et al., 1998). Mutants lacking *spv* require an approximately 100-fold higher dose in order to cause lethal infection in the mouse (Gulig and Curtiss, 1987). A second virulence gene cluster required for growth in the reticuloendothelial system (RES) is located on SPI-2 (Ochman et al., 1996; Shea et al., 1996). This locus encodes a second type III secretion system which is required for survival in macrophages in vitro (Ochman et al., 1996; Cirillo et al., 1998; Hensel et al., 1998). SPI-2 mutants are avirulent (>10,000-fold attenuated) in mice (Hensel et al., 1995; Ochman et al., 1996) and are unable to grow in liver and spleen (Shea et al., 1999). Growth at these systemic sites of infection requires additional adaptations to the environmental conditions encountered by *S. typhimurium* within splenic or hepatic macrophages. For instance, *S. typhimurium* is able to overcome intracellular Mg^{2+} deprivation in this niche by expressing a high affinity Mg^{2+} uptake system, MgtBC, encoded by genes on SPI-3 (Blanc-Potard and Groisman, 1997).

Attenuation in mice can be caused not only by defects in bona fide virulence genes, but also by mutations in genes encoding housekeeping functions required for growth or survival in vivo. This group includes genes required for survival of stress conditions (e.g. *htrA*), synthesis of lipopolysaccharide (LPS) (e.g. *galE, rfaJ*) and biosynthesis of nutrients which are unavailable in host tissues (e.g. *purD, aroA*) (Germanier and Fuerer, 1971; Stocker et al., 1983; Johnson et al., 1991; Bäumler et al., 1994). Finally, the expression of both housekeeping genes and bona fide virulence genes is tightly controlled by regulatory proteins. The genes encoding these regulatory proteins form a third class of virulence determinants, which includes *cya/crp, phoPQ, hilA, rpoS, sirA*, and *slyA* (Fields, 1989; Fang et al., 1992; Bajaj et al., 1995; Johnston et al., 1996; Vescovi et al., 1996; Buchmeier et al., 1997).

3.3. Immunity and Vaccine Development

The literature contains a substantial amount of disagreement regarding the relative importance of humoral and cellular immunity in protection of mice against *S. typhimurium* infection. In a landmark review, Eisenstein and co-workers suggest that this controversy is a result of the genetic diversity of mice used in vaccine studies (Eisenstein and Sultzer, 1983). This retrospective analysis revealed that antibodies alone conferred protection in vaccine studies using inherently resistant mouse strains (e.g. CBA). In contrast, when inherently susceptible mouse lineages were used (e.g. BALB/c, C57BL/6), antibodies were poorly protective and instead cellular immunity was required. One of the major variables influencing the outcome of vaccination experiments is the *Ity* (Immunity to Typhimurium) locus, which occurs as a dominant resistant (*Ity^r*) or recessive susceptible (*Ity^s*) allele located on mouse chromosome 1 (Plant and Glynn, 1979). The *Ity* gene is expressed exclusively in macrophages and encodes a protein, designated Nramp1 (natural-resistance-associated macrophage protein), located in the membrane of the phagosome (Vidal et al., 1993; Gruenheid et al., 1997). Susceptible mice carry a point mutation in the *Ity* gene (G169D), which prevents proper membrane integration of Nramp1 (Vidal et al., 1996). Nramp1 is thought to mediate a bacteriocidal mechanism of host macrophages, possibly by pumping Fe^{2+} into the phagosome, and thereby catalyzing the formation of oxygen radicals within the *Salmonella* containing vacuole (Gunshin et al., 1997). In addition to their effect on innate resistance, *Ity* alleles influence antigen processing (Lang et al., 1997). For instance, when leishmanial gp63 antigen is delivered by a *S. typhimurium* live attenuated vaccine, mice carrying the *Ity^r* allele mount a predominantly T-helper-1 (Th_1) response whereas congenic *Ity^s* mice mount a T-helper-2 (Th_2) response (Soo et al., 1998). Thus, the genetic background of mice used in vaccine studies should be considered before extrapolating data to the relevant host.

The mouse model has been used to develop live attenuated vaccine strains carrying defined mutations in two classes of virulence determinants, regulatory genes and house keeping genes. Attenuating mutations in regulatory genes used for vaccine development include *cya/crp* (Curtiss et al., 1988), *ompR* (Dorman et al., 1989), and *phoP* (Miller et al., 1993). House keeping genes whose inactivation results in optimal attenuation in mice include *aroA* (Hoiseth and Stocker, 1981), *htrA* (Strahan et al., 1992), and *galE* (Germanier, 1970; Germanier and Fuerer, 1971). The above mutations have in common that they markedly reduce the ability of *S. typhimurium* to grow in liver and spleen of mice. This is in fact an essential property of any *Salmonella* mouse vaccine, because death in this animal model results from damage of liver and spleen induced by bacterial multiplication at these sites (Khan et al., 1998). Thus, only mutants with marked growth defect at systemic sites of infections are expected to be avirulent in mice and safe as vaccine strains.

4. TYPHOID FEVER

4.1. Course of Infection

Current knowledge of the pathogenesis of *S. typhi* infections is based on observations from clinical cases of typhoid fever, experimental infections of volunteers, and a limited number of experimental infections using primates. The small intestine and particularly the Peyer's patches of the terminal ileum provide the portal of entry facilitating dissemination to systemic sites. *S. typhi* both survives and replicates in the underlying lymphoid tissue of the Peyer's patches since experimentally infected chimpanzees were found to contain as many as 6.2×10^7 bacilli at this site just four days post inoculation (Gaines et al., 1968). By way of this route bacteria may proceed to disseminate via the lymphatics to the regional lymph nodes and pass into the blood via the thoracic duct resulting in a transient primary bacteremia. These events occur rapidly in infected individuals since bacteremia can be detected hours after inoculation (Hornick et al., 1970). The ability of *S. typhi* to survive in human macrophages in vitro suggests that this pathogen resides within an intracellular compartment during growth in liver and spleen. Bacterial growth in liver and spleen leads to splenomegaly and hepatomegaly. Typhoid fever patients are often constipated during the early stages of infection. Subsequent to the onset of fever, about one third of patients develop diarrhea. Other symptoms of typhoid fever include headache, psychosis, malaise, anorexia, and temperature as high as 104°F (Miller et al., 1995). Although fever is a characteristic symptom of *S. typhi* infections, circulating endotoxin appears to play little or no part in its elaboration (Hornick et al., 1970). Butler et al. reported no or low-level bacteremia in the majority of clinical typhoid fever cases (Butler et al., 1978). A transient primary bacteremia shortly after infection and in some cases multiple secondary bacteremias, also transient in nature, were observed in volunteers (Hornick et al., 1970).

Evidence reviewed above shows that the course of *S. typhi* infections in man closely resembles that of *S. typhimurium* in mice. As a result, the use of the mouse model has been extremely effective in identifying virulence factors and in developing vaccine candidates for typhoid fever. However, some notable differences between typhoid fever and murine typhoid are identifiable. The incubation period during clinical cases of typhoid fever is frequently reported as 7–14 days, although in a volunteer study it was found to vary by as much as 3 and 56 days with a median of approximately 7 days (Table 1) (Hornick et al., 1970). This is considerably longer than the 3–7 days

Table 1. Characteristics of different diseases caused by *Salmonella* serotypes

	Murine typhoid	Typhoid fever	Bovine enteritis
Causative agent	*S. typhimurium*	*S. typhi*	*S. typhimurium*
	S. enteritidis	*S. paratyphi A,B,C*	
Incubation period	3–7 days	3–56 days	12–24 hours
Typical symptoms/signs of disease	fever	fever	diarrhea, fever
Mortality resulting from	organ failure	intestinal perforation, organ	dehydration, intestinal
	(liver, spleen)	failure	lesions

observed for murine typhoid in both innately resistant and susceptible mice. The reason for the difference with regard to the early progression of these infections is not clear. Since the main site of infection is the reticuloendothelial system in both diseases it is likely that different growth rates at this site may contribute to differences in incubation periods.

A second shortcoming of using mice is that murine typhoid does not accurately model the mechanisms leading to lethality during typhoid fever. Death in mice is caused by tissue damage in liver and spleen (Khan et al., 1998). Although this mechanism may also contribute to lethality during *S. typhi* infections in humans, a large proportion of deaths results from perforation of the small intestine at areas of the Peyer's patches (Bitar and Tarpley, 1985). These differences in killing mechanisms suggest that the infection of innately susceptible mice (eg. Balb/c) with *S. typhmurium* does not model all aspects of typhoid fever pathogenesis. Furthermore, inherently susceptible mice are not able to check bacterial growth in the liver and spleen and die within 6 to 10 days post infection. Consequently, virulence mechanisms operative during typhoid fever at later times during infection may be difficult to study in the mouse model.

4.2. Virulence Factors

All bona fide virulence determinants of *S. typhimurium* were either identified or initially characterized in the mouse model. A number of important bona fide virulence determinants of *S. typhimurium*, including SPI1, SPI2, and SPI3 are also present in *S. typhi* (Galán and Curtiss III, 1991; Hensel et al., 1997; Blanc-Potard et al., 1999). Thus, both serotypes are likely to use related strategies for invasion of intestinal epithelium and survival in host phagocytes. These examples illustrate that the mouse model is a powerful tool to identify and characterize virulence mechanisms important for the pathogenesis of typhoid fever. However, one of the obvious shortcomings of studying the pathogenesis of typhoid fever using the mouse model is that *S. typhimurium* and *S. typhi* do not possess identical sets of bona fide virulence determinants. For instance, the *spv* operon, which is required for growth of *S. typhimurium* in liver and spleen of mice, is not present in *S. typhi* (Woodward, 1989). Similarly, *S. typhimurium* possesses several fimbrial operons which are absent from the *S. typhi* genome (Bäumler et al., 1997). *S. typhi*, on the other hand produces a capsule, the Vi-antigen, encoded by a DNA region, the *viaB* locus, which is not present in *S. typhimurium* (Hashimoto et al., 1991). Using subtractive hybridization it has been estimated that *S. typhimurium* and *S. typhi* differ by approximately 20% of chromosomal DNA (about 900 kb) (Lan and Reeves, 1996), indicating that bona fide virulence mechanisms, including those important for adaptation to humans, may differ substantially between these serotypes.

4.3. Immunity and Vaccine Development

The apparent differences between *S. typhimurium* and *S. typhi* regarding bona fide virulence determinants seem to have little impact on the usefulness of the mouse model for the development of typhoid fever vaccines. The utility of the mouse model is in part due to the fact that vaccine candidates developed in mice carry mutations in house keeping genes or regulatory genes. In contrast to bona fide virulence determinants, house keeping, and regulatory genes are highly conserved between *Salmonella* serotypes and thus their inactivation produces similar phenotypes in related pathogens. A second strength of the mouse model is that reduced growth in liver and spleen is required for both, sufficient attenuation in mice and safety of typhoid fever vaccines. As a result, the involvement of the mouse model in developing live attenuated typhoid fever vaccines has been extensive and in many cases extremely effective. Our current knowledge about the genetics of *S. typhi* virulence is largely derived from volunteer studies using live attenuated vaccine candidates carrying mutations in house keeping or regulatory genes. Mutations identified in *S. typhimurium*, which have been used to attenuate *S. typhi* for vaccination of humans, include *aroC aroD* (Tacket et al., 1992), *cya/crp* (Tacket et al., 1992), *phoPQ* (Hohmann et al., 1996), and *aroC aroD htrA* (Tacket et al., 1997). *S. typhi* strains attenuated by these mutations have been shown to be safe and immunogenic in volunteers.

Although the development of typhoid fever vaccines using the mouse model has been a success story, there is one notable exception. *S. typhimurium* mutants defective for the biosynthesis of uridine-5′-diphosphate galactose epimerase (GalE) are deficient in the biosynthesis of the outer core of LPS when grown in the absence of galactose. A mutation in *galE* renders *S. typhimurium* avirulent and immunogenic for mice (Germanier, 1970; Germanier and Fuerer, 1971). Using chemical mutagenesis, a *galE* mutant of *S. typhi* (strain Ty21a) was derived and licensed as live oral vaccine (Germanier and Fürer, 1975). However, attenuation of Ty21a is probably due to defects other than those in LPS biosynthesis since a defined *S. typhi galE* mutant is not avirulent for human volunteers (Hone, 1988). Thus, in case of a *galE* mutation, the degree of attenuation observed in the mouse was not predictive of that in the human host.

Interest in live oral vaccines comes in part from their potential for expression of heterologous antigens and the resulting possibility for multivalent vaccine strains providing immunity against a wide range of diseases (Chatfield et al., 1995). A second motivation for the development of live attenuated *S. typhi* vaccines is the assumption that live oral vaccines provide better protection against intracellular pathogens than killed vaccines. This conclusion is based on vaccine studies in innately susceptible mice, which require cellular immunity in order to be protected against challenge with *S. typhimurium*. A large number of experiments using innately resistant mice, however, indicated that killed *S. typhimurium* vaccines, which only elicit a humoral response, elicit a protective immune response (Eisenstein and Sultzer, 1983). In fact, a recent analysis of 17 field trials involving nearly 2 million subjects found that protection conferred by a killed whole cell *S. typhi* vaccine was higher and of greater duration than that provided by the live oral Ty21a vaccine or the Vi-antigen subunit vaccine (Engels et al., 1998). This evidence suggests that disease in resistant mice more closely resembles human typhoid fever than that in susceptible mice (Eisenstein and Sultzer, 1983; Cabello, 1998; Eisenstein, 1998; Pang, 1998).

5. BOVINE ENTERITIS

5.1. Course of Infection

S. typhimurium and *Salmonella dublin* are the serotypes most commonly associated with disease in cattle (Sojka et al., 1975). Milk-fed, 28-day old Friesian/Holstein bull calves have been used to model *S. typhimurium* induced enteritis (Smith et al., 1979; Watson et al., 1998; Tsolis et al., 1999). After oral infection with a dose of 10^6 CFU of *S. typhimurium* ATCC14028, calves develop diarrhea within 12–48 hours (Table 1). At this dose, the disease is self-limited and does not result in mortality. Lethal infections can be induced by inoculation with 10^9–10^{10} CFU/animal and are caused by dehydration and intestinal lesions. Similar dose responses were obtained using other *S. typhimurium* isolates (Rankin and Taylor, 1966; Wray and Sojka, 1978; Smith et al., 1979). *S. typhimurium* initially invades M cells of the follicle associated epithelium of bovine Peyer's patches. This initial interaction is followed by entry into enterocytes of absorptive villi in the terminal ileum (Frost et al., 1997). Necropsy of calves with severe diarrhea reveals enteritis in the mid- to terminal ileum, with pseudomembranous fibrinopurulent necrotizing enteritis over areas of Peyer's patches. Histopathogical examination of the intestine shows destruction of the mucosal epithelium, purulent inflammation, and depletion of lymphocytes in the germinal centers of intestinal lymphoid follicles (Tsolis et al., 1999). Between 2 and 5 days post infection, bacteria can be recovered in similar numbers (up to 10^6 to 10^8 CFU/g tissue) from ileal tissue samples containing Peyer's patches or villous intestine. *S. typhimurium* can be recovered in 10-fold lower numbers from the ileal mesenteric lymph nodes and the cecum. The majority of *S. typhimurium* infections in calves remain localized to the intestine and mesenteric lymph node. We found that even after oral inoculation with high doses (10^9–10^{10} CFU/animal) *S. typhimurium* colonizes the spleen in only 50% of infected animals where it is found in low numbers (10^2 to 10^5 CFU/g tissue).

The disease in calves resembles *S. typhimurium* infections in man, which manifest as acute self-limited gastroenteritis. *S. typhimurium* causes a localized infection in man and bacteremia is a rare complication which occurs in 1–8% of clinical cases. The course of infection and the signs of disease of *S. typhimurium* infection in mice, on the other hand, are markedly different from human and bovine infections (Table 1). Lethality in mice develops as a result of systemic infection, which is not an important feature of bovine disease. In contrast to its uniform distribution in bovine ileal intestinal tissue, *S. typhimurium* preferentially colonizes murine Peyer's patches, while other intestinal tissues in the mouse contain only low bacterial numbers. Furthermore, diarrhea, the main sign of disease in calves and man, does not develop in mice. The different disease manifestations in mice limit the degree to which data from the murine typhoid model can be extrapolated to diarrheal disease caused by *S. typhimurium* in calves and man.

5.2. Virulence Factors

S. typhimurium causes murine typhoid and bovine enteritis using sets of bona fide virulence genes which overlap but are not identical. Most notably, a mutant in *spiB* (SPI-2), which is more than 10,000-fold attenuated in mice causes diarrhea and mortality at wild type levels in calves infected with 10^{10} CFU/animal, suggesting less than 15-fold attenuation. Similarly, mutations in the *spv* operon do not markedly attenuate *S. typhimurium* or reduce the severity of diarrhea in calves (Tsolis et al., 1999). Since

SPI-2 and the *spv* genes are thought to be required for growth in splenic macrophages, these observations are consistent with the idea that systemic infection is not an essential feature of bovine disease. Furthermore, these data suggest that attenuation in the mouse is not predictive of the degree to which a mutation may reduce the severity of diarrhea in calves.

One niche, which is of relatively greater importance in the calf than the mouse, is the terminal ileum. Mutants carrying transposon insertions in *hilA*, *orgA* or *prgH* (SPI-1), are defective for colonization of the ileal mucosa and Peyer's patches in calves and are unable to cause fatal infection at doses as high as 10^{10} CFU/animal. Furthermore, mutations in SPI-1 result in strongly reduced diarrhea (Tsolis et al., 1999) and reduced fluid secretion in bovine ligated ileal loops (Watson et al., 1998; Ahmer et al., 1999). While in calves, mutations in SPI-1 attenuate *S. typhimurium* to a greater degree than mutations in SPI-2 or *spv*, the converse is true in mice, where SPI-1 mutants are at least 200-fold less attenuated than SPI-2 mutants (Galán and Curtiss III, 1989; Ochman et al., 1996). SPI-1 encodes the invasion associated Type III secretion apparatus of *S. typhimurium*, which mediates translocation of effector proteins into the cytosol of intestinal epithelial cells (Collazo and Galan, 1997; Fu and Galan, 1998). These effectors mediate uptake of *S. typhimurium* by epithelial cells (Hardt et al., 1998) and trigger the release of inflammatory cytokines (Hobbie et al., 1997). Although it is likely that the inflammatory response triggered by SPI-1 leads to fluid secretion, the exact mechanism by which *S. typhimurium* causes diarrhea in calves is currently unknown. Furthermore, it remains elusive why SPI-1 mediated invasion and inflammation in mice does not result in diarrhea.

Some of the effector proteins injected into epithelial cells by the invasion associated type III secretion system are encoded by genes, which are not located on SPI-1. For instance, the *sopB* (*sigD*) gene is located on SPI-5 (Hong and Miller, 1998; Wood et al., 1998) and the encoded protein is translocated by the invasion associated type III secretion apparatus of *S. dublin* into epithelial cells (Wood et al., 1996). It has been suggested that SPI-5 is required for enteropathogenicity since inactivation of *sopB* in *S. dublin* reduces fluid secretion in bovine ligated ileal loops (Wood et al., 1998). However, we have found that a *S. typhimurium sopB* mutant causes diarrhea and mortality at wild type levels when calves are infected orally at a dose of 10^{10} CFU/animal (R.M. Tsolis, R.A. Kingsley, L.G. Adams, and A.J. Bäumler, unpublished results). These data suggest that reduced fluid secretion in bovine intestinal loops is not always predictive of the degree to which a mutation reduces virulence during an oral infection in calves. This apparent discrepancy may result from the fact, that ligated intestinal loops model early steps in infection, and that small defects in the initial interaction with the intestinal epithelium may be overcome later in the course of a natural infection.

5.3. Immunity and Vaccine Development

While inhibition of growth at systemic sites of infection is essential for safety of typhoid fever vaccines, reduced growth in the intestine appears to be required for sufficient attenuation in calves. Thus, mutations in SPI-2 or the *spv* operon, which reduce only growth at systemic sites of infection, do not cause sufficient attenuation of *S. typhimurium* for oral vaccination of calves (Tsolis et al., 1999). Similarly, the *S. typhimurium galE* vaccine has been associated with renal lesions when administered parenterally (Wray et al., 1977) and resulted in mortality when administered orally to calves at a dose of 10^{10} CFU/animal (Clarke and Gyles, 1986). Hence, a *S. typhimurium galE* mutant appears to be unsafe for vaccination of calves. A *S. typhimurium aroA* mutant, on the other hand, is attenuated sufficiently to be used as vaccine in both mice and calves (Hoiseth and Stocker, 1981; Stocker et al., 1983). Therefore, despite striking differences in the course of infection and the signs of disease observed during *S. typhimurium* infections of mice and calves, the mouse model has been used successfully to identify safe and efficacious vaccines for cattle. The usefulness of the *aroA* vaccine for immunization in animals developing diarrheal disease likely results from the pleiotrophic effect of this mutation on the growth of *S. typhimurium* in different host environments. *S. typhimurium aroA* mutants are unable to multiply in internal organs of mice because they require 2,3-dihydroxybenzoic acid for growth, a metabolite which is not available in murine tissues (Hoiseth and Stocker, 1981; Benjamin et al., 1990). Furthermore, the generation time of a *S. typhimurium aroA* mutant in the mouse intestine is approximately 24 hours, as compared to less than 3 hours determined for the wild type (Norris et al., 1999). This markedly reduced growth in the intestine may account for the attenuation of *S. typhimurium aroA* mutants in calves.

The ideal vaccine for calves should produce no clinical signs of disease resulting in mortality or reduced weight gain, be shed for only a short time to minimize the possibility of environmental contamination, and elicit protection in young calves since this is the age group most at risk for *S. typhimurium* infection. *S. typhimurium aroA aroD* mutants fulfill most of these requirements. In one study, 10 one week-old calves were vaccinated with a dose of 10^{10} CFU, of which four developed diarrhea, and none shed the vaccine strain for longer than 7 days. Vaccination protected 7/8 calves against a challenge dose, which caused fatal disease in unvaccinated calves (Jones et al., 1991). Thus, the *aroA aroD* vaccine appears promising as an oral vaccine for calves. Since genes involved in enteropathogenicity have now been identified, future designs for vaccine strains may include mutations, which reduce the severity of diarrhea in calves, thereby limiting reduction in weight gain following immunization.

ACKNOWLEDGMENTS

Work in AJB's laboratory is supported by Public Health Service grant #AI40124, grant #9802610 from the U.S. Department of Agriculture and USDA Formula Animal Health Funding to TAF and AJB. RMT is supported by USDA/NRICGP #9702568.

REFERENCES

Ahmer, B.M., J. van Reeuwijk, P.R. Watson, T.S. Wallis, and F. Heffron, 1999, Salmonella SirA is a global regulator of genes mediating enteropathogenesis, Mol. Microbiol. 31:971–982.

Bajaj, V., C. Hwang, and C.A. Lee, 1995, hilA is a novel ompR/toxR family member that activates the expression of Salmonella typhimurium invasion genes, Molecular Microbiology 18:715–727.

Bäumler, A.J., A.J. Gilde, R.M. Tsolis, A.W.M. van der Velden, B.M.M. Ahmer, and F. Heffron, 1997, Contribution of horizontal gene transfer and deletion events to the development of distinctive patterns of fimbrial operons during evolution of *Salmonella* serotypes, J. Bacteriol. 179:317–322.

Bäumler, A.J., J.G. Kusters, I. Stojiljkovic, and F. Heffron, 1994, *Salmonella typhimurium* loci involved in survival within macrophages, Infect. Immun. 62:1623–1630.

Bäumler, A.J., R.M. Tsolis, and F. Heffron, 1996, The *lpf* fimbrial operon mediates adhesion to murine Peyer's patches, Proc. Natl. Acad. Sci. USA. 93:279–283.

Bäumler, A.J., R.M. Tsolis, P.J. Valentine, T.A. Ficht, and F. Heffron, 1997, Synergistic Effect of Mutations in *invA* and *lpfC* on the Ability of *Salmonella typhimurium* to Cause Murine Typhoid, Infect. Immun. 65:2254–2259.

Benjamin, W.H., P. Hall, S.J. Roberts, and D.E. Briles, 1990, The primary effect of the Ity locus is on the growth rate of *Salmonella typhimurium* that are relatively protected from killing, J. Immunol. 144:3143–3151.

Bitar, R. and J. Tarpley, 1985, Intestinal perforation and typhoid fever: a historical and state-of-the-art review, Rev. Infect. Dis. 7:257.

Blanc-Potard, A.B., F. Solomon, J. Kayser, and E.A. Groisman, 1999, The SPI-3 pathogenicity island of salmonella enterica [In Process Citation], J. Bacteriol. 181:998–1004.

Blanc-Potard, A.-B. and E.A. Groisman, 1997, The *Salmonella selC* locus contains a pathogenicity island mediating intramacrophage survival, EMBO J. 16:5376–5385.

Buchmeier, N., S. Bossie, C.Y. Chen, F.C. Fang, D.G. Guiney, and S.J. Libby, 1997, SlyA, a transcriptional regulator of Salmonella typhimurium, is required for resistance to oxidative stress and is expressed in the intracellular environment of macrophages, Infection & Immunity 65:3725–3730.

Butler, T., W.R. Bell, J. Levin, N.N. Linh, and K. Arnold, 1978, Typhoid fever. Studies of blood coagulation, bacteremia, and endotoxemia, Arch. Intern. Med. 138:407–410.

Cabello, F., 1998, Salmonella typhi infections are also modulated by antibodies, Trends Microbiol. 6:470–472.

Carter, P.B. and F.M. Collins, 1974, The route of enteric infection in normal mice, J. Exp. Med. 139:1189–1203.

Chatfield, S.N., M. Roberts, G. Dougan, C. Hormaeche, and C.M. Khan, 1995, The development of oral vaccines against parasitic diseases utilizing live attenuated Salmonella, Parasitology 110:S17–S24.

Cirillo, D.M., R.H. Valdivia, D.M. Monack, and S. Falkow, 1998, Macrophage-dependent induction of the Salmonella pathogenicity island 2 type III secretion system and its role in intracellular survival, Mol. Microbiol. 30:175–188.

Clarke, R.C. and C.L. Gyles, 1986, Galactose epimeraseless mutants of Salmonella typhimurium as live vaccines for calves, Can. J. Vet. Res. 50:165–173.

Collazo, C.M. and J.E. Galan, 1997, The invasion-associated type III system of Salmonella typhimurium directs the translocation of Sip proteins into the host cell, Mol. Microbiol. 24:747–756.

Curtiss, R.D., R.M. Goldschmidt, N.B. Fletchall, and S.M. Kelly, 1988, Avirulent Salmonella typhimurium delta cya delta crp oral vaccine strains expressing a streptococcal colonization and virulence antigen, Vaccine 6:155–160.

Dorman, C.J., S. Chatfield, C.F. Higgins, C. Hayward, and G. Dougan, 1989, Characterization of porin and ompR mutants of a virulent strain of Salmonella typhimurium: ompR mutants are attenuated in vivo, Infect. Immun. 57:2136–2140.

Dunlap, N.E., W.H. Benjamin Jr., R.D. McGall, A.B. Tilden, and D.E. Briles, 1991, A "safe-site" for *Salmonella typhimurium* is within splenic cells during the early phase of infection in mice, Microb. Pathogen. 10:297–310.

Edwards, P.R. and D.W. Bruner, 1943, The occurence and distribution of *Salmonella* types in the United States, J. Infect. Dis. 72:58–67.

Eisenstein, T.K., 1998, Intracellular pathogens: the role of antibody-mediated protection in Salmonella infection, Trends Microbiol. 6:135–136.

Eisenstein, T.K. and B.M. Sultzer, 1983, Immunity to Salmonella infection, Adv. Exp. Med. Biol. 162:261–296.

Engels, E.A., M.E. Falagas, J. Lau, and M.L. Bennish, 1998, Typhoid fever vaccines: a meta-analysis of studies on efficacy and toxicity, Bmj. 316:110–116.

Falkow, S., 1988, Molecular Koch's postulates applied to microbial pathogenicity, Rev. Infect. Dis. 10(Suppl.):274–276.

Fang, F.C., S.J. Libby, N.A. Buchmeier, P.C. Loewen, J. Switala, J. Harwood, and D.G. Guiney, 1992, The alternative sigma factor katF (rpoS) regulates Salmonella virulence, Proc. Natl. Acad. Sci. USA 89:11978–11982.

Fields, P.I., Swanson, R.V., Haidaris, C.G., and Heffron, F., 1986, Mutants of *Salmonella typhimurium* that cannot survive within the macrophage are avirulent, Proc. Natl. Acad. Sci. USA 83:5189–5193.

Fields, P.I., Groisman, E.G., and Heffron, F., 1989, A *Salmonella* locus that controls resistance to microbicidal proteins from phagocytic cells, Science 243:1059–1062.

Frances, C.L., T.A. Ryan, B.D. Jones, S.J. Smith, and S. Falkow, 1993, Ruffles induced by *Salmonella* and other stimuli direct macropinocytosis of bacteria, Nature 364:639–642.

Frost, A.J., A.P. Bland, and T.S. Wallis, 1997, The early dynamic response of the calf ileal epithelium to Salmonella typhimurium, Vet. Pathol. 34:369–386.

Fu, Y. and J.E. Galan, 1998, The Salmonella typhimurium tyrosine phosphatase SptP is translocated into host cells and disrupts the actin cytoskeleton, Mol. Microbiol. 27:359–368.

Gaines, S., H. Sprinz, J.G. Tully, and W.D. Tigertt, 1968, Studies on infection and immunity in experimental typhoid fever. VII. The distribution of Salmonella typhi in chimpanzee tissue following oral challenge, and the relationship between the numbers of bacilli and morphologic lesions, J. Infect. Dis. 118:293–306.

Galán, J.E. and R. Curtiss III, 1989, Cloning and molecular characterization of genes whose products allow *Salmonella typhimurium* to penetrate tissue culture cells, Proc. Natl. Acad. Sci. USA 86:6383–6387.

Galán, J.E. and R. Curtiss III, 1991, Distribution of the *invA*, -*B*, -*C*, and -*D* genes of *Salmonella typhimurium* among other *Salmonella* serovars: *invA* mutants of *Salmonella typhi* are deficient for entry into mammalian cells, Infect. Immun. 59:2901–2908.

Germanier, R., 1970, Immunity in experimental salmonellosis. I. Protection iduced by rough mutants of *Salmonella typhimurium*, Infect. Immun. 2:309–315.

Germanier, R. and E. Fuerer, 1971, Immunity in experimental salmonellosis. II. Basis for avirulence and protective capacity of *galE* mutants of *Salmonella typhimurium*, Infect. Immun. 4:663–673.

Germanier, R. and E. Fürer, 1975, Isolation and Characterization of *galE* mutant Ty21a of *Salmonella typhi*: a candidate strain for a live, oral typhoid vaccine, J. Infect. Dis. 131:553–558.

Groisman, E.A. and H. Ochman, 1997, How Salmonella became a pathogen, Trends Microbiol. 5:343–349.

Gruenheid, S., E. Pinner, M. Desjardins, and P. Gros, 1997, Natural resistance to infection with intracellular pathogens: the Nramp1 protein is recruited to the membrane of the phagosome, J. Exp. Med. 185:717–730.

Gulig, P.A. and R. Curtiss, 1987, Plasmid-associated virulence of *Salmonella typhimurium*, Infect. Immun. 1987:2891–2901.

Gulig, P.A. and T.J. Doyle, 1993, The *Salmonella typhimurium* virulence plasmid increases the growth rate of salmonellae in mice, Infect. Immun. 61:504–511.

Gulig, P.A., T.J. Doyle, J.A. Hughes, and H. Matsui, 1998, Analysis of host cells associated with the Spv-mediated increased intracellular growth rate of Salmonella typhimurium in mice, Infect. Immun. 66:2471–2485.

Gunshin, H., B. Mackenzie, U.V. Berger, Y. Gunshin, M.F. Romero, W.F. Boron, S. Nussberger, J.L. Gollan, and M.A. Hediger, 1997, Cloning and characterization of a mammalian proton-coupled metal-ion transporter, Nature 388:482–488.

Hardt, W.D., L.M. Chen, K.E. Schuebel, X.R. Bustelo, and J.E. Galan, 1998, S. typhimurium encodes an activator of Rho GTPases that induces membrane ruffling and nuclear responses in host cells, Cell 93:815–826.

Hashimoto, Y., T. Ezaki, N. Li, and H. Yamamoto, 1991, Molecular cloning of the ViaB region of Salmonella typhi, FEMS Microbiol. Lett. 69:53–56.

Hensel, M., J.E. Shea, A.J. Bäumler, C. Gleeson, F. Blattner, and D.W. Holden, 1997, Analysis of the boundaries of *Salmonella* pathogenicity island 2 and the corresponding chromosomal region of *Escherichia coli* K-12, J. Bacteriol. 179:1105–1111.

Hensel, M., J.E. Shea, C. Gleeson, M.D. Jones, E. Dalton, and D.W. Holden, 1995, Simultaneous identification of bacterial virulence genes by negative selection, Science 269:400–403.

Hensel, M., J.E. Shea, S.R. Waterman, R. Mundy, T. Nikolaus, G. Banks, A. Vazquez-Torres, C. Gleeson, F.C. Fang, and D.W. Holden, 1998, Genes encoding putative effector proteins of the type III secretion system of Salmonella pathogenicity island 2 are required for bacterial virulence and proliferation in macrophages, Mol. Microbiol. 30:163–174.

Hobbie, S., L.M. Chen, R.J. Davis, and J.E. Galan, 1997, Involvement of mitogen-activated protein kinase pathways in the nuclear responses and cytokine production induced by Salmonella typhimurium in cultured intestinal epithelial cells, J. Immunol. 159:5550–5559.

Hohmann, A.W., G. Schmidt, and D. Rowley, 1978, Intestinal colonization and virulence of *Salmonella* in mice, Infect. Immun. 22:763–770.

Hohmann, E.L., C.A. Oletta, K.P. Killeen, and S.I. Miller, 1996, phoP/phoQ-deleted Salmonella typhi (Ty800) is a safe and immunogenic single-dose typhoid fever vaccine in volunteers, J. Infect. Dis. 173:1408–1414.

Hoiseth, S.K. and B.A.D. Stocker, 1981, Aromatic-dependent *Salmonella typhimurium* are non-virulent and effective as live oral vaccines, Nature 291:238–239.

Hone, D.M., S.R. Attridge, B. Forrest, R. Morona, D. Daniels, J.T. LaBrooy, R.C. Bartholomeusz, D.J. Shearman, and J. Hackett, 1988, A *galE via* (Vi antigen-negative) mutant of *Salmonella typhi* Ty2 retains virulence in humans, Infect. Immun. 56:1326–1333.

Hong, K.H. and V.L. Miller, 1998, Identification of a novel Salmonella invasion locus homologous to Shigella ipgDE, J. Bacteriol. 180:1793–1802.

Hopkins, S.A. and J.P. Kraehenbuhl, 1997, Dendritic cells of the murine Peyer's patches colocalize with Salmonella typhimurium avirulent mutants in the subepithelial dome, Adv. Exp. Med. Biol. 417:105–109.

Hormaeche, C.E., 1980, The in vivo division and death rates of Salmonella typhimurium in the spleens of naturally resistant and susceptible mice measured by the superinfecting phage technique of Meynell, Immunology 41:973–979.

Hornick, R.B., S.E. Greisman, T.E. Woodward, H.L. DuPont, A.T. Dawkins, and M.J. Snyder, 1970, Typhoid fever:Pathogenesis, and immunologic control, N. Engl. J. Med. 283:686–691.

Johnson, K., I. Charles, G. Dougan, D. Pickard, P. O'Gaora, G. Costa, T. Ali, I. Miller, and C. Hormaeche, 1991, The role of a stress-response protein in Salmonella typhimurium virulence, Mol. Microbiol. 5:401–407.

Johnston, C., D.A. Pegues, C.J. Hueck, A. Lee, and S.I. Miller, 1996, Transcriptional activation of Salmonella typhimurium invasion genes by a member of the phosphorylated response-regulator superfamily, Mol. Microbiol. 22:715–727.

Jones, B.D., N. Ghori, and S. Falkow, 1994, *Salmonella typhimurium* initiates murine infection by penetrating and destroying the specialized epithelial M cells of the Peyer's patches, J. Exp. Med. 180:15–23.

Jones, P.W., G. Dougan, C. Hayward, N. Mackensie, P. Collins, and S.N. Chatfield, 1991, Oral vaccination of calves against experimental salmonellosis using a double aro mutant of Salmonella typhimurium, Vaccine 9:29–34.

Khan, S.A., P. Everest, S. Servos, N. Foxwell, U. Zahringer, H. Brade, E.T. Rietschel, G. Dougan, I.G. Charles, and D.J. Maskell, 1998, A lethal role for lipid A in Salmonella infections, Mol. Microbiol. 29:571–579.

Kubori, T., Y. Matsushima, D. Nakamura, J. Uralil, M. Lara-Tejero, A. Sukhan, J.E. Galan, and S.I. Aizawa, 1998, Supramolecular structure of the Salmonella typhimurium type III protein secretion system, Science 280:602–605.

Lan, R. and P.R. Reeves, 1996, Gene transfer is a major factor in bacterial evolution, Mol. Biol. Evol. 13:47–55.

Lang, T., E. Prina, D. Sibthorpe, and J.M. Blackwell, 1997, Nramp1 transfection transfers Ity/Lsh/Bcg-related pleiotropic effects on macrophage activation: influence on antigen processing and presentation, Infect. Immun. 65:380–386.

Maw, J. and G.G. Meynell, 1968, The true division and death rates of *Salmonella typhimurium* in the mouse spleen determined with superinfecting phage P22, British Journal of Experimental Pathology 49:597–613.

Miller, S.I., E.L. Hohmann, and D.A. Pegues, 1995, *Salmonella* (including *Salmonella typhi*), Priciples and practice of infectious diseases. G.L. Mandell, J.E. Bennett, and R. Dolin. New York, Churchill Livingstone. 2:2013–2033.

Miller, S.I., W.P. Loomis, C. Alpuche-Aranda, I. Behlau, and E. Hohmann, 1993, The PhoP virulence regulon and live oral Salmonella vaccines, Vaccine 11:122–125.

Mills, D.M., V. Bajaj, and C.A. Lee, 1995, A 40 kb chromosomal fragment encoding *Salmonella typhimurium* invasion genes is absent from the corresponding region of the *Escherichia coli* K-12 chromosome, Mol. Microbiol. 15:749–759.

Norris, T.L., L.M. Harrison, and A.J. Bäumler, 1999, Phase variation of the *lpf* operon is a mechanism to evade cross immunity between *Salmonella* serotypes, Submitted for publication.

Ochman, H., F.C. Soncini, F. Solomon, and E.A. Groisman, 1996, Identification of a pathogenicity island for *Salmonella* survival in host cells, Proc. Natl. Acad. Sci. USA 93:7800–7804.

Ørskov, J. and O. Moltke, 1929, Studien über den Infektionsmechanismus bei verschiedenen Paratyphus-Infektionen in weien Mäusen, Zeitschrift für Immunitätsforschung 59:357–405.

Pang, T., 1998, Vaccination against intracellular bacterial pathogens, Trends Microbiol. 6:433.

Plant, J. and A.A. Glynn, 1979, Locating salmonella resistance gene on mouse chromosome 1, Clin. Exp. Immunol. 37:1–6.

Rankin, J.D. and R.J. Taylor, 1966, The estimation of Doses of *Salmonella typhimurium* Suitable fot the Experimental Production of Disease in Calves, Vet. Rec. 78:706–707.

Richter-Dahlfors, A., A.M.J. Buchan, and B.B. Finlay, 1997, Murine salmonellosis studied by confocal microscopy: *Salmonella typhimurium* resides intracellularly inside macrophages and excerts a cyto-toxic effect on phagocytes in vivo., J. Exp. Med. 186:569–580.

Shea, J.E., C.R. Beuzon, C. Gleeson, R. Mundy, and D.W. Holden, 1999, Influence of the Salmonella typhimurium Pathogenicity Island 2 Type III Secretion System on Bacterial Growth in the Mouse, Infect. Immun. 67:213–219.

Shea, J.E., M. Hensel, C. Gleeson, and D.W. Holden, 1996, Identification of a virulence locus encoding a second type III secretion system in *Salmonella typhimurium*, Proc. Natl. Acad. Sci. USA 93:2593–2597.

Smith, B.P., F. Habasha, M. Reina-Guerra, and A.J. Hardy, 1979, Bovine salmonellosis: experimental production and characterization of the disease in calves, using oral challenge with Salmonella typhimurium, Am. J. Vet. Res. 40:1510–1513.

Sojka, W.J., C. Wray, E.B. Hudson, and J.A. Benson, 1975, Incidence of salmonella infection in animals in England and Wales, 1968–73, Vet. Rec. 96:280–284.

Soo, S.S., B. Villarreal-Ramos, C.M. Anjam Khan, C.E. Hormaeche, and J.M. Blackwell, 1998, Genetic control of immune response to recombinant antigens carried by an attenuated Salmonella typhimurium vaccine strain: Nramp1 influences T-helper subset responses and protection against leishmanial challenge, Infect. Immun. 66:1910–1917.

Stocker, B.A., S.K. Hoiseth, and B.P. Smith, 1983, Aromatic-dependent "Salmonella sp." as live vaccine in mice and calves, Developments in Biological Standardization 53:47–54.

Strahan, K., S.N. Chatfield, J. Tite, G. Dougan, and C.E. Hormaeche, 1992, Impaired resistance to infection does not increase the virulence of Salmonella htrA live vaccines for mice, Microb. Pathog. 12:311–317.

Tacket, C.O., D.M. Hone, R.d. Curtiss, S.M. Kelly, G. Losonsky, L. Guers, A.M. Harris, R. Edelman, and M.M. Levine, 1992, Comparison of the safety and immunogenicity of delta aroC delta aroD and delta cya delta crp Salmonella typhi strains in adult volunteers, Infect. Immun. 60:536–541.

Tacket, C.O., D.M. Hone, G.A. Losonsky, L. Guers, R. Edelman, and M.M. Levine, 1992, Clinical acceptability and immunogenicity of CVD 908 Salmonella typhi vaccine strain, Vaccine 10:443–446.

Tacket, C.O., M.B. Sztein, G.A. Losonsky, S.S. Wasserman, J.P. Nataro, R. Edelman, D. Pickard, G. Dougan, S.N. Chatfield, and M.M. Levine, 1997, Safety of live oral Salmonella typhi vaccine strains with deletions in htrA and aroC aroD and immune response in humans, Infect. Immun. 65:452–456.

Tsolis, R.M., S.M. Townsend, T.A. Ficht, L.G. Adams, and A.J. Bäumler, 1999, Attenuation in the mouse does not predict the ability of *Salmonella typhimurium* mutants to cause enteritis, submitted for publication.

Tsolis, R.M., S.M. Townsend, T.A. Ficht, L.G. Adams, and A.J. Bäumler, 1999, Identification of *Salmonella typhimurium* host range factors by signature tagged mutagenesis, submitted for publication.

Vazquez-Torres, A., J. Jones-Carson, A.J. Bäumler, S. Falkow, W. Brown, M. Le, R. Breggen, T. Parks, and F.C. Fang, 1999, Extraintestinal dissemination of *Salmonella* via CD18-expressing phagocytes, Submitted for publication.

Vescovi, E.G., F.C. Soncini, and E.A. Groisman, 1996, Mg^{2+} as an extracellular signal: environmental regulation of Salmonella virulence, Cell 84:165–174.

Vidal, S.M., D. Malo, K. Vogan, E. Skamene, and P. Gros, 1993, Natural resistance to infection with intracellular parasites: isolation of a candidate for Bcg, Cell 73:469–485.

Vidal, S.M., E. Pinner, P. Lepage, S. Gauthier, and P. Gros, 1996, Natural resistance to intracellular infections: Nramp1 encodes a membrane phosphoglycoprotein absent in macrophages from susceptible (Nramp1 D169) mouse strains, J. Immunol. 157:3559–3568.

Watson, P.R., E.E. Galyov, S.M. Paulin, P.W. Jones, and T.S. Wallis, 1998, Mutation of invH, but not stn, reduces salmonella-induced enteritis in cattle, Infection & Immunity 66:1432–1438.

Wood, M.W., M.A. Jones, P.R. Watson, S. Hedges, T.S. Wallis, and E.E. Galyov, 1998, Identification of a pathogenicity island required for Salmonella enteropathogenicity, Mol. Microbiol. 29:883–891.

Wood, M.W., R. Rosqvist, P.B. Mullan, M.H. Edwards, and E.E. Galyov, 1996, SopE, a secreted protein of *Salmonella dublin*, is translocated into the target eukaryotic cell via a *sip*-dependent mechanism and promotes bacterial entry, Mol. Microbiol. 22:327–338.

Woodward, M.J., McLaren, I., and Wray, C., 1989, Distribution of virulence plasmids within salmonellae, J. Gen. Microbiol. 135:503–511.

Wray, C. and W.J. Sojka, 1978, Experimental Salmonella typhimurium infection in calves, Res. Vet. Sci. 25:139–143.

Wray, C., W.J. Sojka, J.A. Morris, and M.W. Brinley, 1977, The immunization of mice and calves with gal E mutants of Salmonella typhimurium, Journal of Hygiene 79:17–24.

29

SIPS, SOPS, AND SPIs BUT NOT *STN* INFLUENCE SALMONELLA ENTEROPATHOGENESIS

T. S. Wallis, M. Wood, P. Watson, S. Paulin, M. Jones, and E. Galyov

Institute for Animal Health
Compton, Berkshire, RG20 7NN United Kingdom

1. SUMMARY

The virulence factors influencing Salmonella-induced enteropathogenesis remain poorly characterised. The interactions of different serotypes of Salmonella with bovine ileal mucosa have been characterised in the ligated ileal loop model. In a quantitative intestinal invasion assay *Salmonella dublin*, *S. choleraesuis*, *S. gallinarum*, and *S. abortusovis* strains were all recovered from ileal mucosa, either with or without Peyer's patches in similar numbers. This observation suggests that the magnitude and route of intestinal invasion does not mediate Salmonella serotype host specificity. Despite being equally invasive there was a clear hierarchy in the enteropathogenicity of these serotypes. The magnitude of the enteropathogenic responses did not correlate to serotype host specificity. These observations implicate undefined serotype specific factors in influencing enteropathogenicity independently of intestinal invasion. Disruption of genes in *Salmonella Pathogenicity Island* (SPI) 1 of *S. typhimurium* and *S. dublin* blocked the secretion of *Salmonella Invasion Proteins* (Sips) and *Salmonella Outer Proteins* (Sops). These mutants were significantly less invasive and enteropathogenic then the wild type strain in ligated ileal loops. Disruption of *sopB* and *sopD* significantly reduced enteropathogenesis, but without influencing intestinal invasion. These two genes appear to act in concert. Surprisingly, disruption of *stn*, the Salmonella enterotoxin gene cloned on the basis of its homology to cholera toxin, did not influence enteropathogenesis. *SopB* was mapped to the 20 centisome of *S. typhimurium* and is flanked by 5 genes that are organised in a manner typical of a pathogenicity island, which we have termed SPI-5. Mutation of the other genes in SPI-5 also attenuated enteropathogenesis but not virulence for mice, suggesting SPI-5 is a key locus specifically influencing Salmonella enteropathogenesis.

Mechanisms in the Pathogenesis of Enteric Diseases 2, edited by Paul and Francis.
Kluwer Academic / Plenum Publishers, New York, 1999.

2. INTRODUCTION

Over the past decade considerable progress has been made in our understanding of the pathogenesis of salmonellosis, with the identification of numerous virulence genes and distinct pathogenicity islands. However as the majority of these virulence factors have only been characterised in mice, which do not exhibit the enteric form of disease, factors influencing enteritis remain poorly defined.

Following oral ingestion it is widely accepted that virulent salmonellas invade the intestinal mucosa to initiate infection of the host. This process has been primarily studied in mice in which the main portal of entry of salmonellas into the host is via M cells overlaying the Peyer's Patches (Jones et al., 1994). Studies in mice have also suggested that Salmonella serotype host specificity is influenced by the ability of different serotype to invade and damage intestinal mucosa (Pascopella et al., 1995). Several studies in other species have demonstrated that salmonellas are also capable of directly penetrating the apical membrane of enterocytes (Takeuchi, 1968; Wallis et al., 1986; Watson et al., 1995; Frost et al., 1997). Thus apparently the route and magnitude of intestinal invasion by salmonellas depends on both host and serotype specific factors.

The work of many groups has demonstrated that the genes mediating invasion of epithelial cells are clustered at a specific locus called SP1-1 (for a detailed review see Collazo et al., 1997). SPI-1 encodes a type III secretion system, associated regulatory genes and the Salmonella invasion proteins (Sips). Together SPI-1 encoded proteins facilitate the translocation of proteins from within Salmonellas into target eukaryotic cells. Recently 5 Salmonella outer proteins (Sops) have been identified and shown to be secreted by Salmonellas by a SPI-1-dependent mechanism. One such protein, SopE is translocated into epithelial cells *in vitro* and facilitates the invasion of epithelial cells (Wood et al., 1996) by stimulating the reorganisation of the cell cytoskeleton (Hardt et al., 1998). While Sips and Sops have been characterised *in vitro* the role of these virulence determinants in the enteropathogenesis of salmonellosis is less clear.

The role of toxins in Salmonella induced enteropathogensis is also unclear. Over the past 20 years there have been numerous reports describing various cytotoxic, cytotonic and enterotoxic activities expressed by different Salmonella serotypes. More recently *stn*, a putative enterotoxin gene was cloned on the basis of its homology to cholera toxin (Chopra et al., 1994), although its role in Salmonella-induced enteropathogenesis was not demonstrated.

The aims of this study were first to characterise the intestinal invasiveness and enteropathogenesis of different Salmonella serotypes and second to assess the roles of SPI-1, Sops and *stn* on enteropathogenesis.

3. RESULTS AND DISCUSSION

Cattle are useful animals for studying Salmonella pathogenesis, because unlike mice, they are susceptible to both enteric and systemic forms of salmonellosis. The bovine ligated ileal loop model allows the study of the interactions of several Salmonella strains with intestinal mucosa within one animal. We have developed this model to quantify both bacterial invasion in a gentamicin protection assay (Watson et al., 1995) and enteropathogenic responses including fluid secretion and intestinal inflammation (Wallis et al., 1995). Intestinal invasiveness was assessed 2 h after loop inoculation with a dose of *circa* 10^9 cfu (the minimum dose which will induce potent enteropathogenic responses by virulent *S. typhimurium* strains within 12 h). Wild type strains of *S. typhimurium*, *S. dublin*, *S. choleraesuis*, *S. gallinarum*, and *S. abortusovis* were all recovered from mucosal biopsies, either with or without Peyer's Patch mucosa in similar numbers. This result indicates Salmonella-serotype host specificity cannot be explained solely by the inability of serotypes that are avirulent for cattle being unable to invade the intestines. These observations are in marked contrast to previous studies characterising the invasiveness of *S. typhimurium*, *S. typhi*, and *S. gallinarum* for murine intestine; *S. gallinarum* was non-invasive for murine intestine (Pascopella et al., 1995). These observations clearly demonstrate that both host and serotype specific factors influence intestinal invasion and that what occurs in one host serotype combination is not predictive of the phenotype of the same or different serotypes in other host species.

The role of SPI-1 in mediating intestinal invasion was assessed by comparing the intestinal invasiveness of isogenic mutants of *invH* and *sipB* in *S. typhimurium* and *S. dublin* strains. Disruption of *invH* or *sipB* resulted in a reduction of between 1.0 and 3.0 Log_{10} cfu in the recoveries from ileal mucosa of the mutants compared to the wild type parental strains (Watson et al., 1995; Galyov et al., 1997). These results show SPI-1 contributes to intestinal invasion *in vivo* in cattle. This is in agreement with qualitative observations in mice. In contrast, a *S. dublin sopB* mutant (which does not express the secreted SopB protein), was fully invasive for intestinal mucosa suggesting this protein is not involved in the invasion process (Galyov et al., 1997). Recently a homologue for *sopB* was identified in *S. typhimurium* which does influence invasion for epithelial cells *in vitro* (Hong and Miller, 1998). The reasons for the discrepancies of these observations are unclear and warrant further investigation.

The enteropathogenicity of wild type and mutant strains was also assessed by measuring secretory and inflammatory responses in bovine ileal ligated loops. The different serotypes showed a hierarchy in the ability to elicit enteropathogenic responses despite all strains being invasive for intestinal mucosa. *S. typhimurium* and *S. gallinarum* induced significantly greater secretory and inflammatory responses than *S. dublin* which in turn induced greater responses than *S. choleraesuis*. *S. abortusovis* failed to elicit any detectable secretory and inflammatory responses. Therefore the induction of enteropathogenic responses does not correlate to serotype-host specificity. For example, *S. gallinarum* is avirulent for cattle but can induce potent enteropathogenic responses in the artificially confined environment of ligated ileal loops. Thus the reasons for the avirulence of this serotype for cattle lie elsewhere in the interaction of this organism in cattle. It is also interesting to note the lack of enteropathogenic responses induced by *S. abortusovis*. This is despite intestinal invasion and therefore the introduction of endotoxin into the intestinal sub-mucosa which would be expected to induce an inflammatory response.

The effect of defined mutations on Salmonella enteropathogenesis was also assessed. Disruption of the *stn* gene in both *S. typhimurium* and *S. dublin* had no effect on the enteropathogenicity of these strains (Fig. 1), suggesting this gene plays no major role in Salmonella enteropathogenesis (Watson et al., 1998). In contrast, disruption of *invH* (Fig. 1) and *sipB* (Fig. 2) abolished the ability of *S. typhimurium* and *S. dublin* respectively to elicit secretory and inflammatory responses. This demonstrates that SPI-1 plays a major role in Salmonella enteropathogenesis. Disruption of either *sopB* or *sopD* also resulted in a significant reduction of *S. dublin*-induced secretory and

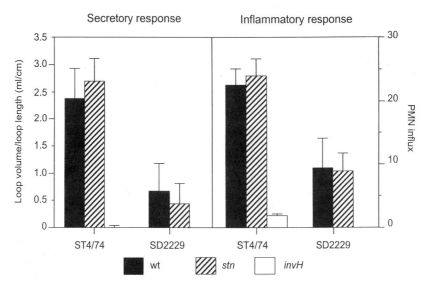

Figure 1. Roles of *invH* and *stn* in Salmonella-induced enteritis. Disruption of *invH* abolishes *S. typhimurium* induced enteropathogenesis. Disruption of *stn* has no effect on enteropathogenesis induced by either *S. typhimurium* or *S. dublin* strains.

inflammatory responses (Fig. 2) implicating genetic loci in addition to SPI-1 in this process. The *sopB sopD* double mutant elicited lower enteropathogenic responses than the two single mutations suggesting SopB and SopD together act in concert (Jones et al., 1998). Sequence analysis of SopB identified a functional domain homologous to mammalian inositol polyphosphate 4-phosphatases. Recently we have shown that SopB has inositol phosphate phosphatase activity *in vitro* (Norris et al., 1998). This activity

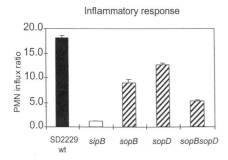

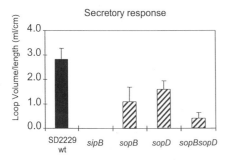

Figure 2. Roles of *sipB*, *sopB*, and *sopD* in *S. dublin* induced enteropathogenesis. *sopB* and *sopD* act in concert to induce enteropathogenic responses.

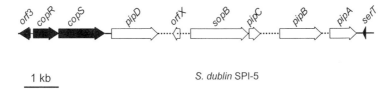

1 kb   *S. dublin* SPI-5

Figure 3. The structure of the SPI-5 pathogenicity island of *S. dublin*. The solid lines and arrows (ORFs) indicate DNA sequences common to both *S. dublin* and *E. coli* K12. The dotted line and unfilled ORFs indicate SPI-5 which is only present in salmonellas and maps to the 20 centisome of *S. typhimurium*.

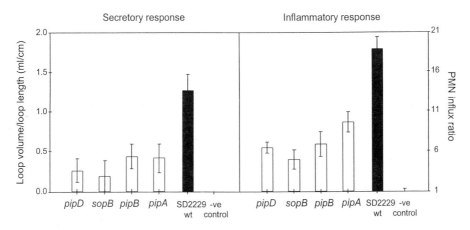

Figure 4. SPI-5 influences *S. dublin*-induced enteropathogenesis. Secretory and inflammatory responses induced by wild type and SPI-5 mutants in ligated ileal loops 12h after loop inoculation. LB broth was used as a negative control.

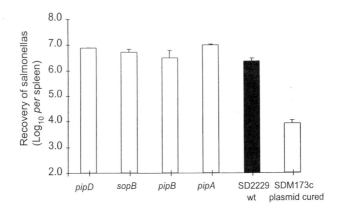

Figure 5. SPI-5 does not influence the virulence of *S. dublin* for Balb/c mice. Spleen counts 4 days after intraperitoneal challenge with approximately 30cfu of wild type of SPI-5 mutants. A plasmid cured derivative of SD2229 was used as an attenuated control strain.

in vivo is likely to modulate inositol phosphate intracellular signalling pathways within enterocytes, including Ca^{2+}-dependant chloride secretion. This could account for the reduction in enteropathogenicity of the *sopB* mutant.

Sequence analysis of the DNA flanking *sopB* identified features characteristic of a pathogenicity island that we have named SPI-5 (Wood et al., 1998). SPI-5 contains 5 genes, unique to Salmonella flanked by the *serT* and *copS* genes that are also present in *E. coli* K12 (Fig. 3). Mutation of *pipA*, *pipB*, and *pipC* all resulted in a significant reduction of enteropathogenic responses in ligated ileal loops (Fig. 4). The same mutants were fully virulent in mice following intraperitoneal challenge (Fig. 5). Together these results suggest that SPI-5 be involved in the enteric but not systemic phase of salmonellosis. The specific function of PipA, B, and C remain uncharacterised and is the subject of ongoing studies.

REFERENCES

Chopra, A.K., Peterson, J.W., Chary, P., and Prasad, R. 1994, Molecular characterization of an enterotoxin from *Salmonella typhimurium*. Microbiol. Pathog. 16:85–98.

Collazo, C.M. and Galan, J.E. 1997, The invasion-associated type-III protein secretion system in Salmonella—a review. Gene 192:51–59.

Frost, A.J., Bland, A.P., and Wallis, T.S. 1997, The early dynamic response of the calf ileal epithelium to *Salmonella typhimurium*. Vet. Pathol. 34:369–386.

Galyov, E.E., Wood, M.W., Rosqvist, R., Mullen, P.B., Watson, P.R, Hedges, S., and Wallis, T.S. 1997, A secreted effector protein of *Salmonella dublin* is translocated into eukaryotic cells and mediates inflammation and fluid secretion in infected ileal mucosa. Mol. Microbiol. 25:903–912.

Hardt, W.D., Chen, L.M., Schuebel, K.E., Bustelo, X.R., and Galan, J.E. 1998, *S. typhimurium* encodes an activator of Rho GTPases that induces membrane ruffling and nuclear responses. Cell 93:815–826.

Hong, K.H. and Miller, V.L. 1998, Identification of a novel *Salmonella* invasion locus homologous to Shigella *ipgDE*. J. Bacteriol. 180:1793–1802.

Jones, B.D., Ghori, N., and Falkow, S. 1994, *Salmonella typhimurium* initiates murine infection by penetrating and destroying the specialized epithelial M cells of the Peyer's patches. J. Exp. Med. 180:15–23.

Jones, M.A., Wood, M.W., Mullen, P.B., Watson, P.R., Wallis, T.S., and Galyov, E.E. 1998, Secreted effector proteins of *Salmonella dublin* act in concert to induce enteritis. Infect. Immun. 66:5799–5804.

Norris, F.A., Wilson, M.P., Wallis, T.S., Galyov, E.E., and Majerus, P. 1998, SopB, a protein required for virulence of *Salmonella dublin*, is an inositol phosphate phosphatase. P.N.A.S. 95:14057–14059.

Pascopella, L., Raupach, B., Ghori, N., Monack, D., Falkow, S., and Small, P. 1995, Host restriction phenotypes of *Salmonella typhi* and *Salmonella gallinarum*. Infect. Immun. 63:4329–4335.

Takeuchi, A. 1967, Electron microscope studies of experimental salmonella infection. Am. J. Pathol. 50:109–136.

Wallis, T.S., Starkey, W.G., Stephen, J., Osborne, M.P.O., and Candy, D.C.A. 1986, The nature and role of mucosal damage in relation to *Salmonella typhimurium*-induced fluid secretion in the rabbit ileum. J. Med. Microbiol. 22:390–349.

Wallis, T.S., Paulin, S., Plested, J., Watson, P.R., and Jones, P.W. 1995, *Salmonella dublin* virulence plasmid mediates systemic but not enteric phases of Salmonellosis in cattle. Infect. Immun. 63:2755–2761.

Watson, P.R., Paulin, S., Jones, P.W., and Wallis, T.S. 1995, Characterisation of intestinal invasion by *Salmonella typhimurium* and *Salmonella dublin* and effect of a mutation in the *invH* gene. Infect. Immun. 63:2743–2754.

Watson, P.R., Galyov, E.E., Paulin, S., Jones, P.W., and Wallis, T.S. 1998, *invH*, but not *stn*, influences *Salmonella*-induced enteritis in cattle. Infect. Immun. 66:1432–1438.

Wood, M.W., Rosquist, R., Mullen, P., Edwards, M., and Galyov, E.E. 1996, SopE, a secreted protein of *Salmonella dublin* is translocated into the target eukaryotic cell via a *sip*-dependent mechanism and promotes bacterial entry. Mol. Microbiol 22:327–338.

Wood, M.W., Jones, M.A., Watson, P.R, Hedges, S., Wallis, T.S., and Galyov, E.E. 1998, Identification of a pathogenicity island required for Salmonella enteropathogenicity. Mol. Microbiol. 29:883–891.

30

PHASE VARIABLE SWITCHING OF *IN VIVO* AND ENVIRONMENTAL PHENOTYPES OF *SALMONELLA TYPHIMURIUM*

R. E. Isaacson, C. Argyilan, L. Kwan, S. Patterson, and K. Yoshinaga

Department of Veterinary Pathobiology
University of Illinois
2001 S. Lincoln Ave.
Urbana, Illinois 61802

1. SUMMARY

Previously it was shown that S. typhimurium strain 798, which is known to cause persistent asymptomatic infections in pigs, exists in two phenotypes. One phenotype, which is called adhesive, was shown to produce pili, is adhesive to porcine enterocytes, is readily phagocytized, and then survives intracellularly in phagocytes. The other phenotype, termed non-adhesive, does not produce pili, does not attach to enterocytes, is phagocytized less efficiently, and does not survive within the phagocyte. Cells in each phenotype can freely switch to the other phenotype at a fairly high frequency and thus the shift between each phenotype is phase variation. Further analysis of these phenotypes identified 4 additional characteristics that were co-regulated by phase variation. The first is the enterocyte-specific adhesin, which was shown to be type 1 fimbriae. Mutations in *fimA*, the major pilin molecule, led to a decreased ability to colonize the gut of pigs and mice. The second characteristic is O-antigen production. Adhesive cells produce a long O-antigen (up to 18 subunits) while non-adhesive cells do not (only 1–2 subunits). The long O-antigen produced by the adhesive cells leads to resistance to serum and appears to be the result of phase variable expression of *rfaL*. A third locus, *ebu*, has been identified based on differential color production of colonies growing on Evans blue-Uranine plates. The relationship of this trait to in vivo survival or virulence is not known but *ebu* is genetically related to a family of transcriptional activators. The fourth locus, *prv* is located on the virulence plasmid and a mutation in *prv* results in delayed time to death in mice. It is hypothesized that the adhesive phenotype is the in vivo, virulent form, while the non-adhesive phenotype is the environmental, avirulent form. By modulating the fraction of cells in each phase, persistent asymptomatic infections can be promoted.

Mechanisms in the Pathogenesis of Enteric Diseases 2, edited by Paul and Francis.
Kluwer Academic / Plenum Publishers, New York, 1999.

2. INTRODUCTION

Salmonella enterica is one of the leading causes of food poisoning in man (Bean and Potter, 1992). In 1996 it was estimated that there were between 0.7 and 4 million cases of salmonellosis in the United States resulting in close to 3800 deaths (Buzby and Roberts, 1996). The costs associated with disease were estimated to be between $0.6 and 3.5 billion. A major outbreak of salmonellosis in Denmark caused by *S. enterica* associated with the consumption of pork has stimulated renewed interest in Salmonella and food safety by pork producers, consumers, and the government (Wegener and Baggesen, 1996). A combination of many factors including the outbreak in Denmark has prompted the United States Department of Agriculture to place *S. enterica* at the top of its priority list of food borne pathogens (Davies, 1997). In Denmark, *S. typhimurium* is the most common serotype isolated from pigs (78.2%) and is the second most common cause of food borne salmonellosis in humans (27.8%) (Baggesen, Wegener et al., 1996; Wegener and Baggesen, 1996). In the United States *S. typhimurium* is of similar significance. Thus, the study of *S. typhimurium* in swine as a potential food borne pathogen is warranted.

The introduction of *S. typhimurium* into the food chain appears to be manifested by the early exposure of pigs to this organism which results in long term persistent, but sub-clinical infections. Wood et al. (1989) demonstrated that when post-weanling pigs were challenged with *S. typhimurium*, they remained infected for as long as 28 weeks. However, after an initial bout of moderate to severe diarrhea, the infected pigs remained clinically healthy. We have replicated these experiments using lower doses (10^8) with similar results (Isaacson, Firkins et al., In press). With lower doses, disease is much milder and only 50% or less of challenged pigs get any signs of diarrhea. Pigs challenged with the lower dose of *S. typhimurium* do not continually shed *S. typhimurium* in their feces but at slaughter most (~85%) were still infected. Parenthetically, this makes the identification of carrier animals difficult. Infected animals can serve as reservoirs of *Salmonella* that can be spread to other animals or to contaminate food products at harvest. This is particularly true after shipment of pigs from the farm to the slaughter plant. The stress associated with shipment increases shedding of Salmonella in the feces of infected pigs (Isaacson, Firkins et al., In press).

The pathogenesis of salmonellosis caused by *S. typhimurium* requires the expression of unique sets of virulence genes that are coordinately regulated. Specific environmental cues most likely act as signals that trigger the expression of these genes (Miller, Kukrail et al., 1989; Miller and Mekalanos, 1990; Mekalanos, 1992). The first step in pathogenesis is the colonization of the intestinal tract. This process is mediated by the attachment of *S. typhimurium* to the mucosal surface in the intestines (Gahring, Heffron et al., 1990). Once attached to these tissues, *S. typhimurium* invades these cells. Invasion is mediated through an elaborate process that includes dependence on a type III protein secretion system and the coordinate expression of unique sets of genes. The primary route of invasion is believed to be via M-cells (Clark, Jepson et al., 1994; Jones, Ghori et al., 1994). Attachment to M-cells appears to be mediated by long polar fimbriae (Lpf) (Baumler, Tsolis et al., 1996). *S. typhimurium* subsequently escape from the M-cells and enter macrophages located in the Peyer's patches. Once in the macrophage, they express other virulence associated genes that allow them to replicate and survive within the macrophage. The ability to survive within phagocytes is an important attribute that contributes to virulence. Invasion of macrophages leads to spread of *S. typhimurium* to either regional lymph nodes or throughout the body causing life-threatening septicemia. Attachment to and invasion of enterocytes also occurs (Takeuchi, 1967). However, it is not clear whether this route can lead to wide spread dissemination. As will be discussed below, we believe that enterocytes may be important for long-term colonization.

For *S. typhimurium* to survive the array of host defense mechanisms, they must express sets of genes that lead to a variety of resistances including resistance to oxidative destruction, hydrolytic enzymes, cationic peptides, and serum complement. As already stated, the expression of these virulence/resistance mechanisms is tightly regulated. At least 2 well-described global regulatory systems have been identified that appear to control the virulence/resistance-related genes. The PhoP/PhoQ two-component regulatory system is involved in either the activation or repression of at least 40 bacterial genes known to be involved in invasion and intracellular survival in leukocytes (Groisman, Chiao et al., 1989; Miller and Mekalanos 1990; Vescovi, Soncini et al., 1994). The alternative sigma factor, RpoS, is known to positively regulate genes encoding stress response proteins expressed in stationary phase (Small, Blankenhor et al., 1994). RpoS also regulates expression of the plasmid encoded <u>S</u>almonella <u>p</u>lasmid <u>v</u>irulence (*spv*) genes that are required for systemic infections. We have been studying a third important global regulatory mechanism, phase variation (Isaacson and Kinsel, 1992). Phase variation appears to modulate expression of virulence genes controlling adhesion to enterocytes, production of O-antigen, resistance to serum complement, intracellular survival in enterocytes, and several others that have not been characterized (Isaacson and Kinsel, 1992; Kwan and Isaacson, 1998).

3. PHASE VARIATION

Phase variation is a well described meta-stable regulatory mechanism employed for the transient expression of many bacterial surface proteins. The most intensively studied phase variation system in *S. typhimurium* controls expression of the H1 and H2 flagellar antigens (Silverman and Simon, 1980; Simon, Zieg et al., 1980). In this system, the promoter for the H1 antigen and the repressor of the H2 antigen is encoded on a small invertible DNA element. In one orientation, the H1 antigen is expressed along with the H2 repressor. When the DNA sequence containing the promoter inverts, the H1 antigen and the H2 repressor are no longer expressed because the promoter is oriented in the "wrong" direction. Since the H2 repressor is not expressed, the H2 antigen is expressed. The model of an invertible DNA sequence is a common, although non-exclusive, theme in phase variation. Type 1 pili of *Escherichia coli* are controlled by this system (Eisenstein, 1981). On the other hand, other mechanisms of phase variation are known including differential methylation of GATC boxes (Braaten, Blyn et al., 1991; Hale, van der Woude et al., 1994), strand slippage replication in relevant promoters (Isaacson and Patterson, 1994), and cassette insertion adjacent to active promoters (Haas, Veit et al., 1992; Zhang, Deryckere et al., 1992). The mechanism of phase variation controlling virulence/resistance genes in *S. typhimurium* has not yet been determined.

3.1. Virulence Genes Associated with Phase Variation

Previously, we showed that *S. typhimurium* 798, which is a clinical isolate obtained from a pig, could be grown in two phases (Isaacson and Kinsel, 1992). The phases can be distinguished by various phenotypic traits. The phases were originally identified as having distinctly different colonial morphologies on blood agar and these differences correlated with ability to attach to porcine enterocytes in vitro. Cells that were adhesive formed colonies that were "large", while non-adhesive cells came from "small" colonies. Using electron microscopy, it was shown that adhesive cells produced fimbriae while non-adhesive cells did not. In addition, the adhesive cells produced between 10 and 15 unique envelope associated proteins absent in the non-adhesive cells. Because intracellular survival in leukocytes is an important process in the pathogenesis of salmonellosis, cells of both phenotypes were tested for their abilities to enter leukocytes and then to resist killing within the leukocyte. Adhesive cells were more readily phagocytized than non-adhesive cells, and the adhesive cells were resistant to killing while the non-adhesive cells were rapidly killed.

Using colony morphology (Isaacson and Kinsel, 1992), and later a detection system employing Evan Blue-Uranine agar plates (Patterson, Yoshinaga et al., 1998), the rates of transition from adhesive phase to non-adhesive phase and back were measured. The in vitro rate of transition from non-adhesive to adhesive phase was 10^{-3}/cell/generation. The in vitro rate of transition from adhesive to non-adhesive phase was 10^{-5}/cell/generation. In analyzing several of the phenotypic traits associated with the two phases, it was shown that when cells undergo phase variation, they acquire all of the traits associated with the new phenotype (Isaacson and Kinsel, 1992). Thus, this particular phase variation mechanism has global regulatory properties.

3.1.1. New Genes Associated with Phase Variation. To discover specific genes that were regulated by phase variation, a collection of mutations was prepared. Because it was expected that factors associated with virulence would frequently be associated with exported proteins, the transposon Tn*phoA* was used to create the mutations. The mutants then were screened in two assays. The first was an in vitro adhesion assay (Isaacson and Kinsel, 1992) and the second was an electrophoresis assay. In the in vitro adhesion assay, mutants were assessed for their abilities to attach to porcine enterocytes. Four mutants were selected as non-adhesive. Two of those mutants represented phase variants in adhesion and were not analyzed. The other two did not appear to be phase variants and were analyzed (see below). In the electrophoresis assay, mutants that lacked one of the unique proteins present in the adhesive phase cells but absent from non-adhesive phase cells were sought. To do this, envelope extracts were prepared from each of the mutants and compared to non-mutant adhesive and non-adhesive phase cells by SDS-gel electrophoresis (Kwan and Isaacson, 1998). Two mutants were selected for further analysis: mutant #55 and mutant #59.

3.1.2. Analysis of Mutants. Using the kanamycin resistance gene encoded by Tn*phoA*, as a selective marker, the Tn*phoA* in the two mutants identified in the electrophoresis screen were cloned and DNA flanking the transposon sequenced. Two unique sequences were identified. Mutant #55 was shown to contain a mutation in *rfaL* (Kwan and Isaacson, 1998), while mutant #59 had a mutation in the virulence plasmid located in the 20 kb region between *spv* and *pef* (plasmid encoded fimbriae). This locus has been tentatively called plasmid-encoded virulence (*prv*). The two non-adhesive mutants also were analyzed and both contained mutations in a fimbrial gene that will be reported elsewhere.

3.1.3. Analysis of the rfaL *Mutant.* The gene *rfaL* encodes an enzyme that serves as the O-antigen ligase (Kadam et al., 1991; Klena, Ashford et al., 1992). This enzyme is responsible for the linkage of the O-antigen to the core in the lipopolysaccharide. Thus, it is important in the final assembly stage of the O-antigen. Assuming that expression of *rfaL* indeed was phase variable it would be expected that the *rfaL* mutant and the non-adhesive phase cells would be defective in O-antigen production while the adhesive phase cells would produce a complete O-antigen. This prediction was correct. When lipopolysaccharide was analyzed by SDS-gel electrophoresis followed by staining with silver, adhesive phase cells were shown to produce a long O-antigen with oligomeric repeats up to 18, while the non-adhesive cells produced a short O-antigen (2–4 oligomeric repeats) and the *rfaL* mutant failed to produce O-antigen. The expression of O-antigen has been linked to smooth colony formation and resistance to serum complement. Colonies containing adhesive phase cells were smooth consistent with the production of a long O-antigen, while colonies containing either non-adhesive cells or the *rfaL* mutant were rough. The rough colony morphology was particularly apparent after prolonged incubation at 37°C (Kwan and Isaacson, 1998). Likewise, cultures containing adhesive cells were resistant to porcine complement while the non-adhesive cells and *rfaL* mutant were sensitive to complement (Fig. 1). When 200 to 400 viable cells were adjusted to 10% whole serum, adhesive cells grew, while the non-adhesive cells and the *rfaL* mutant not only failed to grow but were killed.

3.1.4. Phagocytic Uptake and Intracellular Survival. To determine if either mutant #55 (*rfaL*) or #59 (*prv*) had any role in entry into leukocytes or intracellular survival, both mutants were tested as previously described using the gentamicin selection protocol. Neither *rfaL* nor *prv* affected uptake (Fig. 2) or intracellular survival (Fig. 3). This indicates that O-antigen and the product encoded by *prv* are not involved in either of these leukocyte related virulence functions.

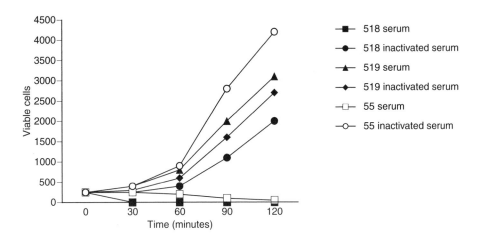

Figure 1. Growth of *S. typhimurium* in porcine serum. *S. typhimurium* was adjusted to 400–500 cells per ml and mixed with an equal volume of 20% porcine serum or 20% porcine serum that was heat inactivated. At intervals, an aliquot was removed and the number of viable *S. typhimurium* cells determined by culturing on LB agar. *S. typhimurium* 518 is in the non-adhesive phase and 519 is in the adhesive phase. Mutants #55 and #59 were described above.

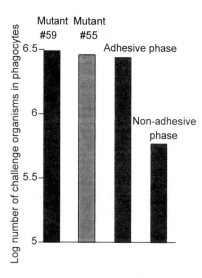

Figure 2. Uptake of *S. typhimurium* by porcine leukocytes. Approximately 10^8 bacterial cells were mixed with 10^6 leukocytes and incubated for 60 minutes. Extracellular bacteria were removed by centrifugation and adherent bacteria killed by exposure to gentamicin. The leukocytes were lysed and viable cells determined by plating on LB agar.

3.1.5. Effect of prv *on Mouse Virulence.* Preliminary experiments were performed to determine if *prv* had any effects on mouse virulence. No difference in mortality (LD_{50}) was detected when the *prv* mutant was compared to its parent in balbC mice. However, at a high challenge dose of 10^{10} orally, there was a consistent delay to death by the *prv* mutant. While it took 5 days to maximum lethality in the mice challenged with the parent, it took until day 12 to achieve the same level of mortality (Fig. 4). Although the number of mice challenged was not sufficient to achieve statistical

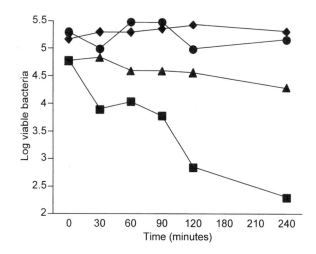

Figure 3. Intracellular survival in porcine leukocytes. Approximately 10^8 bacterial cells were mixed with 10^6 leukocytes and incubated for 60 minutes. Extracellular bacteria were removed by centrifugation and adherent bacteria killed by exposure to gentamicin. The leukocytes containing intracellular *S. typhimurium* were incubated in the presence of gentamicin for various times, aliquots removed and the number of viable bacteria determined by plating on LB agar. ■—■, non-adhesive phase cells; ●—●, adhesive phase cells; ▲—▲, mutant #55; ◆—◆, mutant #59.

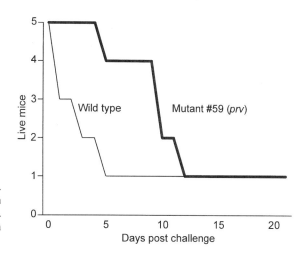

Figure 4. Lethality of mutant #59 in mice. BalbC mice were challenged orally with 10^{10} of the wild type parent or mutant #59. Time to death was recorded for each mouse.

significance in this experiment, this result was a reproducible result achieved with this and several other mutants containing mutated virulence genes.

3.1.6. Preliminary Characterization of the Nonadhesive Mutant. In preliminary experiments, one of the non-adhesive mutants was used to challenge both balbC mice and pigs. In mice, there was a small increase in the dose required to achieve an LD_{50}. Whether this difference was statistically significant was not determined. However, when the concentration of non-adhesive mutant cells in different tissue sites was compared to its parent, it was noted that the non-adhesive mutant did not colonize intestinal sites as well as its isogenic parent. These differences were statistically significant. The mutant was able to invade and spread beyond the intestinal tract. On the other hand, systemic spread did not appear to be altered in the non-adhesive mutant. That is, the concentration of the mutant did not differ from its parent in peripheral sites such as lung, liver, and spleen. In pigs, the mutant was less able to colonize the intestinal tract compared to its parent. Thus, the non-adhesive mutant exhibited altered colonization patterns in both animal species, but the mutation did not affect its ability to invade and disseminate throughout the body.

4. DISCUSSION

Initially we hypothesized that part of the mechanism that mediated the development and maintenance of persistent, asymptomatic *S. typhimurium* infections in animals was dependent on an adhesive/colonization process. To that end, it was possible to demonstrate that *S. typhimurium* strain 798 attached to enterocytes isolated from pigs (Isaacson and Kinsel, 1992). Furthermore, it was demonstrated that expression of adhesiveness was phase variable and correlated with differences in colonial morphology (Isaacson and Kinsel, 1992, Isaacson and Kinsel, 1992). In addition to the ability to attach to enterocytes, adhesive cells also were shown to produce fimbriae, to have 10–15 unique envelope associated proteins, to be resistant to intracellular killing by phagocytes but were more readily phagocytized, to be resistant to the killing action of complement, and produced a long O-antigen (Kwan and Isaacson, 1998). The expression of all of these traits was coordinately regulated and shown to shift between the two phases (or phenotypes) at a rate between 10^{-3}–10^{-5} per cell/generation (Isaacson and Kinsel, 1992; Patterson, Yoshinaga et al., 1998). This all or none global regulation allows cells to express a variety of virulence related attributes (adhesive phase) when they are needed in animals. Thus, we would assume that adhesive phase cells were virulent while non-adhesive phase cells would be non-virulent. Since the non-virulent cells would either be killed in animals or rapidly shed because of their inability to attach to enterocytes, we also would assume that the adhesive cells were adapted to in animal growth while the non-adhesive cells were adapted to growth outside of the animal. If the non-adhesive mutant used to challenge animals indeed was only defective in its ability to colonize the intestinal tract, the lack of long-term intestinal colonization would occur. However, since that mutant still retained the ability to produce the other virulence factors, it would not be killed. Thus, if M-cell specific adhesins were produced, the mutant still could invade and disseminate like the wild type strain, cause a high degree of mortality, but be rapidly cleared from the intestines. Therefore, it could cause septicemia but not cause persistent infections. Based on the preliminary animal studies using mice and pigs, that is exactly what occurs.

Since the production of disease is dose dependent, it would be expected that if the population size of the adhesive, and thus virulent cells, was maintained at a concentration that was below the threshold required to cause disease, it might result in a non-clinical, persistent infection. A mechanism would be required that maintained this population below that threshold. By modulating the fraction of total *S. typhimurium* cells in each of the two phases, it would be possible to satisfy these conditions. By continually undergoing phase variation, the population of adhesive cells could be maintained at a level that was sufficient to colonize the intestines, but insufficient to cause disease. Cells that transitioned to the non-adhesive phase would either no longer be able to colonize the intestines and would either be shed in feces, or if recognized by phagocytes, killed. Thus, phase variation may be an important controlling factor mediating persistent infections.

A second hypothesis developed based on this data is that long term persistent infections are based on adhesion to enterocytes not M-cells. M-cells are believed to be the preferred route of systemic invasion (Clark, Jepson et al., 1994; Jones, Ghori et al., 1994). The loss of adhesive capacity to enterocytes correlates with the inability to effectively colonize the intestines. Since the non-adhesive mutant is still capable of invading via M-cells and causing lethal infections, the loss of adhesiveness only seems to affect local intestinal colonization.

ACKNOWLEDGMENT

This work was supported by a grant from the United States Department of Agriculture, National Research Initiative number 9503296.

REFERENCES

Baggesen, D.L., H.C. Wegener, et al., 1996. Typing of *Salmonella enterica* serovar Saintpaul: an outbreak investigation. APMIS **104**. 411–418.

Baumler, A.J., R.M. Tsolis, et al., 1996. The *lpf* fimbrial operon mediates adhesion of *Salmonella typhimurium* to murine peyer's patches. Proc Natl Acad Sci USA **93**. 279–283.

Bean, N.H. and M.E. Potter, 1992. *Salmonella* serotypes from human sources, January 1991 through December. US Anim. Health Assoc., Louisville, Kentucky.

Braaten, B.A., L.B. Blyn, et al., 1991. Evidence for a methylation-blocking factor (mbf) locus involved in pap pilus expression and phase variation in *Escherichia coli*. J. Bacteriol. **173**. 1789–1800.

Buzby, J. and T. Roberts, 1996. Microbial foodborne illness. Choices **First Quarter**. 14–17.

Clark, M.A., M.A. Jepson, et al., 1994. Preferential interaction of *Salmonella typhimurium* with mouse Peyer's patch M cells. Res Microbiol **145**. 543–552.

Davies, P., 1997. Food safety and its impact on domestic and export markets. Swine Health and Production **5**. 13–20.

Eisenstein, B.I., 1981. Phase variation of type 1 fimbriae in *Escherichia coli* is under transcriptional control. Science **214**. 337–339.

Gahring, L.C., F. Heffron, et al., 1990. Invasion and replication of *Salmonella typhimurium* in animal cells. Infect. Immun. **58**. 443–448.

Groisman, E.A., E. Chiao, et al., 1989. *Salmonella typhimurium* phoP virulence gene is a transcriptional regulator. Proc. Natl. Acad. Sci. USA **86**. 7077–7081.

Haas, R., S. Veit, et al., 1992. Silent pilin genes of *Neisseria gonorrhoeae* MS11 and the occurrence of related hypervariant sequences among other gonococcal isolates. Molec. Microbiol **6**. 197–208.

Hale, W.B., M.W. van der Woude, et al., 1994. Analysis of nonmethylated GATC sites in the *Escherichia coli* chromosome and identification of sites that are differentially methylated in response to environmental stimuli. J. Bacteriol **176**. 3438–3441.

Isaacson, R.E., L.D. Firkins, et al., In press. Effect of transportation and feed withdrawal on shedding os *Salmonella* Typhimurium among experimentally infected pig. Am. J. Vet. Res.

Isaacson, R.E. and M. Kinsel, 1992. Adhesion of *Salmonella typhimurium* to porcine intestinal epithelial surfaces—identification and characterization of 2 phenotypes. Infect Immun **60**. 3193–3200.

Isaacson, R.E. and S. Patterson, 1994. Analysis of a naturally occurring K99(+) enterotoxigenic *Escherichia coli* strain that fails to produce K99. Infect Immun **62**. 4686–4689.

Jones, B.D., N. Ghori, et al., 1994. *Salmonella typhimurium* initiates murine infection by penetrating and destroying the specialized epithelial M cells of the Peyer's patches. J Exp Med **180**. 15–23.

Klena, J.D., R.S. Ashford, et al., 1992. Role of *Escherichia coli* K-12 *rfa* genes and the *rfp* gene of *Shigella dysenteriae*1 in the generation of lipopolysaccharide core heterogeneity and attachment of O antigen. J. Bacteriol. **174**. 7297–7303.

Kwan, L.Y. and R.E. Isaacson, 1998. Identification and characterization of a phase-variable nonfimbrial *Salmonella typhimurium* gene that alters O-antigen production. Infec. Immun. **66**. 5725–5730.

Mekalanos, J.J., 1992. Environmental signals controlling expression of virulence determinants in bacteria. J. Bacteriol. **174**. 1–7.

Miller, S.I., A.M. Kukrail, et al., 1989. A two-component regulatory system (phoP/phoQ) controls *Salmonella typhimurium* virulence deteriminats in bacteria. Proc. Natl.Acad. Sci. USA **86**. 5054–5058.

Miller, S.I. and J.J. Mekalanos, 1990. Constitutive expression of the *phoP* regulon attenuates S. *typhimurium* virulence and survival within macrophages. J. Bacteriol. **170**. 2575–2583.

P.R., M., S.K. Kadam, et al., 1991. Cloning and characterization and DNA sequence of the *rfaLK* region for lipopolysaccharide synthesis in *Salmonella typhimurium* LT-2. J. Bacteriol **173**. 7151–7163.

Patterson, S.K., K. Yoshinaga, et al., 1998. Phase variation of *Salmonella typhimurium* detectable on Evans blue-uranine plates. Second International Rushmore Conference on Mechanisms in the Pathogenesis of Enteric Diseases, Rapid City, SD.

Silverman, M. and M. Simon, 1980. Phase variation: genetic analysis of switching mutants. Cell **19**. 845–854.

Simon, M., J. Zieg, et al., 1980. Phase variation: evolution of a controlling element. Science **209**. 1370–1374.

Small, P., D. Blankenhor, et al., 1994. Acid and base resistance in *Escherchia coli* and *Shigella flexneri*: role of *rpoS* and growth pH. J. Bacteriol. **176**. 1729–1737.

Takeuchi, A., 1967. Electron microscopic studies of experimental *Salmonella* infection. I. Penetration into the intestinal epithelium by *Salmonella typhimurium*. Am. J. Pathol. **50**. 109–136.

Vescovi, E.G., F.C. Soncini, et al., 1994. The role of the PhoP/PhoQ regulon in *Salmonella* virulence. Res Microbiol **145**. 473–480.

Wegener, H.C. and D.L. Baggesen, 1996. Investigation of an outbreak of human salmonellosis caused by *Salmonella enterica* ssp. enterica serovar Infantis by use of pulsed field gel electrophoresis. Int J Food Microbiol **32**. 125–31.

Zhang, Q.Y., D. Deryckere, et al., 1992. Gene conversion in *Neisseria gonorrhoeae*—evidence for Its role in pilus antigenic variation. Proc Natl Acad Sci USA **89**. 5366–5370.

31

A PRELIMINARY SURVEY OF ANTIBIOTIC RESISTANCE OF *SALMONELLA* IN MARKET-AGE SWINE

Leigh A. Farrington,[*][1] Roger B. Harvey,[2] Sandra A. Buckley,[2] Larry H. Stanker,[2] and Peter D. Inskip[1]

[1] Department of Veterinary Anatomy and Public Health
Texas A&M University
College Station, Texas
77843
[2] Food Animal Protection Research Laboratory
USDA, ARS
College Station, Texas
77845

1. SUMMARY

We conducted an epidemiological survey of antibiotic resistance in *Salmonella* recovered from market-age swine at five different Texas farms. These farms, which were visited between October 1997 and June 1998, were completely integrated, farrow-to-finish operations. Samples were taken from the lymph nodes and cecal contents at the time of slaughter. The *Salmonella* samples that were recovered were sent to the National Veterinary Services Laboratory for serotyping. Antibiotic resistance was determined using the Dispens-O-Disc Susceptibility Test System using 13 different antimicrobial agents that have been utilized in either veterinary medicine, human medicine, or both. Preliminary analysis of the first 183 samples out of approximately 400 *Salmonella* samples recovered indicated that 183 (100%) of the *Salmonella* samples were resistant to penicillin G, and 122 (66.7%) were resistant to chlortetracycline. Six (3.3%) were resistant to four antibiotics (chlortetracycline, penicillin G, streptomycin, and sulfisoxazole), and 25 (13.7%) were resistant to three antibiotics (chlortetracycline, penicillin G, and either streptomycin, sulfisoxazole, or ampicillin). Variation was seen between serotypes, with four out of five *S. agona* samples (80.0%) and two out of eight *S. derby* samples (25.0%) resistant to four antibiotics. Variation in antibiotic resistance also was seen between farms. There is an increasing concern about the prevalent usage

Mechanisms in the Pathogenesis of Enteric Diseases 2, edited by Paul and Francis.
Kluwer Academic / Plenum Publishers, New York, 1999.

291

of antibiotics in medicine and agriculture and the relationship this may have on emerging microbial resistance patterns; therefore, continued surveillance on antibiotic resistance in animal production is warranted.

2. INTRODUCTION

The issue of antibiotic resistance in bacteria has raised concerns for health and safety worldwide. Resistance was first noted in 1940 when an enzyme capable of hydrolyzing penicillin was detected in *E. coli* (Tenover and Hughes, 1996). Since that time antibiotic resistance has become common in many genera of bacteria (Swartz, 1997; Tenover and Hughes, 1996; Witte, 1998). Today many *Salmonella* serotypes have been isolated that demonstrate resistance to multiple antibiotics (D'Aoust et al., 1992; Epling and Carpenter, 1990; Threlfall et al., 1997). *S. typhimurium* strain DT104, which is found in many places including the United States and Europe, has demonstrated resistance to ampicillin, tetracycline, streptomycin, chloramphenicol, and sulfonamides (Glynn et al., 1998; Witte, 1998). Resistance can create a problem in both human and veterinary medicine. Since many *Salmonella* species are not host-specific, *Salmonella* in food-producing animals becomes a possible source of infection for humans. If an infection becomes systemic, serious illness and even death can occur if the antibiotics used for treatment are not effective (D'Aoust et al., 1992). Vast amounts of antibiotics are used each year, not only in the treatment of illness in humans and animals, but also subtherapeutically in food-producing animals for prophylaxis and growth promotion (D'Aoust et al., 1992; Witte, 1998). In the early 1980's approximately 14.3 million kg of antibiotics were produced annually in the United States. Approximately 40% of that was used as a feed additive for livestock and poultry (Swartz, 1997). It has been theorized that the widespread use of antibiotics in human and veterinary medicine, as well as in animal production, has acted as a selective agent for antibiotic resistance in bacteria (D'Aoust et al., 1992; Epling and Carpenter, 1990; Swartz, 1997; Tenover and Hughes, 1996; Witte, 1998). This study was initiated to determine the extent of antibiotic resistance in various *Salmonella* serotypes isolated from swine and to identify the resistance patterns that occur.

3. MATERIALS AND METHODS

All media, antibiotic disks and test reagents used in this study were manufactured by Difco with the exception of the brilliant green agar (Oxoid).

3.1. Sample Collection

Ileo-cecal lymph nodes and cecal contents were collected from market-age swine at the time of slaughter from October 1997 to June 1998. Sampling occurred multiple times at each of five completely integrated, farrow-to-finish Texas farms. Pre-enrichment for lymph nodes and cecal contents was performed in both GN broth, Hajna and tetrathionate broth base with added iodine. Following post-enrichment of all of the samples in Rappaport-Vassiliadis R10 broth, each sample was streaked on brilliant green agar with novobiocin. Samples that appeared positive for *Salmonella* were biochemically characterized using lysine iron agar and triple sugar iron agar. *Salmonella* positives were confirmed by slide agglutination using *Salmonella* O antiserum poly A–I and Vi and Group C_1 factors 6,7. Approximately 400 *Salmonella* positive samples were sent to the National Veterinary Services Laboratory for serotyping. Each sample was stored in pure culture on tryptic soy agar.

3.2. Antibiotic Resistance

Antibiotic resistance patterns were determined for 183 of the *Salmonella* samples. Thirteen pair of *Salmonella* isolates (26 isolates) were recovered from the lymph node and cecal contents of the same pig and were of the same serotype. Of the 13 pair, 92.3% showed different resistance patterns; therefore, *Salmonella* isolates from the lymph node and cecal contents of the same pig were treated as different samples. Thirteen different antimicrobial agents were utilized—amikacin (30µg), ampicillin (10µg), cephalothin (30µg), chloramphenicol (3µg), chlortetracycline (30µg), enrofloxacin (5 µg), gentamicin (10µg), kanamycin (30µg), nitrofurantoin (300µg), penicillin G(10 units), streptomycin (10µg), sulfisoxazole (300µg), and trimethoprim (5µg). Antibiotic resistance testing was carried out according to the disk diffusion procedure described by the National Committee for Clinical Laboratory Standards, NCCLS (NCCLS, 1997; NCCLS, 1998). Each *Salmonella* sample was grown overnight on blood agar. Five mL of tryptic soy broth was inoculated with four to five *Salmonella* colonies to achieve turbidity similar to that of a 0.5 McFarland standard (direct colony suspension method). This suspension was streaked on a 150mm Mueller Hinton plate, and after five to ten minutes the antibiotic disks were placed on the plate using the 12-cartridge semi-automatic dispenser. The 13th antibiotic disk was manually placed in the center of the plate. The plates were incubated for 18–20 hours at 37°C (rather than at the NCCLS recommendation of 35°C). The zone of inhibition was measured as the diameter of the circle without bacterial growth surrounding each antibiotic disk. Each sample was classified as susceptible, intermediate or resistant to each of the 13 antimicrobial agents using the NCCLS zone diameter interpretive standards based on clinical efficacy (NCCLS, 1997; NCCLS, 1998).

4. RESULTS AND DISCUSSION

A preliminary analysis of 183 samples was performed (Fig. 1). Resistance was found to several antimicrobial agents used extensively in the past. 100% of the samples were resistant to penicillin G, an antibiotic introduced in both human and veterinary medicine in the 1940's and still used today primarily in large animal medicine (Adams, 1995; Kucers et al., 1997). Ampicillin and cephalothin, both related to penicillin, are often active against penicillin G-resistant bacteria (Kucers et al., 1997). 1.1% of the samples were classified as resistant to ampicillin, and 1.1% were classified as intermediate. 0.6% of the samples were intermediate to cephalothin. Reduced sensitivity to chlortetracycline was seen in 100% of the samples with 66.7% of the samples resistant to and 33.3% of the samples intermediate to chlortetracycline. Chlortetracycline was first introduced into veterinary medicine in 1948 and now is used as a feed and water additive for food-producing animals (Adams, 1995). Resistance also has developed against the aminoglycoside streptomycin, which was first used in human and veterinary medicine in the 1940's (Kucers et al., 1997). 13.1% of the samples were classified as resistant to streptomycin and 79.2% of the samples were classified as intermediate.

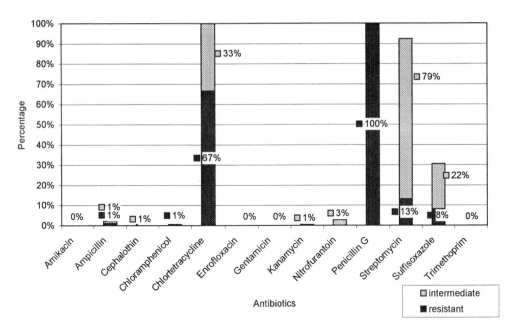

Figure 1. Percentage of samples classified as resistant and intermediate to each antibiotic.

Virtually no resistance was observed to the other three aminoglycosides, kanamycin, gentamicin, and amikacin. Only 0.6% of the samples were classified as intermediate to kanamycin. Sulfisoxazole, a sulfonamide, has been used clinically for about 50 years. It is now used almost exclusively in combination with another drug, such as trimethoprim, in both human and veterinary medicine (Adams, 1995; Kucers et al., 1997). Resistance to sulfisoxazole was observed with 8.2% of the samples considered resistant and 22.4% of the samples considered intermediate. No resistance to trimethoprim was seen. Chloramphenicol, introduced in 1947, and nitrofurantoin, introduced in 1953, have been banned from use in food-producing animals but are still used in human and small animal medicine (Adams, 1995; Allen et al., 1998; Kucers et al., 1997). 0.6% of the samples were resistant to chloramphenicol. 2.7% of the samples were intermediate to nitrofurantoin. No resistance was observed to the fluoroquinolone, enrofloxacin.

Multidrug-resistance (resistance to two or more antibiotics) was found in 69.5% of the samples. Resistance to two, three, and four antibiotics was found in 52.5%, 13.7% and 3.3% of the samples, respectively. Four of the six (66.7%) resistant to four antibiotics were *S. agona* and two of the six (33.3%) were *S. derby*. Both *S. agona* and *S. derby* are somatic serogroup B. All six samples were resistant to the same four antibiotics—chlortetracycline, penicillin G, streptomycin, and sulfisoxazole. Out of the 13.7% (25 samples) resistant to three antibiotics, all were resistant to chlortetracycline, penicillin G, and either streptomycin (68%), sulfisoxazole (24%) or ampicillin (8%). The antibiotic resistance patterns by serotype and somatic serogroup can be seen in Table 1 and Table 2. A significant difference (p < 0.05) was found between serotypes in their antibiotic resistance patterns, with *S. derby* showing increased resistance to streptomycin and *S. derby*, *S. schwarzengrund* and the "other" category showing increased resistance to sulfisoxazole when compared to the remaining serotypes. A significant difference (p < 0.05) also was detected between somatic serogroups in their resistance patterns.

Table 1. Antibiotic resistance of *Salmonella* by serotype[a]

Antibiotics	*anatum* 11 occurrences	*derby* 8 occurrences	*livingstone* 21 occurrences	*montevideo* 41 occurrences	*schwarzengrund* 59 occurrences	other[b] 43 occurrences representing 19 serotypes	p-value[c]
Amikacin	0/0	0/0	0/0	0/0	0/0	0/0	—
Ampicillin	0/0	0/0	0/0	0/0	0/1.7	4.7/2.3	P = 0.69
Cephalothin	0/0	0/0	0/0	0/0	0/1.7	0/0	P = 1.00
Chloramphenicol	0/0	0/0	0/0	0/0	0/0	2.3/0	P = 0.68
Chlortetracycline	63.6/36.4	87.5/12.5	76.2/23.8	61.0/39.0	72.9/27.1	55.8/44.2	P = 0.29
Enrofloxacin	0/0	0/0	0/0	0/0	0/0	0/0	—
Gentamicin	0/0	0/0	0/0	0/0	0/0	0/0	—
Kanamycin	0/0	0/0	0/0	0/0	0/1.7	0/0	P = 1.00
Nitrofurantoin	0/0	0/0	0/0	0/2.4	0/1.7	0/7.0	P = 0.73
Penicillin G[d]	100/—	100/—	100/—	100/—	100/—	100/—	—
Streptomycin	0/90.9	37.5/62.5	19.0/81.0	7.3/87.8	11.9/83.1	16.3/65.1	P < 0.01
Sulfisoxazole	0/45.5	25.0/25.0	0/0	0/4.9	10.2/40.7	16.3/18.6	P < 0.01
Trimethoprim	0/0	0/0	0/0	0/0	0/0	0/0	—

[a]Percent of resistant samples/percent of intermediate samples for each serotype.
[b]The "other" category represents serotypes that occurred less than 6 times in the 183 samples analyzed. These serotypes and the number of times they each occurred are as follows: 4,5,12:I-monophasic(5), *S. agona*(5), *S. braenderup*(1), *S. havana*(5), *S. johannesburg*(1), *S. mbandaka*(2), *S. meleagridis*(2), *S. menhaden*(1), *S. muenchen*(1), *S. muenster*(3), multiple serotypes(1), *S. newbrunswick*(1), *S. orion*(1), *S. tennessee*(1), *S. thompson*(3), *S. typhimurium*(5), *S. typhimurium* strain copenhagen(3), *S. urbana*(1), and *S. worthington*(1).
[c]Fisher's exact test for association between serotypes and antibiotic resistance.
[d]An intermediate category for penicillin G is not defined.

Table 2. Antibiotic resistance of *Salmonella* by somatic serogroup[a]

Antibiotics	B 80 occurrences	C_1 69 occurrences	E_1 17 occurrences	G_2 6 occurrences	other[b] 11 occurrences representing 6 groups	p-value
Amikacin	0/0	0/0	0/0	0/0	0/0	—
Ampicillin	0/1.3	0/0	0/0	0/0	18.2/9.1	P < 0.01
Cephalothin	0/1.3	0/0	0/0	0/0	0/0	P = 1.00
Chloramphenicol	0/0	0/0	0/0	0/0	9.1/0	P = 0.09
Chlortetracycline	75.0/25.0	68.1/31.9	52.9/47.1	50.0/50.0	27.3/72.7	P = 0.01
Enrofloxacin	0/0	0/0	0/0	0/0	0/0	—
Gentamicin	0/0	0/0	0/0	0/0	0/0	—
Kanamycin	0/1.3	0/0	0/0	0/0	0/0	P = 1.00
Nitrofurantoin	0/1.3	0/2.9	0/0	0/0	0/18.2	P = 0.10
Penicillin G	100/—	100/—	100/—	100/—	100/—	—
Streptomycin	21.3/75.0	10.1/85.5	0/70.6	0/66.7	0/90.9	P < 0.01
Sulfisoxazole	15.0/33.8	2.9/5.8	0/35.3	0/16.7	9.1/27.3	P < 0.01
Trimethoprim	0/0	0/0	0/0	0/0	0/0	—

[a]Refer to footnotes of Table 1.
[b]The "other" category represents somatic serogroups that occurred less than 6 times in the 183 samples analyzed. These serogroups and the number of times they each occurred are as follows: C_2(1), E_2(1), E_3(1), N(1), R(1), and an undefined group containing the 4,5,12:I-monophasic and multiple serotypes classifications that have no defined somatic serogroup(6).

Table 3. Antibiotic resistance of *Salmonella* by apramycin exposure[a]

Aminoglycosides	Exposed to Apramycin 83 occurrences	Not Exposed to Apramyein 100 occurrences	p-value
Amikacin	0/0	0/0	—
Gentamicin	0/0	0/0	—
Kanamycin	0/0	0/1.0	P = 0.58
Streptomycin	13.3/78.3	13.0/80.0	P = 0.80

[a]Refer to footnotes of Table 1.

Somatic serogroups B and C_1 expressed increased resistance to streptomycin, and somatic serogroup B and the "other" category expressed increased resistance to sulfisoxazole. The "other" category also showed increased resistance to ampicillin but showed decreased resistance and increased intermediate susceptibility to chlortetracycline when compared to the remaining serogroups.

Two of the farms sampled in this study used the aminoglycoside, apramycin, subtherapeutically. It was used as a feed and water additive for the sows and as creep feed for their piglets for the first 21 days after birth. As seen in Table 3, no significant difference (p > 0.05) was found in resistance to the aminoglycosides, amikacin, gentamicin, kanamycin, and streptomycin, between the group that was exposed to apramycin, and the group that was not. A significant difference (p < 0.05) was detected among farms in resistance of the *Salmonella* spp. isolated to the antibiotics chlortetracycline and sulfisoxazole as seen in Table 4. The highest rate of resistance to chlortetracycline was found in the samples from farm A, and the lowest rate of resistance was found in the samples from farm E. Conversely, the samples from farm A had the lowest rate of intermediate susceptibility to chlortetracycline while those from farm E had the highest rate. The samples from farm E showed an increased rate of resistance to sulfisoxazole when compared to the remaining farms. All of the farms sampled in this study infrequently administered chlortetracycline as a therapeutic agent. Subtherapeutic admin-

Table 4. Antibiotic resistance of *Salmonella* by farm[a]

Antibiotics	A 62 occurrences	B[b] 77 occurrences	C 13 occurrences	D 25 occurrences	E[b] 6 occurrences	p-value
Amikacin	0/0	0/0	0/0	0/0	0/0	—
Ampicillin	0/0	2.6/0	0/0	0/4.0	0/16.7	P = 0.06
Cephalothin	0/1.6	0/0	0/0	0/0	0/0	P = 0.58
Chloramphenicol	0/0	0/0	0/0	4.0/0	0/0	P = 0.24
Chlortetracycline	79.0/21.0	66.2/33.8	46.2/53.8	56.0/44.0	33.3/66.7	P = 0.02
Enrofloxacin	0/0	0/0	0/0	0/0	0/0	—
Gentamicin	0/0	0/0	0/0	0/0	0/0	—
Kanamycin	0/1.6	0/0	0/0	0/0	0/0	P = 0.58
Nitrofurantoin	0/3.2	0/2.6	0/0	0/0	0/16.7	P = 0.32
Penicillin G	100/—	100/—	100/—	100/—	100/—	—
Streptomycin	12.9/82.3	13.0/79.2	7.7/76.9	16.0/76.0	16.7/66.7	P = 0.80
Sulfisoxazole	12.9/40.3	3.9/11.7	0/30.8	8.0/8.0	33.3/16.7	P < 0.01
Trimethoprim	0/0	0/0	0/0	0/0	0/0	—

[a]Refer to footnotes of Table 1.
[b]Farms B and E used the aminoglycoside, apramycin, subtherapeutically.

istration of chlortetracycline was discontinued on all of the farms approximately five years prior to this study.

5. CONCLUSIONS

Reduced susceptibility was observed to nine of the thirteen antibiotics tested. Resistance was found to ampicillin, chloramphenicol, chlortetracycline, penicillin G, streptomycin, and sulfisoxazole. Intermediate resistance to cephalothin, kanamycin, and nitrofurantoin also was seen. Multidrug-resistance was found in over two-thirds of the samples with chlortetracycline and penicillin G common to all of these resistance patterns. Although no trend was detected between subtherapeutic administration of apramycin and resistance to the four aminoglycosides tested, additional studies are necessary to provide insight into the relationship between antibiotic usage in medicine and agriculture and the emergence of microbial resistance.

REFERENCES

Adams, H.R., ed., 1995, *Veterinary Pharmacology and Therapeutics*, 7th ed., Iowa State University Press, Ames, Iowa.

Allen, D.G., et al., 1998, *Handbook of Veterinary Drugs*, 2nd ed., Lippincott-Raven, Philadelphia, Pa.

D'Aoust, J., et al., 1992, Antibiotic Resistance of Agricultural and Foodborne *Salmonella* Isolates in Canada: 1986–1989, *J Food Prot* 55(6):428–434.

Epling, L.K. and Carpenter, J.A., 1990, Antibiotic Resistance of *Salmonella* Isolated from Pork Carcasses in Northeast Georgia, *J Food Prot* 53(3):253–254.

Glynn, M.K., et al., 1998, Emergence of Multidrug-Resistant *Salmonella Enterica* Serotype Typhimurium DT104 Infections in the United States, *N Engl J of Med* 338(19):1333–1338.

Kucers, A., et al, 1997, *The Use of Antibiotics: A Clinical Review of Antibacterial, Antifungal and Antiviral Drugs*, 5th ed., Butterworth-Heinemann, Oxford.

National Committee for Clinical Laboratory Standards, 1997, Performance Standards for Antimicrobial Disk Susceptibility Tests—Sixth Edition, Approved Standard, M2-A6, National Committee for Clinical Laboratory Standards 17(1).

National Committee for Clinical Laboratory Standards, 1998, Performance Standards for Antimicrobial Susceptibility Testing—Eighth Informational Supplement, M100-S8, National Committee for Clinical Laboratory Standards 18(1).

Swartz, M.N, 1997, Use of Antimicrobial Agents and Drug Resistance, *N Engl J of Med* 337(7):491–492.

Tenover, F.C. and Hughes, J.M., 1996, The Challenges of Emerging Infectious Diseases: Development and Spread of Multiply- Resistant Bacterial Pathogens, *JAMA* 275(4):300–304.

Threlfall, E.J., et al., 1997, Increase in Multiple Antibiotic Resistance in Nontyphoidal *Salmonellas* from Humans in England and Wales: A Comparison of Data for 1994 and 1996, *Microbial Drug Resistance* 3(3):263–266.

Witte, W., 1998, Medical Consequences of Antibiotic Use in Agriculture, *Science* 279:996–997.

32

PROPHYLACTIC ADMINISTRATION OF IMMUNE LYMPHOKINE DERIVED FROM T CELLS OF *SALMONELLA ENTERITIDIS-* IMMUNE PIGS

Protection against *Salmonella Choleraesuis* Organ Invasion and Cecal Colonization in Weaned Pigs

Kenneth J. Genovese,[1] Robin C. Anderson,[2,3] David E. Nisbet,[3]
Roger B. Harvey,[3] Virginia K. Lowry,[1*] Sandra Buckley,[3]
Larry H. Stanker,[3] and Michael H. Kogut[3]

[1] Department of Veterinary Pathobiology
[1*] Department of Veterinary Anatomy and Public Health
Texas A&M University
College Station, Texas 77843
[2] Milk Specialties Company, Dundee, Illinois 60118
[3] USDA ARS FAPRL
College Station, Texas 77845

SUMMARY

Experiments involving 132 weaned piglets were conducted to evaluate the efficacy of a *Salmonella enteritidis*-immune lymphokine (PILK) derived from the T cells of *Salmonella enteritidis* (SE)-immunized pigs to protect weaned piglets from *Salmonella choleraesuis* (SC) infection. Fourteen-to-seventeen day-old piglets were weaned and randomly placed into 1 of 5 groups: (1) noninfected controls, (2) PILK 3X noninfected, (3) SC infected controls, (4) PILK 1X SC infected, and (5) PILK 3X SC infected. PILK was given orally either one time (PILK 1X) or three times (PILK 3X) over 14 days. One hour after the first PILK administration on day 0, piglets were orally challenged with 10^7 cfu of SC. Weights were recorded on day 0, day 7, and day 14. On day 14, pigs in groups 3, 4, and 5 were sacrificed and organs and lymph tissue were cultured

Mechanisms in the Pathogenesis of Enteric Diseases 2, edited by Paul and Francis.
Kluwer Academic / Plenum Publishers, New York, 1999.

for the presence of SC. Three replicates of this experiment were pooled and analyzed. A significant reduction in the number of pigs positive for SC in the liver, lung, and spleen was found in group 5 (PILK 3X) when compared to group 3 (inf. cont. [p < 0.001]). The number of SC positive cecal contents was dramatically reduced in group 5 group when compared to group 3, with the PILK 3X group showing 13% positive pigs versus 55.2% in the infected controls (p < 0.05). Weight gain over the 14 day study in the infected PILK 3X group (group 5) was found to be comparable to the gain observed in the group 1 (noninfected controls). The pigs receiving PILK 3X (group 2) with no SC challenge gained significantly more weight than all other groups, including the noninfected controls (group 1 [p < 0.05]). The results of these experiments indicate that PILK protects against SC infection in weaned pigs while enhancing performance in the presence of an SC infection.

1. INTRODUCTION

Recently weaned pigs have an increased susceptibilty to infectious diseases in comparison to mature and suckling swine (Blecha et al., 1983; Wilcock and Schwartz, 1992). This increase in susceptibilty to infectious agents post-weaning may be comprised of multiple factors, including loss of maternally derived antibodies, developmental deficiencies of the immune response, and stress-induced susceptibility due to increased glucocorticoids in these pigs (Blecha et al., 1983; Wilcock and Schwartz, 1992; Blecha et al., 1985; Aurich et al., 1990; Abughali et al., 1994; El-Awar and Hahn, 1991). With the trend leaning towards weaning piglets from sows earlier, 8–10 days of age in some cases, the influence of developmental deficiencies of the immune system on increased susceptibility to infectious diseases becomes an even more important concern (Blecha et al., 1983).

Developmental deficiencies in immune functions and subsequent susceptibility to infectious diseases have been well documented in neonatal mammalian species. Human, equine, and bovine neonates exhibit deficient or impaired neutrophil and T cell functions for the first weeks of life (Coignal et al., 1984; Hauser et al., 1986; Hill, 1987; Miller, 1979; Rosenthal and Cairo, 1995; Higuchi et al., 1997; Lee and Roth, 1992; Lee and Kehrli, 1998; Zwahlen et al., 1992). Susceptibility to gram negative bacteria has also been well documented in equine, porcine, and bovine neonates (Carter and Martens, 1986; Drieson et al., 1993; Selim et al., 1995). Young pigs exhibit developmental deficiencies within both the humoral and cellular arms of the immune system. Development of B and T cell compartments in neonatal pigs takes several weeks to become stable and the different classes of immunoglobulins in various sites change with the age of the pig (Bianchi et al., 1992; McCauley and Hartmann, 1984). Decreased mitogenic responses of T cells from young pigs have also been observed (Blecha et al., 1983; El-Awar and Hahn, 1991; Shi et al., 1994; Hoskinson et al., 1990).

Our laboratory has focused on developmental deficiencies of the immune response of neonatal avian species during the first 4-to-7 days post-hatch and the possibility of augmenting the immune response during the first week post-hatch and at other times of increased susceptibility to disease. Heterophils, the avian counterpart of the mammalian neutrophil, from 1-to-7 day-old chickens and turkeys have been shown to be functionally deficient when compared to the heterophils of immunologically mature birds, exhibiting deficiencies in the phagocytosis and intracellular killing of bacteria (Wells et al., 1998; Lowry et al., 1997). T cell functions in chickens have also been characterized as functionally deficient during the first days post-hatch (Kline and Sanders, 1980; Lehtonin et al., 1989; Lowenthal et al., 1994). Accompanying these deficiencies in immune functions is an increased susceptibility to bacterial infections (Ziprin et al., 1989).

We have demonstrated that the administration of immune lymphokines (ILK) derived from the splenic T cells of *Salmonella enteritidis* (SE)-immune chickens protects both chickens and turkeys from SE organ invasion at one day-of-age (McGruder et al., 1993; Ziprin et al., 1996; Genovese et al., 1998). Further, heterophils isolated from the peripheral blood of day-old chickens and turkeys treated with ILK exhibit increased functional capabilities, showing increased phagocytic and bactericidal activities (Lowry et al., 1997; Kogut et al., 1995; Wells et al., 1998; Genovese et al., 1998).

Considering the use of immune lymphokine in neonatal poultry for augmentation of the immune response and subsequent disease resistance, we have postulated that an immune lymphokine (PILK) derived from the T cells of SE-immune swine would protect weaned pigs from *Salmonella choleraesuis* (SC) organ invasion. The purpose of the present study was to observe the effects of PILK on SC organ invasion, cecal colonization by SC, and weight gain in weaned piglets.

2. MATERIALS AND METHODS

2.1. Experimental Animals

Fourteen-to-17 day-old piglets (Landrace X Yorkshire X Hampshire/Duroc) (average weight 13.5 pounds) were acquired from a commercial swine operation. Piglets were checked for general good health, ear-tagged, and randomly placed into pens in an isolation facility on the grounds of the USDA ARS FAPRL in College Station, TX. Rectal swabs were obtained from all piglets upon arrival and were cultured for the presence of any *Salmonella* species (Andrews et al., 1978). Pens were equiped with nipple watering systems and feed was provided *ad libitum* using self-feeders. Additional warmth was provided by heating pads on the floor of each pen. For the first 7 days post-weaning, piglets were fed a Phase I diet (formulation provided by Dr. Knabe, Department of Animal Science, Texas A&M University) and for the last 7 days of the study were fed a Phase II diet (Dr. Knabe).

2.2. Bacteria

A porcine isolate of *Salmonella choleraesuis* (SC) var. Kunzendorf χ3246 was selected for novobiocin-nalidixic acid (NONA) resistance in our laboratory and maintained in tryptic soy broth (TSB). Inocula for challenge with SC was prepared using sterile phosphate-buffered saline (PBS) and adjusted to a stock concentration of 10^9 colony forming units (CFUs) per milliliter using a spectrophotometer with a 625 nm reference wavelength. The viable cell concentration of the inocula was determined by colony counts on brilliant green agar (BGA) with NONA (Difco Laboratories, Detroit, MI). The 10^9 stock of SC was serially diluted to 1×10^7 CFU/ml using PBS.

2.3. Porcine Salmonella Enteritidis-Immune Lymphokine Preparation

Two gilts (Landrace × Yorkshire) weighing approximately 180 pounds each, and determined to be *Salmonella* species-free were used for immune lymphokine (PILK) production. Pigs were fed a nonmedicated finisher diet *ad libitum*. Pigs were challenged three times weekly for four weeks with 10 ml of 10^9 CFU *Salmonella enteritidis* (SE). Five ml of SE were given by oral gavage and 5 ml were given intranasally. During the fifth week pigs were not challenged with SE, and at the end of the fifth week pigs were euthanized and spleens were obtained aseptically. Splenic T cells were isolated as previously described (Tellez et al., 1993). T cells were placed in 175 cm^2 T flasks at a concentration of 5×10^6 cells/ml in serum-free RPMI 1640 (Sigma) with 7.5 µl of concanavalin A (Con A) and incubated for 48 hours at 37 C in a 5% CO_2 incubator. After incubation, supernatants were collected and centrifuged at $2000 \times g$ for 15 minutes to remove all cells. Supernatants were treated with α-mannopyrannoside to inactivate any residual Con A and concentrated five-fold using YM-100 and YM-10 membranes (Amicon Corp.). The retentate was then sterile filtered using 0.22 µm filters (Corning) and stored at −20 C.

2.4. Experimental Design

Pigs were randomly assigned to one of five groups: Group (1) = noninfected controls (n = 7), Group (2) = noninfected PILK 3X (n = 7), Group (3) = SC infected controls (n = 10), Group (4) = SC infected PILK 1X (n = 10), Group (5) = SC infected PILK 3X (n = 10), Pigs were acclimated to their surroundings for three days prior to the study. During the acclimation period, rectal swabs were taken from individual pigs to determine the presence of any *Salmonella* species and all piglets were determined to be free of any *Salmonella* species. On day 0, pigs were weighed and administered respective treatments. Pigs in groups 2, 4, and 5 were administered 5 ml of PILK by oral gavage. Pigs in groups 1 and 3 were administered 5 ml of RPMI 1640 via oral gavage. One hour post-administration, pigs in groups 3, 4, and 5 were challenged with 1×10^7 CFU SC by oral gavage. Daily rectal swabs from individual pigs in groups 3, 4, and 5 were obtained and weights for all groups were recorded on days 7 and 14. Pigs in Groups 2 and 5 were administered PILK twice more, on days 5 and 10 for a total of 3 PILK treatments (3X). Pigs in groups 1, 3, and 4 received RPMI 1640 on these days. On day 14, pigs in groups 3, 4, and 5 were euthanized, weighed, and tissue samples were aseptically collected. Tissue samples from the tonsil, liver, lung, spleen, ileocolic lymph nodes, ileocolic junction, and cecal contents were cultured for the presence of SC using previously described methods (Gray et al., 1995). Briefly, samples were inoculated into GN Hajna broth (Difco Laboratories, Detroit, MI) for 24 hr at 37 C; 100 µl of GN Hajna broth was then placed into Rappaport-Vassiliadas (RV) (Difco Laboratories) broth for 24 hr at 37 C. RV broth was then streaked onto BGA NONA plates using sterile inoculation loops and incubated at 37 C for 24 hr. Plates were scored positive or negative for the presence of SC. Random colonies from BGA NONA plates were tested using SC antisera. Three repetitions of this experiment were performed.

2.5. Statistics

Statistical analysis was performed using Sigma Stat software (Jandel Scientific, San Rafael, CA). Differences between groups were analysed using the paired t test. All analysis were performed using pooled data from three replicates of this experiment.

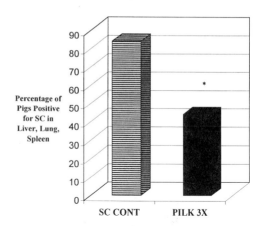

Figure 1. SC Organ Invasion: Pigs were challenged with 1×10^7 cfu SC orally on Day 0. Organ invasion (liver, lung, spleen) data for SC infected control and SC infected PILK 3X groups shown. Significant differences indicated with an asterisk (P < 0.001).

3. RESULTS

3.1. Organ Invasion by SC

In Fig. 1, results are presented as the mean percentage of three replicate experiments to determine the effects of PILK on SC organ invasion in weaned pigs. The PILK 3X group had a highly significant (P < 0.001) reduction in the number of pigs in which SC was recovered from the liver, lung, and spleen. The PILK 1X infected group had a biological reduction in organ invasion, but not a statistical reduction. Culture of lymphoid tissue, including tonsil, ileocolic junction, and ileocolic lymph nodes for the presence of SC did not reveal any differences between any of the infected groups; all SC infected groups had high levels (80–90%) of positive lymph tissue (data not shown).

3.2. Weight Gain

Pigs in the SC infected PILK 3X group gained weight comparable to pigs in the noninfected control group (Fig. 2). Pigs in the PILK 3X noninfected group gained a significant amount more than even the noninfected control group (P < 0.01) and the SC infected control group (P < 0.001). No statistical differences were noted between the PILK 1X infected group and infected control pigs.

3.3. SC Recovered From Cecal Contents

There was a highly significant reduction in the number of pigs positive for SC in cecal contents in the PILK 3X group (P < 0.001; Fig. 3). Only 13% of pigs in the PILK 3X infected group had SC recovered from the cecal contents while the SC infected control group had over 55% of pigs positive for SC in the cecal contents. The PILK 1X group was not statistically different from the SC infected control pigs in the isolation of SC from cecal contents.

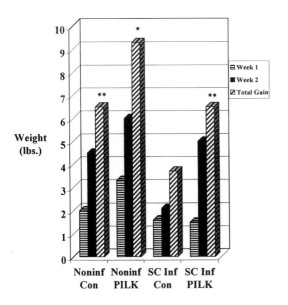

Figure 2. Average Weight Gain: Pigs were weighed on Day 0, Day 7 (Week 1), and Day 14 (Week 2). Total gain represents the sum of week 1 and week 2 gains for each group. Data for each group for each time point represent the mean of 3 experiments. A single asterisk represents a significant difference from all groups and a double asterisk indicates a significant difference from SC infected controls only (P < 0.001).

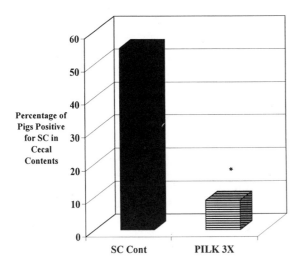

Figure 3. SC in Cecal Contents: Pigs were challenged with 1×10^7 cfu SC on Day 0 orally. Data for SC infected controls and SC infected PILK 3X groups shown (±SEM). Significant differences indicated with an asterisk (P < 0.05).

4. DISCUSSION

The purpose of these experiments was to determine if lymphokines (PILK) obtained from the T cells of SE-immune pigs would protect weaned piglets from SC organ invasion and cecal colonization and whether this protection would translate into higher weight gains even in the presence of an infection with SC. Results presented here indicate that PILK given multiple times reduces SC organ invasion significantly (P < 0.001), significantly decreases SC cecal colonization (P < 0.001), and improved weight gain by pigs in the presence of an SC infection.

Previous reports from our laboratory have demonstrated the effectiveness of lymphokines derived from the T cells of SE-immune hens in protecting day-old chickens and turkeys from SE organ invasion (McGruder et al., 1993; Ziprin et al., 1996; Genovese et al., 1998). Additional work has shown that these lymphokines (ILK) are also able to protect day-old chickens from mortality, organ invasion, and cecal colonization by *Salmonella gallinarum* (SG) (Kogut et al., 1996). *Escherichia coli* (EC) air-sacculitis and mortality have also been shown to be reduced by the prophylactic treatment of chickens with ILK (McGruder et al., 1998). Kogut and colleages have observed that the protection attained with ILK in day-old chickens and turkeys against gram negative bacteria is mediated by the avian heterophil, the avian counterpart of the mammalian neutrophil (Kogut et al., 1994). This cross-species protection against different gram negative bacteria in chickens by ILK led us to believe that lymphokines from the T cells of pigs challenged with SE would protect pigs against an SC infection. If, indeed, the response to the administration of PILK to pigs is similar to that of ILK in chickens, the effector cell activated would be the porcine neutrophil and, thus, would help to explain why the protection conferred by PILK, lymphokine derived from SE-immunized pigs, against SC is non-species specific. Studies are currently underway in our laboratory to identify the specific effector(s) of the protection observed in weaned pigs with PILK.

Susceptibility to infectious diseases at weaning may be attributed to several factors, including loss of maternally derived antibodies, developmental deficiencies in the immune response, and elevated glucocorticoid levels in animals during weaning. Production pressures on the swine industry force producers to look for ways to increase production. One possible means to attain increased production would be to wean piglets from sows earlier (Lecce et al., 1979). However, weaning pigs and other species at an early age has been shown to have deleterious effects on the health and survivability of these animals, most likely due to a deficient immune response and subsequent inability to fight off infections (Blecha, 1983; Wilcock and Schwartz, 1992; El-Awar et al., 1991; Carter and Martens, 1986; Drieson et al., 1993; Selim et al., 1995; Shi et al., 1994; Hoskinson et al., 1990). If loss of maternal antibodies and developmental deficiencies in the immune response of young pigs are at least partially responsible for the increased susceptibility to bacterial disease observed at weaning, early weaning of pigs leaves these animals at an even greater defensive disadvantage, immunologically speaking, than pigs weaned at older ages.

The present work has shown that prophylactic administration of PILK to weaned pigs may provide a way to eleviate the susceptibility to infectious agents, such as SC, that is associated with early weaning of pigs. This preliminary work has led to many questions which our laboratory is currently attempting to answer. Further studies to identify the cell(s) responsible for the protection from SC organ invasion and SC cecal colonization in weaned pigs are currently underway. Early evidence has suggested that the cell responsible is the neutrophil and work in poultry also suggests that the neutrophil would be the prime target for PILK action. Once the effector cell(s) is identified, the mechanism of action of PILK on these cells, whether a direct or indirect action, will be investigated. Experiments designed to understand the weight gains observed in PILK-treated pigs will also be conducted. Studies on the colonization or harboring of SC in lymph tissue will be conducted to ascertain if PILK has any effect on long-term carrier status of SC in infected pigs and whether PILK may shorten the carrier state in infected animals.

Salmonella species in swine production are a major concern to producers and consumers of pork products. We have demonstrated that a product derived from the T cells of SE-immune swine, when administered prophylactically to weaned piglets, protects these pigs from *Salmonella choleraesuis* infection, causing reductions in SC organ invasion and SC in the cecum, and improves weight gain in the presence or absence of a SC infection.

REFERENCES

Abughali N., Berger M., and Tosi M.F., 1994, Deficient total cell content of CR3 (CD11b) in neonatal neutrophils. Blood. 83:1086–1092.

Andrews W.H., Poelma P.L., Wilson C.R., et al., 1978, Isolation and identification of Salmonella. In: Bacteriological Analytical Manual. 5th ed. Association of Official Analytical Chemists, Washington, D.C.

Aurich J.E., Dobrinski I., Happen H.O., et al., 1990, ω-endorphin and met-enkephalin in plasma of cattle during pregnancy, parturition, and the neonatal period. J Reprod Fert. 89:605–612.

Bianchi A.T.J., Zwart R.J., Jeurissen S.H.M., et al., 1992, Development of the B- and T-cell compartments in porcine lymphoid organs from birth to adult life: an immunohistological approach. Vet Immun Immunopath. 33:201–222.

Blecha F., Pollman S., and Nichols, D.A., 1985, Immunologic reactions of pigs regrouped at or near weaning. Am J Vet Res. 46:1934–1937.

Blecha F., Pollmann D.S., and Nichols D.A., 1983, Weaning pigs at an early age decreases cellular immunity. J Anim Sci. 56:396–400.

Carter G.K. and Martens R.J., 1986, Septicemia in the neonatal foal. Comp Cont Educ Pract Vet. 8:S256–S270.

Coignal F.L., Bertram T.A., Roth J.A., et al., 1984, Functional and ultrastructural evaluations of neutrophils from foals and lactating and nonlactating mares. Am J Vet Res. 45:898–901.

Drieson S.J., Carland P.J., and Fahy V.A., 1993, Studies on preweaning diarrhea. Aust Vet J. 70:259–262.

El-Awar F.Y. and Hahn E.C., 1991, Sources of antibody-dependent cellular cytotoxicity deficiency in young pig leukocytes. J Leuk Biol. 49:227–235.

Genovese K.J., Moyes R.B., Wells L.L., et al., 1998, Resistance to Salmonella enteritidis organ invasion in day-old turkeys and chickens by transformed t cell line produced lymphokines. Avian Dis. (in press).

Genovese K.J., Lowry V.K., Stanker L.H., et al., 1998, Administration of Salmonella enteritidis-immune lymphokines to day-old turkeys by subcutaneous, oral, and nasal routes: a comparison of effects on Salmonella enteritidis liver invasion, peripheral blood heterophilia, and heterophil activation. Avian Path. (in press).

Gray J.T., Fedorka-Cray P.J., Stabel T.J., et al., 1995, Influence of inoculation route on the carrier state of Salmonella choleraesuis in swine. Vet Microbiol. 47:43–59.

Hauser M.A., Koob M.D., and Roth J.A., 1986, Variation of neutrophil function with age in calves. Am J Vet Res. 47:152–153.

Higuchi H., Nagahata H., Hiroki M., and Noda H., 1997, Relationship between age-dependent changes of bovine neutrophil functions and their intracellular Ca^{2+} concentrations. J Vet Med Sci. 59: 271–276.

Hill H.R., 1987, Biochemical, structural and functional abnormalities of polymorphonuclear leukocytes in the neonate. Pediatric Research. 22:375–382.

Hoskinson C.D., Chew B.P., Wong T.S., 1990, Age-related changes in mitogen-induced lymphocyte proliferation and polymorphonuclear neutrophil function in the piglet. J Anim Sci. 68:2471–2478.

Kline K. and Sanders B.G., 1980, Developmental profile of chicken splenic lymphocyte responsiveness to con A and PHA and studies on chicken splenic and bone marrow cells capable of inhibiting mitogen stimulated blastogenic responses of adult splenic lymphocytes. J Immunology. 125:1992–1997.

Kogut M.H., Tellez G.I., McGruder E.D., et al., 1996, Evaluation of Salmonella-enteritidis-immune lymphokines on host resistance to Salmonella enterica ser. gallinarum infection in broiler chicks. Avian Path. 25:737–749.

Kogut M.H., McGruder E.D., Hargis B.M., et al., 1994, Dynamics of the avian inflammatory response to Salmonella enteritidis immune lymphokines: changes in avian blood leukocytes populations. Inflammation. 18:373–388.

Kogut M.H., McGruder E.D., Hargis B.M., et al., 1995, In vivo activation of heterophil function in chickens following injection with Salmonella enteritidis-immune lymphokines. J Leuk Biol. 57:56–62.

Lecce J.G., Armstrong W.D., Crawford P.C., et al., 1979, Nutrition and management of early weaned piglets. I. liquid vs. dry feeding. J Anim Sci. 48:1007.

Lee C.-C. and Roth J.A., 1992, Differences in neutrophil function in young and mature cattle and their response to IFN γ. Comp Haem Intern. 2:140–147.

Lee E.-K. and Kehrli M.E., 1998, Expression of adhesion molecules on neutrophils of periparturient cows and neonatal calves. Am J Vet Res. 59:37–43.

Lehtonin L., Vanio O., and Toivanen P., 1989, Ontogeny of alloreactivity in the chicken as measured by mixed lymphocyte reaction. Dev Comp Immun. 13:187–195.

Lowenthal J.W., Connick T.E., McWaters P.G., et al., 1994, Development of t cell immune responsiveness in the chicken. Immun Cell Biol. 72:115–122.

Lowry V.K., Genovese K.J., Bowden L.L., et al., 1997, Ontogeny of the phagocytic and bactericidal activities of turkey heterophils and their potentiation by Salmonella enteritidis-immune lymphokines. FEMS Immun Micro. 19:95–100.

McCauley I. and Hartmann P.E., 1984, Changes in piglet leucocytes, B lymphocytes, and plasma cortisol from birth to three weeks after weaning. Res Vet Sci. 37:234–241.

McGruder E.D., Ray P.M., Tellez G.I., et al., 1993, Salmonella enteritidis immune leukocyte-stimulated soluble factors: effects on increased resistance to Salmonella organ invasion in day-old leghorn chicks. Poult Sci. 72:2264–2271.

McGruder E.D., Kogut M.H., Genovese K.J., et al., 1998, Salmonella enteritidis-immune lymphokine prevents colibacillosis in an induced Escherichia coli infection model in broiler chicks. Res Vet Sci. (submitted).

Miller M.E., 1979, Phagocyte function in the neonate: selected aspects. Pediatrics. (suppl.) 709–712.

Rosenthal J. and Cairo M.S., 1995, Use of cytokines in combination with antibiotics in neonatal sepsis: a review of the role of adjunctive therapy in the management of neonatal sepsis. Intern J Ped Hem/Onc. 2:477–487.

Selim S.A., Cullor J.S., Smith B.P., et al., 1995, The effect of Eschericia coli J5 and modified live Salmonella dublin vaccines in artificially reared neonatal calves, Vaccine. 13:381–390.

Shi J., Goodband R.D., Chengappa M.M., et al., 1994, Influence of interleuken-1 on neutrophil function and resistance to Streptococcus suis in neonatal pigs, J Leuk Biol. 56:88–94.

Tellez G.I., Kogut M.H., and Hargis B.M., 1993, Immunoprophylaxis of Salmonella enteritidis infection by lymphokines in leghorn chicks. Avian Dis. 37:1062–1070.

Wells L.L., Lowry V.K., DeLoach J.R., et al., 1998, Age-dependent phagocytosis and bactericidal activities of the chicken heterophil. Dev Comp Immun. 22:103–109.

Wells L.L., Lowry V.K., Genovese K.J., et al., 1998, Enhancement of phagocytosis and bacterial killing by heterophils from neonatal chicks after administration of Salmonella enteritidis-immune lymphokines. Vet Microbiol. (in press).

Wilcock B.P. and Schwartz K.J., 1992, Salmonellosis. In: Leman A.D., Straw B.E., Mengeling W.L., D'Allaire S., and Taylor D.J., eds. Diseases of Swine. 7th ed. Ames, IA: Iowa State University Press, 570–583.

Ziprin R.L., Corrier D.E., and Ellissalde M.H., 1989, Maturation of resistance to salmonellosis in newly hatched chicks: inhibition by cyclosporin. Poult. Sci. 68:1637–1642.

Ziprin R.L., Kogut M.H., McGruder E.D., et al., 1996, Efficacy of Salmonella enteritidis (SE)-immune lymphokines from chickens and turkeys on SE liver invasion in one-day-old chicks and turkey poults. Avian Dis. 40:186–192.

Zwahlen R.D., Wyder-Walther M., and Roth D.R., 1992, Fc receptor expression, concanavalin A capping, and enzyme content of bovine neonatal neutrophils: a comparative study wth adult cattle. J Leuk Biol. 51:264–269.

33

SIALIC ACID DEPENDENCE AND INDEPENDENCE OF GROUP A ROTAVIRUSES

Theresa B. Kuhlenschmidt, William P. Hanafin, Howard B. Gelberg, and Mark S. Kuhlenschmidt

Department of Pathobiology
College of Veterinary Medicine
University of Illinois
Urbana, Illinois 61802

1. SUMMARY

We have found (1), in contrast to previous reports, the human rotavirus Wa strain is sialic acid-dependent for binding to and infectivity of MA-104 cells and (2), a dual carbohydrate binding specificity is associated with both human Wa and Porcine OSU rotaviruses. One carbohydrate binding activity is associated with triple-layered virus particles (TLP) and the other with double-layered virus particles (DLP). In binding and infectivity studies, we found that gangliosides were the most potent inhibitors of both the human and porcine rotavirus TLP. Furthermore, glycosylation mutant cells deficient in sialylation or neuraminidase-treated MA104 cells, did not bind rotavirus TLP from either strain. Our results show that human Wa binding and infectivity cannot be distinguished from the porcine OSU strain and appears to be sialic acid-dependent. Direct binding of human or porcine TLP to a variety of intact gangliosides was demonstrated in an thin-layer chromatographic (TLC) overlay assay. Human or porcine rotavirus DLP did not bind to any of the intact gangliosides but surprisingly bound asialogangliosides. This binding was abolished by prior treatment of the glycolipids with ceramide glycanase suggesting the intact asialoglycolipid was required for DLP binding. After treatment of either human or porcine TLP with EDTA to remove the outer shell, virus particles bound only to the immobilized asialogangliosides. These results suggest that rotavirus sugar binding specificity can be interpreted either as sialic acid-dependent or independent based on whether the virus preparation consists primarily of triple-layered or double-layered particles. Of perhaps greater interest is the

Mechanisms in the Pathogenesis of Enteric Diseases 2, edited by Paul and Francis.
Kluwer Academic / Plenum Publishers, New York, 1999.

possibility that sialic acid-independent carbohydrate binding activity plays a role in virus maturation or assembly.

2. INTRODUCTION

Rotaviruses are a major cause of viral diarrhea in the young of most mammalian species. Their significance in terms of individual mortality is well documented (for review see, Kapikian and Chanock, 1990). They are a major cause of morbidity in infants and young children in developed countries and of morbidity and mortality in developing countries. Rotavirus infections are also of prime agricultural importance since they frequently cause serious neonatal diarrheal diseases of many animal species, most notably neonatal and post-weaning pigs and calves. Morbidity due to rotavirus infections in these species often reaches 80% while mortality can be as high as 60% (Bohl, 1979). In order to establish a firm scientific basis for the ultimate prevention and control of rotavirus disease, a greater understanding of the molecular mechanisms of rotavirus host cell interaction is required.

Rotaviruses are composed of three layers of structural proteins surrounding a dsRNA core. The complete rotavirus particle is defined as a triple layer particle (TLP). Depletion of calcium from TLP results in removal of the outermost layer and exposing the double layer particle (DLP) which does not normally enter host cells and is thus not infective.

The earliest and requisite step for productive viral infection is recognition and binding of TLP to villous tip enterocytes. The tissue and cell tropism displayed by rotaviruses is consistent with the hypothesis that a specific host cell-surface receptor(s) mediates recognition. Our recent work characterized the structure and function of a porcine intestinal GM_3 ganglioside receptor for porcine rotavirus. As an extension of these studies, the binding requirements of the human rotavirus are examined in this present review. We found, contrary to previous reports (Fukudome, 1989; Willoughby, 1990) of sialic acid independency for binding and infectivity, the human Wa strain rotavirus TLP is dependent on sialic acid for these activities. In addition, we discovered a sialic acid independent carbohydrate binding specificity for the DLP prepared from either porcine or human rotavirus.

3. MATERIALS AND METHODS

3.1. Cells and Virus

Group A (OSU) porcine rotavirus was propagated in MA-104 cells using modifications of standard techniques (Rolsma, 1994). Human Wa strain rotavirus was obtained from American Type Culture Collection (ATTC) and was propagated in Caco-2 cells using standard techniques. Following extraction from cellular material, the virus was purified by isopycnic centrifugation on a cesium chloride gradient. Double and triple layered virus particles were separately collected and radioiodinated as previously described (Rolsma, 1994).

CHO-KI and glycosylation-deficient mutant cells, Lec-1, Lec-2, and Pro-5, originally described by Stanley (Stanley, Caillibot, and Siminovitch, 1975; Stanley, Narasimhan et al., 1975; Stanley and Siminovitch, 1977), were obtained from ATTC.

3.2. Binding Assay

Binding of radiolabeled rotavirus particles to host cells in suspension was measured as previously described (Rolsma, 1994). Briefly, cells were washed three times with modified Eagle's medium (MEM) by centrifugation at $200 \times g$ and adjusted to a concentration of 2×10^6 cells/ml. One ml of cells in MEM were mixed with 15 μl (75 ng) of $[^{125}I]$-TLP or $[^{125}I]$-DLP and rotated end-over-end at 5 RPM at 4°C. Aliquots were removed at appropriate time intervals and immediately overlaid onto 0.2 ml of a silicone/mineral oil mixture in a 0.4 ml microcentrifuge tubes and centrifuged at $15,600 \times g$ for 30 seconds in a microcentrifuge. Radioactivity in the pellets was enumerated in a gamma counter and virus binding was defined as the pellet cpm divided by the input cpm $\times 100$.

3.3. Competitive Binding Assay

A variety of biomolecules typically found enriched on eukaryotic cell surfaces, particularly glycoconjugates, were evaluated for the ability to block rotavirus binding to host cells. Radiolabeled virus was preincubated with putative competitor molecules for 30 minutes prior to the addition of cells and virus binding measured following 30 min incubation as described above.

3.4. TLC Overlay Assay

Direct binding of $[^{125}I]$ TLP or DLP to individual gangliosides was measured using modifications of a TLC blot overlay assay as previously described (Rolsma, 1998). Briefly, gangliosides were chromatographed on plastic-backed TLC plates, the plate thoroughly dried by air evaporation and then overlaid with 1×10^6 to 1×10^7 cpm of $[^{125}I]$ TLP or DLP in 14 ml of TNC buffer (Rolsma, 1994), and allowed to incubate for 2.5 hour at 4°C. The plates were washed 7 times with TNC buffer and dried. Virus binding was visualized by autoradiography.

3.5. Focus Forming Infectivity Assay

Focus forming infectivity assays were conducted using neuraminidase or sham-treated cells as previously described (Rolsma, 1998). Purified TLP were trypsinized and diluted in MEM to achieve a final concentration of 300–1000 ffu/75 μl. Virus infectivity was quantified using an peroxidase immunohistochemical assay.

3.6. Chemical and Enzymatic Treatments

3.6.1. EDTA Treatment of Rotavirus TLP Was Performed as Previously Described (Rolsma, 1994)

3.6.2. Ceramide Glycanase Digestion of Asialogangliosides Was Performed as Follows. Asialogangliosides (10 μg) were dissolved in 50 μl of buffer (0.5 mg/ml sodium taurodeoxy-cholate, 2 mg/ml sodium cholate, 50 μmoles/ml sodium acetate, pH 5) and incubated at 37°C for 72 hr with 0.5 U of ceramide glycanase (V-labs). Following incubation the mixture was evaporated to dryness, redissolved in choroform : methanol (2 : 1 v/v), and applied to thin-layer plates for chromatographic analyses and overlay assays.

4. RESULTS

4.1. Cell Binding Assays

As we previously reported (Rolsma, 1994) for the porcine OSU rotavirus, infectious TLP from the human Wa strain rapidly bound to MA-104 cells in suspension while non-infectious DLP did not. Approximately 50% of input TLP bound to MA-104 cells within 30 minutes contrasting to less than 5% of input DLP. Figure 1 shows that in addition to MA-104 cells, other cells such as CHO-K1 also bind comparable amounts of TLP isolated from either porcine OSU or human Wa rotavirus strains. The Lec-1 mutant cells, deficient only in sialylation of N-linked glycoproteins bound nearly the same amount of porcine or human TLP as the Pro-5 parental and MA104 control cells. Interestingly, Lec-2 cells, CHO mutant cells deficient in sialylation of all glycoconjugates, do not support porcine OSU or human Wa TLP binding. However, the parent CHO cell line, Pro-5, which displays a normal complement of sialoglycoconjugates, exhibits good binding by both virus strains.

In other cell binding experiments (data not shown), MA-104 cells pretreated with neuraminidase to remove surface sialic acid, bound only 16% of input porcine TLP compared to control treated cells (Rolsma, 1994). Likewise, human TLP did not bind well to neuraminidase treated cells; only 6.0% of TLP from the human strain bound to the neuraminidase-treated cells compared to untreated cells. Taken together, these data suggest that sialic acid expressed on the cell surface is required for TLP binding by both human and porcine rotavirus strains.

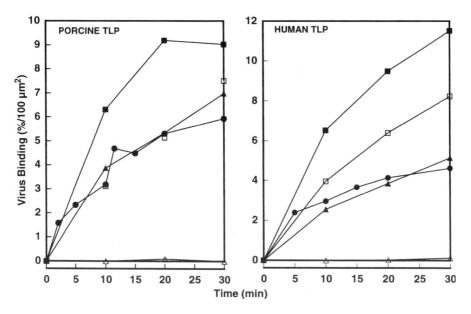

Figure 1. Comparison of binding of porcine and human ^{125}I TLP to normal and glycosylation-defective cells. CHO-K1 cells, two lectin-resistant mutants (Lec-1 and Lec-2), and their parental Pro-5 cells and MA104 cells were harvested from tissue culture, suspended to a density of 2×10^6/ml, and tested for their ability to bind ^{125}I TLP as described in Materials and Methods. The percentage bound at each time point divided by the surface area of the respective cell type is plotted versus time of incubation. □, Pro-5; ■, CHO-K1; ●, MA104; ▲, Lec-1; △, Lec-2.

4.2. Competitive Binding Assay

Using a blocking assay to measure the effect of various glycoconjugates on human rotavirus binding to MA-104 cells, it was found that purified porcine intestinal gangliosides $NeuAcGM_3$ and $NeuGcGM_3$ inhibited the binding of human TLP by 50% at concentrations of 5 and 1.5 µM respectively (Table 1). These I_{50} values are of the same magnitude found for the porcine rotavirus. This finding prompted us to survey a range of natural and synthetic glycoconjugates as potential receptors for human rotavirus. Using the competitive binding assay as described in Materials and Methods, the

Table 1. Relative Inhibitory Capacity of Various Glycoconjugates on Porcine and Human Rotavirus Binding to MA104 Cells. ^{125}I human or porcine TLP were preincubated with the indicated glycoconjugates and virus binding was measured using the competitive binding assay as described in Materials and Methods. Unless where otherwise noted, binding data are listed as µM sialic acid concentrations required to inhibit virus binding by 50% as compared to control incubations in the absence of added inhibitor

Compound	Porcine	Human
GANGLIOSIDES	µM (I_{50})	µM (I_{50})
GD1A	>11	<0.74
GM2 (bovine)	0.7	1.4
$NeuGcGM_3$	0.6	1.5
GT1B	>14	3.4
$NeuAcGM_3$	1.5	5
GM1 (bovine)	6.5	30
ASIALOGANGLIOSIDES		
GA1	>67	67[b]
GA2	>36	>36[b]
Lactosylceramide	ND	>24[b]
SACCHARIDES		
Colominic acid	>>6.6	>1800
N-acetylneuraminic acid	ND	>2000
3'sialyllactose	2700	4000
Lactose	ND	>20,000
Colominic acid sulfate	ND	>10 mg/ml
GLYCOPROTEINS		
Bovine submaxillary mucin	>2.2	12
Transferrin	ND	>56
Glc40-BSA	NI	>70[a]
Fetuin	ND	>205
Gal40-BSA	NI	>231[a]
Alpha-1-acid glycoprotein	ND	337
GlcNAc44-BSA	NI	>408[a]
GLYCOSAMINOGLYCAN		
Heparin	NI	>2 mg/ml
Chondroitin sulfate	NI	>2 mg/ml

[a]Expressed as µM monosaccharide concentration.
[b]Expressed as µM sphingosine concentration.

relative binding potency (I_{50}) was examined and the results are compared to those obtained for the porcine rotavirus. Gangliosides were the most potent inhibitors of human rotavirus binding, effective in the µM range. Removal of sialic acid from the ganglioside results in a much less effective inhibitor. AsialoGM$_1$ and asialoGM$_2$ (GA$_1$ and GA$_2$ respectively), were not inhibitory at 10 times the concentration of the intact gangliosides. Free sialyllactose was inhibitory but only at 1000 times the level of NeuAcGM$_3$, indicating the intact ganglioside is a far more effective competitor for virus binding than the released oligosaccharide. As has been reported by others (Yolken, 1987), mucins, glycoconjugates rich in sialic acid, are effective inhibitors of human rotavirus binding. Serum glycoproteins with terminal sialic acid were much less inhibitory. For example, α-1-acid glycoprotein inhibited human rotavirus binding at about 200 times that of the NeuGcGM$_3$. Sialic acid polymers, colominic acid and colominic acid sulfate, and glycosaminoglycans were ineffective, suggesting that the virus is not indiscriminately attracted to negatively charged molecules. Neoglycoproteins containing galactose, glucose or N-acetylglucos-amine were also ineffective in blocking rotavirus binding to MA-104 cells.

4.3. Infectivity Studies

Neuraminidase treatment of MA-104 cells rendered these cells less vulnerable to infection by TLP from either the human or porcine rotaviruses. As measured immunologically in a focus forming assay (data not shown), the neuraminidase treated cells had 9% of the focus forming units from the human TLP compared to control treated cells. Similarly, porcine TLP showed 5% the number of focus forming units compared to control, sham-treated cells. These data show that surface sialic acid is critical for infectivity for either the human Wa or porcine OSU TLP.

4.4. TLC Overlay Assay

We recently reported that TLP but not DLP from porcine rotavirus bound to purified porcine intestinal NeuAcGM$_3$ and NeuGcGM$_3$ immobilized on TLC plates (Rolsma, 1998). This result confirms that gangliosides block binding of TLP by direct interaction with the virus and that DLP, which are not infectious, do not recognize host cell-surface receptors or immobilized gangliosides. The data presented in Fig. 2 shows that TLP from either porcine OSU or human Wa bind preferentially to intact, fully sialylated gangliosides and to a much lesser extent to GA$_1$ and GA$_2$. Treatment with EDTA removes the outer shell of the TLP and leaves only the double layer particle remaining. Surprisingly, EDTA-treated TLP bound only to the asialoglycolipids, GA$_1$ and GA$_2$. When purified DLP from either porcine or human strains were tested directly using the TLC overlay assay it was confirmed that they bound specifically to the asialogangliosides rather than gangliosides or other sialoglycoconjugates. This DLP binding activity appears to require the intact glycolipid molecule since ceramide glycanase treatment, which hydrolyses the oligosaccharide from the ceramide portion, abolished binding. Glycosylceramides, lactosylceramide, glucosyl-ceramide, galactosylceramide, and globosides did not support DLP binding. These data demonstrate a dual carbohydrate binding specificity for human and porcine rotavirus particles: TLP bind sialoglycoconjugates and DLP at this point appear to specifically bind GA$_1$ and GA$_2$.

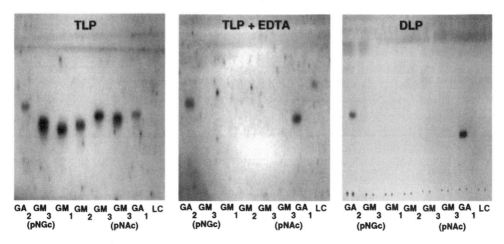

Figure 2. Direct binding of ^{125}I rotavirus preparations to glycolipids immobilized on TLC plates. One nmole each of bovine brain gangliosides, GM_1, GM_2, and GM_3, purified porcine intestinal $NeuAcGM_3$ (pNAc) and $NeuGcGM_3$ (pNGc), lactosylceramide (LC) and GA_1 and GA_2 were applied to each of three TLC plates. The plates were chromatographed, overlaid with TLP (left panel), EDTA-treated TLP (middle panel), and DLP (right panel). Virus binding was detected by autoradiography.

5. DISCUSSION

It has been generally assumed the presence of host cell-surface sialic acids are not required for human rotavirus binding and infectivity. In earlier studies, Fukudome et al. (Fukudome, 1989) reported that adsorption and infection of human rotavirus to MA104 cells is not sensitive to neuraminidase or periodate pretreatment of the cells while other rotaviruses, SA11 or NCDV, showed sensitivity to these treatments. Willoughby et al. (Willoughby, 1990) reported that SA 11 and Wa rotaviruses bound immobilized GA_1 (asialoGM$_1$) but not intact gangliosides. Paradoxically, however, Yolken et al. (Yolken, 1987) showed that sialoglycoproteins and bovine submaxillary mucin inhibited *in vitro* replication of the Wa strain of human rotavirus. The purpose for this study was to further examine the sugar binding specificity of the cellular receptor(s) for the human rotavirus (Wa strain) using our previously established virus cell binding and TLC overlay assays that have proved useful in studying porcine rotavirus host cell recognition (Rolsma, 1998). With a clear understanding of the critical binding epitope required for human rotavirus host cell recognition, it is more likely that an appropriate receptor mimetic can be found that will be therapeutically effective at inhibiting infection and ameliorating rotavirus-mediated infant death especially in developing nations.

Using a blocking assay in which potential candidates for receptors compete with cells for virus binding, we found the same types of sialoglycoconjugates that blocked porcine TLP binding also inhibited human TLP binding. As was the case for porcine rotavirus, the most potent inhibitors of human Wa rotavirus binding to MA104 cells were gangliosides and bovine submaxillary mucin.

Asialoglycoconjugates did not inhibit the binding of human or porcine TLP to MA104 cells. Thus, as tested in our system, inhibition of porcine or human rotavirus TLP binding to host cells required sialic acid epitopes on glycoconjugates and suggested that cell-surface sialic acid was required for host cell recognition.

To further address the question of whether surface sialic acid is required for human Wa rotavirus binding to host cells, we examined a variety of control and glycosylation-defective cell lines for their ability to support porcine OSU and human Wa rotavirus binding. Lec-2 mutant cells, deficient in sialylation of glycolipids, and N-linked glycoproteins, do not bind either porcine or human rotavirus TLP. The Lec-1 mutant cells, deficient only in sialylation of N-linked glycoproteins bound nearly the same amount of porcine or human TLP as the Pro-5 parental and MA104 control cells. These data not only suggest cell surface sialic acid is required for both porcine OSU and human Wa rotavirus binding but that gangliosides are the preferred glycoconjugate receptor.

Using a virus overlay assay, we also investigated the direct interaction of virus and gangliosides immobilized on TLC plates. This study showed that human or porcine rotavirus TLP bound to intact gangliosides, whereas quite unexpectedly, porcine or human rotavirus DLP bound to the asialogangliosides, GA_1 and GA_2. This "recognition" of asialogangliosides was not revealed in the cell virus blocking assay because DLP do not bind to any cells we have tested and GA_1 and GA_2 do not block TLP binding. Presumably, DLP do not bind to cells because there is not sufficient GA_1- or GA_2-type receptors exposed on normal cells. Human and porcine DLP did not bind to any of the glycosylation mutants cells, Lec-1 or Lec-2. Willoughby et al. (Willoughby, 1990) and Srnka et al. (Srnka, 1992) previously showed binding of rotavirus preparations to GA_1 and GA_2 immobilized to TLC plates. However, these authors used metrizamide rather than CsCl gradients to purify their virus. It has been reported that metrizamide is more gentle to the virus but does not separate DLP and TLP as well as CsCl (Chen, 1992). Rotavirus DLP and TLP are difficult to separate completely even during CsCl gradient centrifugation and upon storage (or dilution of calcium concentrations) the TLP can gradually become deshelled to form DLP. It is not known if these other investigators had mostly DLP or TLP virus, but their observation of binding specificity for asialogangliosides could be explained by a preponderance of DLP in their virus preparations. Even small amounts of TLP particles in a predominantly DLP virus preparation will show postive results in infectivity assays. Accordingly, results of experiments aimed at determining whether there is a requirement for sialic acid in human rotavirus binding appear dependent on the relative amounts of DLP and TLP in the preparation as well as the method used to demonstrate activity.

The significance of the finding that the non-infectious rotavirus DLP binds specifically to GA_1 and GA_2 immobilized on TLC plates is not clear. We do not know yet whether our discovery of the asialoganglioside lectin-like activity in DLP is physiologically relevant. It is intriguing to speculate, however, that it may be involved in intracellular trafficking during viral maturation or perhaps as a lectin activity involved in stabilizing TLP structure. Regardless, this finding is significant in that it may explain some sources of contradiction in the requirement for sialic acid for host cell recognition by human rotaviruses.

REFERENCES

Bohl, E.H., 1979, Rotavirus diarrhea in pigs: Brief review, J. Am. Vet. Med. Assoc. 174:613–615.
Chen, D. and Ramig, R.F., 1992, Determinants of rotavirus stability and density during CsCl purification, Virology 186:228–237.
Fukudome, K., Yoshie, O., and Konno, T., 1989, Comparison of human, simian, and bovine rotaviruses for requirement of sialic acid in hemagglutination and cell adsorption, Virology 172:196–205.

Kapikian, A.Z. and Chanock, R.M., 1990, Rotaviruses, In: Virology, Editor: Fields, B.N. and Knipe, D.M., Raven Press, New York, p. 1353–1403.

Rolsma, M.D., Gelberg, H.B., and Kuhlenschmidt, M.S., 1994, Assay for evaluation of rotavirus-cell interactions: Identification of an enterocyte ganglioside fraction that mediates porcine group A rotavirus recognition, J. Virol. 68:258–268.

Rolsma, M.D., Kuhlenschmidt, T.B., Gelberg, H.B., and Kuhlenschmidt, M.S., 1998, Structure and Function of a Ganglioside Receptor for Porcine Rotavirus, Journal of Virology 72:9079–9091.

Srnka, C.A., Teimeyer, M.J.H., Moreland, G.M., Schweingruber, H., deLappe, B.W., James, P.G., Gant, T., Willoughby, R.E., Yolken, R.H., Nashed, M.A., Abbas, S.A., and Laine, R.A., 1992, Cell surface ligands for rotavirus: Mouse intestinal glycolipids and synthetic carbohydrate analogues, Virology 190:794–805.

Stanley, P., Caillibot, V., and Siminovitch, L., 1975, Selection and characterization of eight phenotypically distinct lines of lectin-resistant Chinese hamster ovary cells, Cell 6:121–128.

Stanley, P., Narasimhan, S., Siminovitch, L., and Schachter, H., 1975, Chinese hamster ovary cells selected for resistance to the cytotoxicity of phytohemagglutinin are deficient in a UDP-N-acetylglucosamine-glycoprotein N-acetylglucosaminyltransferase activity, Proc. Natl. Acad. Sci (USA) 72:3323–3327.

Stanley, P. and Siminovitch, L., 1977, Complementation between mutants of CHO cells resistant to a variety of plant lectin, Somatic Cell Genetics 3:391–405.

Willoughby, R.E., Yolken, R.H., and Schnaar, R.L., 1990, Rotaviruses specifically bind to the neutral glycosphingolipid asialo-GM1, J. Virol. 64:4830–4835.

Yolken, R.H., Willoughby, R.E., Wee, S.B., Miskuff, R., and Vonderfecht, S., 1987, Sialic acid glycoproteins inhibit in vitro and in vivo replication of rotaviruses, J. Clin. Invest. 79:148–154.

34

NEW APPROACHES TO MUCOSAL IMMUNIZATION

Lucía Cárdenas-Freytag,[1] Elly Cheng,[1] and Aysha Mirza[2]

Tulane University School of Medicine
Department of Microbiology and Immunology[1]
Department of Pediatrics[2]
1430 Tulane Avenue
New Orleans, Louisiana 70112-2699

SUMMARY

Every year more than 17 million deaths worldwide are caused by infectious diseases. The great majority of these deaths occur in underdeveloped countries and are attributed to diseases preventable by existing vaccines, or diseases that could potentially be prevented with new vaccines. The fact that most human and veterinary pathogens establish infection in the host by initiating contact at a mucosal surface, provide the rationale for the development of mucosal vaccines. An increasing number of strategies have been proposed to facilitate mucosal immunization. Among the most widely investigated strategies are the use of attenuated microorganisms; the inclusion of immunizing antigens in lipid-based carriers, the genetic creation of transgenic plants and the use of mucosal adjuvants derived from bacterial toxins. This review provides a brief summary of the most recent advances in the field of mucosal immunization with an special emphasis on a promising genetically detoxified mucosal adjuvant, LT(R192G), derived from the heat-labile toxin of enterotoxigenic *E. coli*. We present evidence regarding the safety, immunogenicity, and efficacy of LT(R192G) for the development of a new generation of mucosal vaccines.

1. INTRODUCTION

Clearly, in humans as well as in veterinary medicine, the most effective way for the control and eradication of infectious diseases is through vaccination. Preventing an infectious disease rather than treating the disease with antimicrobial agents once the infection is established represents the most cost-effective public health measure,

Mechanisms in the Pathogenesis of Enteric Diseases 2, edited by Paul and Francis.
Kluwer Academic / Plenum Publishers, New York, 1999.

particularly if the vaccine is administered at a young age. The implementation of effective vaccination strategies would lead to improved health worldwide, and to reduced morbidity and mortality of the entire population, resulting in immense savings to society and to the health care system.

The World Health Organization estimates that in 1997, 17.3 million deaths were due to infectious and parasitic diseases. Currently, almost 4 million children die annually from diseases preventable by existing vaccines, while another 8 million die from diseases that could be prevented with new vaccines. Obviously, there is a pressing need to develop immunization strategies for those diseases for which vaccines are not currently available, and to improve the traditional vaccines so their cost is reduced and their effectiveness and ease of administration enhanced.

Traditional vaccine strategies have for the most part relied on the use of parenteral methods of immunization. Although this is an effective method to induce protection against a number of virulent organisms, it is known that parenteral immunization is generally not effective at eliciting secretory IgA responses, or local cell-mediated immunity. In addition, the use of needles in mass immunization is not desirable due to the inherent increase of the risk of transmission of blood-borne pathogens.

A myriad of microbial pathogens enter the host using a mucosal surface as their portal of entry. The mucosal immune system comprises a large accumulation of immunoglobulin producing cells, while the lymphoid tissues present in mucosal surfaces are directly involved in host defenses. Consequently, the design of effective vaccines administered directly on mucosal tissues, and capable of eliciting a protective immune response against mucosal pathogens is very desirable. In the last decade, the search for novel means to achieve effective mucosal immunization has expanded considerably. This review discusses the latest developments in the field of mucosal immunization, and focuses particularly in the use of detoxified bacterial toxins as potent mucosal adjuvants.

2. MUCOSAL IMMUNIZATION STRATEGIES

The majority of human and veterinary pathogens establish disease by initial colonization or invasion of a mucosal surface. Therefore, it is advantageous to design vaccines that induce protective mucosal immune responses and prevent the initial colonization by the pathogen. An ideal vaccine should be effective, affordable, given in single or few doses, administered at a young age, easy to administer, and stable. In theory, these criteria can be met using mucosal vaccines. However, mucosal vaccines need to be delivered in such a way that they do not induce development of tolerance and at the same time the vaccine must elicit protective immune responses at the level of mucosal and systemic compartments. A number of mucosal immunization strategies have been devised to facilitate the delivery, efficacy, and effectiveness of mucosal vaccines. Some of the proposed strategies include, attenuated bacteria or viruses as antigen-delivery vectors, lipid based delivery systems such as liposomes or Iscoms, transgenic plants expressing heterologous antigens and bacterial toxins used as mucosal adjuvants.

2.1. Attenuated Bacteria and Viruses

Attenuated viruses and bacteria can be modified for use as carriers by inserting genes encoding a protein from a heterologous pathogen into their genome. Historically, one of the main obstacles for the use of live vaccines was the potential reversion of attenuated strains to virulence. However, the combination of modern molecular biology techniques and the elucidation of virulence mechanisms of bacterial pathogenesis at the molecular level, have made possible the construction of safe genetically stable bacterial or viral mutants.

The use of genetically attenuated mutants of *Salmonella* as oral delivery vehicles of heterologous antigen strains has been extensively investigated. This system is attractive because it can lead to the development of bivalent vaccines, protecting not only against *Salmonella* infection, but also against the pathogens from which the foreign antigen is derived. The attenuated bacteria retain the capacity to invade the epithelium and in some cases invade deeper tissues, while delivering the relevant antigen to the lymphoid follicles present in the GALT.

Antigens of viral, parasitic, and bacterial origin have been successfully cloned and expressed in attenuated *Salmonella* vectors. Numerous studies have demonstrated that immunization with these recombinant bacteria result in the generation of humoral and cell mediated responses directed not only against the cloned antigen, but also against the delivering *Salmonella* strain (for reviews see (Cardenas and Clements, 1993; Schodel and Curtiss, 1995). The major problems associated with this delivery system are instability of the expressed antigen *in vivo*, low levels of expression of the cloned gene, and over-attenuation of the *Salmonella* strain.

Other bacterial mucosal delivery systems include the use of commensal bacteria to deliver antigens directly to mucosal surfaces (Fischetti et al., 1996); mucosal administration of BCG carrying genes expressing foreign virulence determinants (Langermann et al., 1994) and attenuated *Listeria monocytogenes* as delivery vectors of antigen-encoding plasmid DNA (Dietrich et al., 1998).

Recombinant DNA and RNA viruses have also been explored as vectors for mucosal delivery. Taking advantage of the abundant existing knowledge about the biology, structure, and molecular biology of poliovirus, adenovirus, and poxviruses; these viruses have been used as vectors for mucosal vaccines (for reviews see (Morrow et al., 1996; Rosenthal et al., 1996; Morrow et al., 1999)). Different approaches have been investigated to develop viral vectors. Two of the most promising approaches are the construction of chimeric viruses expressing foreign epitopes (Muster et al., 1995), and the use of encapsidated replicons encoding foreign genes (Moldoveanu et al., 1995). Recent studies illustrate that it is also possible to induce antigen-specific humoral, mucosal, and cell-mediated responses to foreign viral antigens, after mucosal immunization with adenovirus-based vectors encoding foreign genes (Buge et al., 1997).

2.2. Microspheres, Liposomes, and ISCOMs

Biodegradable polymer microspheres offer the advantage of controlled release of antigens for extended periods. A variety of immunogens has been encapsulated in microspheres usually composed of the material used in biodegradable sutures, which is known as poly (DL-lactid-co-glycolide) or DL-PLG. These polymers have been used in drug delivery systems for a number of years and their safety and ease of use have been amply documented. Several bacterial and viral antigens encapsulated into DL-PLG microspheres have been tested in various animal models. It is clear form these studies that oral or intranasal immunization with microencapsulated antigens, induces mucosal and systemic immune responses and in a number of cases protection against challenge with the virulent pathogen (Duncan et al., 1996). One of the hindrances in the creation of microsphere-based vaccines is that the organic solvents used in the microencapsulation process can damage or change the nature of the encapsulated antigen. In that regard a number of other synthetic and natural polymers, such as starch, agarose, and alginate—based microspheres are being investigated for use in vaccines delivered by the mucosal route.

Lipid–based delivery systems such as liposomes and immune stimulating complexes (ISCOMs) are used to deliver antigens in a system designed to protect a concentrated amount of antigen from degradation. Liposomes are aqueous suspensions of phospholipids organized in bilayer structures. ISCOMs are saponin containing lipid mixtures, which associate with protein antigens. Although several published reports point to the fact that Iscoms are effective as mucosal adjuvant carriers of multiple microbial antigens (Smith et al., 1998), others indicate that they are poor immunopotentiators when delivered orally (Ghazi et al., 1995). Liposomes have been mostly used in systemic immunizations, but have also been shown to be effective as components of potential oral and intranasal vaccines (Michalek et al., 1992). A limitation for the use of liposomes is their relative instability in the gut as well as during storage.

2.3. Transgenic Plants

The expression of recombinant molecules in plants is possible by genetic transformation of the plant using *Agrobacterium* T-DNA vectors, or viral vectors in which a plant virus is modified to encode the foreign gene. Both approaches have lead to the production of transgenic plants expressing antigens from pathogenic organisms. In recent studies, mice fed transgenic potatoes expressing the binding subunit of the heat-labile toxin of *E. coli* (LT-B) or capsid proteins from Norwalk virus (Haq et al., 1995; Mason et al., 1996), were able to produce serum and gut mucosal antigen-specific immune responses. More significantly, when adult human volunteers were fed raw potatoes transformed with LT-B, they mounted a specific immune response reflected in production of IgA anti-LT-B antibody secreting cells (ASC) as well as specific serum and mucosal IgA and IgG (Tacket et al., 1998).

There are many advantages inherent to the use of transgenic plants to deliver immunizing antigens to humans and animals. Plants are easy and inexpensive to grow and propagate, and can provide a limitless supply of the antigen of interest. However, because the levels of expression of the foreign gene are relatively low, it remains to be determined if other proteins less immunogenic than LT-B can induce effective immune responses after ingestion of reasonable amounts of transgenic plants.

2.4. Mucosal Adjuvants

Most antigens induce very poor immune responses when given orally. In addition, mucosal administration of antigens can induce immune tolerance. This phenomenon is characterized by the fact that animals fed a protein antigen repeatedly have a reduced ability to develop an immune response to this antigen when exposed to it by a systemic route. A strategy to overcome this problem is to administer the antigen concomitantly with a mucosal adjuvant that abrogates the induction of systemic tolerance.

The most potent mucosal immunogens known are cholera toxin (CT) produced by *Vibrio cholera* and the heat-labile enterotoxin (LT) produced by enterotoxigenic *E. coli*. These two mucosal adjuvants will be discussed in detail below.

The properties of other substances as mucosal adjuvants have been investigated and are the subject of various publications. Certain cytokines, such as IL-12 have immunostimulatory proteins when delivered mucosally. Belyakov and colleagues (Belyakov et al., 1998) observed that cytotoxic T lymphocyte responses (CTL) and resistance to mucosal viral transmission were increased by mucosal vaccination with an HIV peptide co-administered with IL-12. In a more recent study, the ability of IL-12 and IL-6 to act as mucosal adjuvants was investigated. Mice immunized with tetanus toxoid (TT) in conjunction with IL-6 or IL-12 were able to develop increased serum antibody titers to TT, which protected the mice from systemic TT challenge. IL-12 was more efficient than IL-6 at eliciting secretory IgA and Th-1-type cytokine responses (Boyaka et al., 1999). Lymphotaxin which is a chemokine produced by NK cells, has also been reported to have immunomodulatory properties, when co-administered nasally with a proteinaceous antigen (Lillard et al., 1999).

Proteosomes are other mucosal adjuvants derived from bacteria. These adjuvants are vesicles of outer membrane proteins derived from meningococci, which associate forming hydrophobic interactions. Relevant antigens are anchored to these vesicles and the preparations are delivered mucosally. Mice immunized i.n. with influenza peptides combined with proteosomes, produced specific humoral and cellular specific immune responses (Levi et al., 1995). Studies in monkeys have shown that formulations consisting of proteosomes and formalinized staphylococcal enterotoxin B (SEB), are safe, immunogenic and protective against lethal SEB aerosol challenge (Lowell et al., 1996). Another report indicates that HIV-gp160 antigen complexed to proteosomes induces specific humoral and secretory responses in mice after intranasal immunization (Lowell et al., 1997). The mucosal adjuvanticity of other natural and synthetic substances are actively being explored. However, the majority of these systems are yet uncharacterized and, for the most part, have been tested only with few antigens and in a limited number of animal models.

3. ADP-RIBOSYLATING BACTERIAL TOXINS AS MUCOSAL ADJUVANTS

A number of bacterial enterotoxins catalyze the transfer of the ADP-ribose moiety from NAD to an eukaryotic target protein. Among these cholera toxin (CT) and the heat-labile enterotoxin (LT) produced by some enterotoxigenic strains of *Escherichia coli,* are known to be the two bacterial proteins with the greatest potential to function as mucosal adjuvants (Clements et al., 1988; Elson, 1989; Xu-Amano et al., 1993). In 1992 Lycke et al. published a paper demonstrating that the adjuvant effect of CT and LT was linked to their ADP-ribosyltransferase activity (Lycke et al., 1992). A few studies report on the potential of ADP-ribosylating bacterial toxins, other than CT or LT, as mucosal adjuvants. For instance, in a study conducted by Roberts and collaborators (Roberts et al., 1995) a mutant pertussis toxin molecule, devoid of ADP-ribosyltransferase activity, immunopotentiated the immune response to TT- fragment C when administered intranasally. In a more recent publication, a chimeric protein composed of a nontoxic form of *Pseudomonas* Exotoxin combined with an HIV-gp120 antigen, induced antigen specific IgG and IgA titers in serum and saliva of immunized mice, after either vaginal, rectal, oral, or subcutaneous administration (Mrsny et al., 1999). The fact that ADP-ribosylating toxins other that LT and CT can act as mucosal adjuvants is not surprising. Whether or not they can act as effectively as LT and CT in other systems remains to be investigated.

3.1. CT, LT, and Detoxified Mutants

Although LT and CT have many features in common, these are clearly distinct molecules with biochemical and immunologic differences, which make them unique. Both LT and CT are synthesized as multisubunit toxins with A and B components. On thiol reduction, the A component dissociates into two smaller polypeptide chains. One of these, the A1 piece, catalyzes the ADP-ribosylation of the stimulatory GTP-binding protein (GSα) in the adenylate cyclase enzyme complex on the basolateral surface of the epithelial cell resulting in increasing intracellular levels of cAMP. The resulting increase in cAMP causes secretion of water and electrolytes into the small intestine through interaction with two cAMP-sensitive ion transport mechanisms (Field, 1980). The B-subunit binds to the host cell membrane receptor (ganglioside GM1) and facilitates the translocation of the A-subunit through the cell membrane.

Recent studies have examined the potential of CT and LT as mucosal adjuvants against a variety of bacterial and viral pathogens using whole killed organisms or purified subunits of relevant virulence determinants from these organisms. Representative examples include tetanus toxoid (Xu-Amano et al., 1993; Xu-Amano et al., 1994; Yamamoto et al., 1996), inactivated influenza virus (Hashigucci et al., 1996; Katz et al., 1996; Katz et al., 1997), recombinant urease from *Helicobacter* spp. (Lee et al., 1995; Weltzin et al., 1997), pneumococcal surface protein A from *Streptococcus pneumoniae* (Wu et al., 1997), Norwalk virus capsid protein (Mason et al., 1996) synthetic peptides from measles virus (Hathaway et al., 1995), HIV-1 C4/V3 peptide T1SP10 MN(A) (Staats et al., 1996), and the HIV-1 *env* gene (Bruhl et al., 1998). There are many other examples and it is clear from these studies that both LT and CT have significant potential for use as adjuvants for mucosally administered antigens. This raises the possibility of an effective immunization program against a variety of pathogens involving the mucosal administration of killed or attenuated organisms or relevant virulence determinants of specific agents in conjunction with LT or CT. However, the fact that these toxins stimulate a net luminal secretory response may prevent their use for practical vaccine applications. For instance, it was observed that as little as 5 μg of purified CT administered orally was sufficient to induce diarrhea in human volunteers, while ingestion of 25 μg of CT elicited a full 20-liter cholera purge (Levine et al., 1983). In recently conducted volunteer studies with LT administered alone or in conjunction with the *V. cholerae* Whole Cell/B-Subunit Vaccine, LT was shown to induce fluid secretion at doses as low as 2.5 μg when administered in conjunction with the vaccine, while 25 μg of LT elicited up to 6-liters of fluid secretion. While the adjuvant effective dose in humans for either of these toxins has not been established, experiments in animals suggest that it may be a comparable to the toxic dose. Taken together, these studies suggest that while LT and CT may be attractive as mucosal adjuvants, studies in animals do not reflect the full toxic potential of these molecules in humans, and that toxicity may seriously limit their practical use.

A number of attempts have been made to alter the toxicity of LT and CT, most of which have focused on eliminating enzymatic activity of the A-subunit associated with enterotoxicity. The majority of these efforts have involved the use of site-directed mutagenesis to change amino acids associated with the crevice where NAD binding and catalysis is thought to occur. Recently, a model for NAD binding and catalysis was proposed (Domenighini et al., 1994; Pizza et al., 1994) based on computer analysis of the crystallographic structure of LT (Sixma et al., 1991; Sixma et al., 1993). Replacement of any amino acid in CT or LT involved in NAD-binding and catalysis by site-directed mutagenesis has been shown to alter ADP-ribosyltransferase activity with a corresponding loss of toxicity in a variety of biological assay systems (Harford et al., 1989; Tsuji et al., 1990; Burnette et al., 1991; Lobet et al., 1991; Moss et al., 1993; Häse et al., 1994; Pizza et al., 1994; Fontana et al., 1995; Merritt et al., 1995; Yamamoto et al., 1997a; Yamamoto et al., 1997b). The adjuvanticity potential of some of these mutants has been tested in animal models using a variety of coadministered antigens (Lycke et al., 1992; Di Tommaso et al., 1996; Partidos et al., 1996; Yamamoto et al., 1997a; Giuliani et al., 1998). In addition, it has been shown that exchanging K for E at position 112 in LT not only removes ADP-ribosylating enzymatic activity, but cAMP activation and adjuvant activity as well (Lycke et al., 1992). However, when given intranasally, two groups independently showed that LT(E112K) can induce significant levels of serum and mucosal antibody responses against the co-administered antigens (de Haan et al., 1998; Komase et al., 1998). It was also reported that a CT(E112K) mutant not only induced high levels of OVA-specific serum IgG and IgE, but it also selectively induced a Th2 type cytokine response when administered subcutaneously (Yamamoto et al., 1997b).

Dickinson and Clements (Dickinson and Clements, 1995) explored an alternate approach to dissociation of enterotoxicity from adjuvanticity. Like other bacterial toxins that are members of the A-B toxin family, both CT and LT require proteolysis of a trypsin sensitive bond to become fully active. In these two enterotoxins, that trypsin sensitive peptide is subtended by a disulfide interchange that joins the A1 and A2 pieces of the A-subunit. In theory, if the A1 and A2 pieces cannot separate, A1 may not be able to find its target (adenylate cyclase) on the basolateral surface or may not assume the conformation necessary to bind or hydrolyze NAD.

A mutant of LT was constructed using site-directed mutagenesis to create a single amino acid substitution, a glycine instead of an arginine at position 192, within the disulfide subtended region of the A subunit separating A1 from A2. This single amino acid change altered the proteolytically sensitive site within this region, rendering the mutant insensitive to trypsin activation. The physical, biological and functional properties of this mutant, designated LT(R192G), have been extensively investigated (Dickinson and Clements, 1996; Cheng et al., 1999; Freytag and Clements, 1999) and it is obvious form these studies that this adjuvant holds great potential for the development of a new generation of mucosal vaccines.

4. PRACTICAL USES OF LT(R192G) IN THE DEVELOPMENT OF MUCOSAL VACCINES

Efficacy studies for LT(R192G) in appropriate animal models have demonstrated that this molecule can function as an effective mucosal adjuvant for killed whole bacteria, fungi and a number of inactivated viruses of importance to both human and veterinary medicine. In addition, this detoxified adjuvant has recently been evaluated in two Phase I safety studies (Oplinger et al., 1997; Tribble et al., 1997).

4.1. Vaccines against Bacterial Pathogens

A paper published by Chong et al. (Chong et al., 1998) illustrates the efficacy of LT(R192G) as a component of a vaccine protective against lethal oral challenge by *Salmonella* sp. In a murine model. For these studies, mice were immunized orally with killed *Salmonella dublin* in conjunction with LT(R192G). Control groups included animals immunized with either viable attenuated *Salmonella dublin* or with killed *S. dublin*. Following two oral immunizations, mice were challenged with 100 LD_{50} of the virulent wild-type parent strain. Results from these experiments showed that animals orally immunized with viable attenuated *S. dublin* or with killed *S. dublin* co-administered with LT(R192G) were solidly protected against challenge with the virulent parent strain, while animals orally immunized with killed *S. dublin* were not.

Analysis of antibody responses demonstrated that animals immunized orally with viable *S. dublin* had a four-fold or greater increase in both serum anti-LPS IgG and fecal anti-LPS IgA compared to animals immunized orally with killed *S. dublin*, or killed *S. dublin* plus LT(R192G).

The cytokine profiles observed in culture supernatants of mononuclear cells obtained from the spleens or mesenteric lymph nodes (MLN) indicated that significant antigen-induced IL-2 was detected only in supernatants of mononuclear cells from of mice orally immunized with killed Salmonella in conjunction with LT(R192G). More significant was the observation that IFN-gamma levels from MLN were significantly elevated in mice given the killed bacteria-adjuvant combination, while the levels of IFN-gamma from spleen supernatants were similar between the two protected groups.

This study demonstrated that the function of LT(R192G) in protection against typhoid-like disease is to upregulate the Th1 arm of the immune response against killed organisms. Specifically, mice orally immunized with killed *S. dublin* in conjunction with LT(R192G) were protected against lethal challenge and had higher IFN-gamma, IL-2, and IgG responses than mice orally immunized with killed *S. dublin* alone which were not protected. This was also the first demonstration of a role for IFN-gamma in protection against challenge following oral immunization with viable attenuated *Salmonella* spp.

In recent studies conducted in our laboratory (Cheng et al., 1999) we have shown that LT(R192G) immunopotentiates the response against tetanus toxoid (TT). Intranasal or oral immunization of Balb/c mice with TT in conjunction with LT(R192G) resulted in enhanced production of antigen specific serum IgG and vaginal IgA. Moreover, mucosal vaccination with LT(R192G) and TT induced both Th1 and Th2 type cellular immune responses. The observed cytokine levels were comparable to those induced by native LT and by LT (A69G). In these experiments, the role of cAMP in mucosal adjuvanticity was examined by comparing the adjuvanticity properties of several active site mutants with LT(R192G), and with native LT and LT-B. It was clear from our results that there is a strong correlation between the ability of LT or LT mutants to induce cAMP accumulation and their ability to elicit production of antigen specific Th1 and Th1 cytokines.

4.2. Vaccines against Fungal Pathogens

Infections caused by opportunistic fungal pathogens such as *Candida albicans* remain a major cause of morbidity and mortality in immunocompromised individuals. Such infections affect thousands of people and cause severe and sometimes fatal diseases. Currently there are no vaccines available against human mycosis and the development of an effective anti-*Candida* vaccine for use in selected patients would be highly advantageous. Studies using experimental animal models have demonstrated the feasibility of developing protective immunity against fungal infections through vaccination. Most of these studies have used parenterally administered vaccines with purified fungal antigens or oral vaccines with live organisms. In a recent paper we report on a new vaccination strategy for prevention of infections caused by *Candida albicans* using heat inactivated *C. albicans* (HK-CA) administered mucosally in conjunction with LT(R192G) (Cardenas-Freytag et al., 1999).

For these experiments, male CBA/J mice immunized i.n. with HK-CA in conjunction with LT(R192G), and control animals immunized with the heat-killed fungus, the adjuvant, or saline alone, were challenged intravenously (i.v.) with 10^4 viable *C. albicans* two weeks following the last application of immunogen. Survival was monitored over a 28-day period, and then the animals were sacrificed and their kidneys were cultured quantitatively. Animals immunized by other methods of immunization, i.e., by intragastric (i.g.) and/or intradermal (i.d.) inoculations of viable *C. albicans* were included as controls.

As seen in Fig. 1, the results from two independent experiments demonstrated that animals vaccinated i.n. with HK-CA + LT(R192G) were able to eradicate *C. albicans* completely from their kidneys. Animals immunized by i.g. followed by i.d. inoculation of viable *C. albicans* also had significantly ($p \leq 0.05$) reduced levels of the yeast in their kidneys, but the reductions were not nearly as dramatic as those observed in animals immunized i.n. with HK-CA in conjunction with LT(R192G). As expected, control animals immunized with LT(R192G) alone or saline had disseminated candidiasis indicated by the presence of high numbers of *C. albicans* in their kidneys. Moreover, as demonstrated in the experiment depicted in panel A (Fig. 1), animals immunized intragastrically with nonviable *C. albicans* with or without adjuvant, did not develop protective responses. The inability of inactivated *Candida* to induce protection when administered intragastrically had been previously observed in our laboratory.

To determine if the protection against a challenge with 10^4 viable *C. albicans* could be demonstrated with higher and more rapidly lethal doses of *C. albicans*, mice were immunized with either HK-CA + LT(R192G), or with LT(R192G) alone, or mock-vaccinated with saline. All animals were subsequently challenged i.v. with 10^5 or 10^6 viable *C. albicans* two weeks following the last i.n. dose. Survival was monitored for 100 days. Figure 2 shows the mortality pattern observed after i.v. challenge. Twenty days after challenging with 10^5 *C. albicans* there were no surviving mice in the LT(R192G) or saline control groups. In contrast, 90% of the animals in the group that received HK-CA + LT(R192G) survived for the entire length of the experiment (100 days post-challenge), and had no detectable numbers of *C. albicans* in their kidneys at the time of sacrifice.

A less dramatic but no less significant effect was observed when mice were challenged with 10^6 viable *C. albicans*. All animals in the groups that were vaccinated with either LT(R192G) or saline died within 72 hours post-challenge. A greater survival rate was initially observed for those animals immunized with HK-CA + LT(R192G) (60% survival after 5 days); however, by day 15 only 20% of the animals were alive. Clearly, i.n. immunization with killed whole *C. albicans* in conjunction with the mucosal adjuvant LT(R192G) stimulated significant levels of protective immunity, even when animals were challenged with doses of *C. albicans* which were rapidly fatal for unimmunized mice.

In an effort to elucidate the nature of the protective immune response in vaccinated animals, groups of mice were studied for the antibody and cellular immune responses developed after vaccination but before challenge. Delayed hypersensitivity (DTH) was assessed by the footpad assay two weeks following the last of three

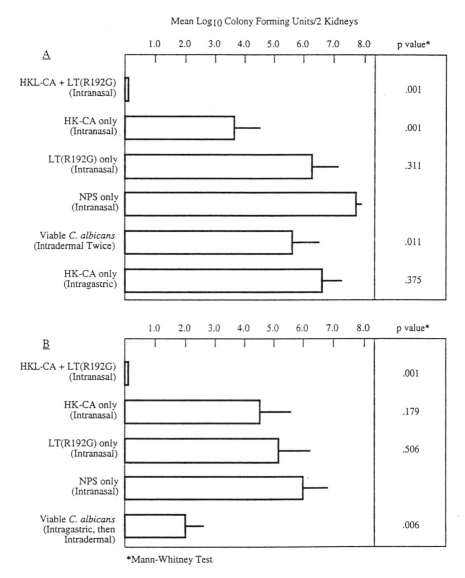

Mean Log$_{10}$ Colony Forming Units/2 Kidneys

Figure 1. Demonstration of protective immunity by culture of kidneys four weeks following i.v. challenge with 10^4 viable *C. albicans*. Animals were immunized i.n. with HK-CA (2×10^7) with or without 10 μg of the adjuvant LT(R192G), adjuvant alone, or saline. Control groups included animals immunized by i.d. exposure to 2×10^6 viable *C. albicans*; animals vaccinated i.g. with 2×10^7 HK-CA or animals given an i.g immunization followed by an i.d. inoculation with live *C. albicans*. Intravenous challenge was performed two weeks following the last exposure to antigen during the immunization protocol.

immunizations with the fungus-adjuvant mixture. The results depicted in Fig. 3 indicate that mice immunized with adjuvant alone developed no DTH response whereas those immunized with HK-CA alone developed only minimal responses. Those responses were not statistically-significant. In contrast, animals immunized with HK-CA + LT(R192G) developed substantial and highly-significant DH responses. The responses of the latter group of animals were comparable to those detected in animals inoculated i.d. or i.g-i.d. The immunological reactivity observed in the HK-CA + LT(R192G) group

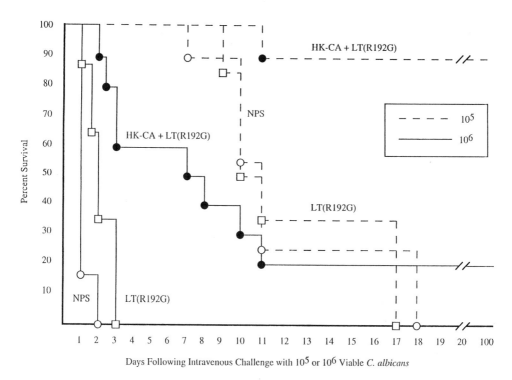

Figure 2. Survival of mice immunized with HK-CA plus LT(R192G), LT(R192G) alone, or saline and challenged i.v. two weeks following the last exposure to antigen with 10^5or 10^6 viable *C. albicans*.

indicates the development of a vigorous antigen-specific T cell response, which correlated with protection and was elicited marginally by inactivated *C. albicans* in the absence of the mucosal adjuvant.

The levels of specific anti-*Candida* antibodies in serum were determined following i.n. immunization of mice with the LT(R192G)-containing vaccine. These animals were challenged i.v. with 10^4 viable *C. albicans* two weeks following the last application of vaccine and then sacrificed four weeks following the i.v. challenge. A control group consisting of animals immunized i.g.-i.d. with viable *Candida* and challenged intravenously with viable *C. albicans* was included in these experiments. As shown in Fig. 4.A, the highest levels of serum IgG against soluble cytoplasmic substances form *C. albicans* (SCS) occurred in those animals that had been immunized with HK-CA in conjunction with LT(R192G) and then challenged i.v. with viable *C. albicans*. These animals had the highest level of protection of any of the vaccine groups examined. Animals immunized with HK-CA alone and then challenged i.v. with viable *C. albicans*, also developed antibodies to SCS, but the levels were much lower than those in animals that received the heat-killed organism with adjuvant. No antibodies were detected in the negative control animals, i.e., those animals given only adjuvant or saline as immunogen and then challenged i.v. with viable *C. albicans*. Interestingly, the positive control group, i.e., those animals immunized by the i.g.-i.d. route with viable *C. albicans* and then challenged i.v. with viable *C. albicans*, had lower total IgG levels, with higher levels of IgG1 when compared to the HK-CA + LT(R192G) group.

Levels of IgG1 and IgG2a were analyzed in the animals immunized with HK-CA plus LT(R192G) that survived challenge with a ten-fold higher dose (10^5) of viable *C.*

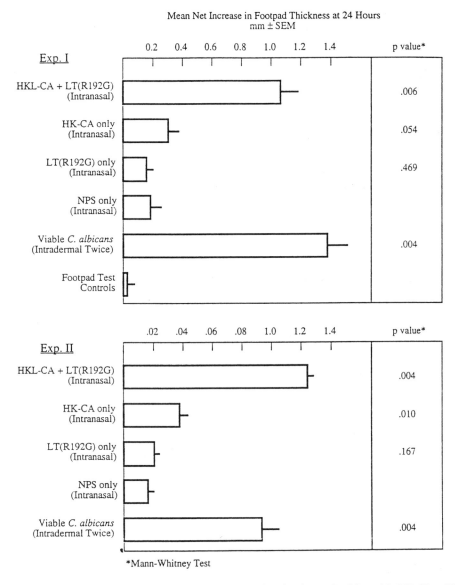

Figure 3. Delayed hypersensitivity to *C. albicans* mannan in mice immunized i.n. with HK-CA with or without LT(R192G), saline, LT(R192G) only, or 10^6 viable C. albicans administered i.d.

albicans. As seen in Fig. 4, animals immunized with HK-CA combined with LT(R192G) and challenged with 10^5 viable *C. albicans* had significant increases in anti-SCS total IgG. This increase was mostly due to a dramatic shift in the levels of anti-SCS IgG2a (Fig. 4B).

Western blot experiments were done to examine the total IgG response to cytoplasmic (SCS) extracts in animals immunized in various ways (Fig. 5). The most interesting observation was that all of the animals immunized with HK-CA plus adjuvant (Lanes 2–9) developed an antibody response to a number of SCS antigens. As seen a strong antibody response in these animals was directed against an antigen with a molecular mass of approximately 29 kDa. These were the animals that were completely

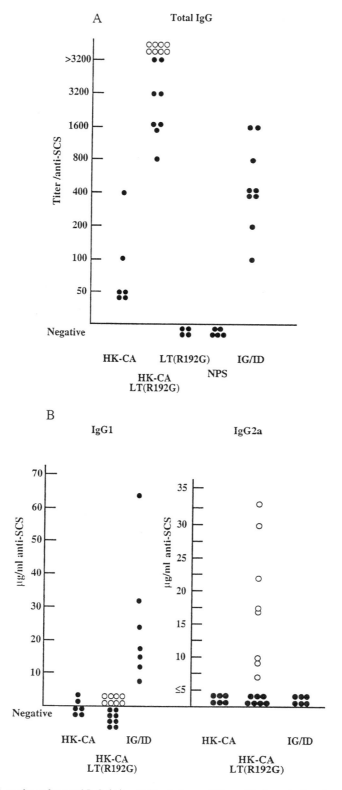

Figure 4. ELISA analyses for total IgG (A) or IgG subclasses (B) specific for cytoplasmic antigens (SCS) of *C. albicans* in sera from animals immunized i.n. with HK-CA with or without LT(R192G), LT(R192G) or saline alone, or with viable *C. albicans* administered i.g./i.d. Sera were obtained at the time of sacrifice i.e., 4 weeks following i.v. challenge with 10^4 viable *C. albicans* (closed circles), or 100 days following i.v. challenge with 10^5 viable *C. albicans* (open circles).

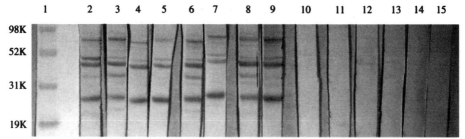

Figure 5. Western blot analyses of sera from animals immunized i.n. with HK-CA with or without LT(R192G). Lane 1—MWM markers, Lanes 2–9—sera from mice immunized with HK-CA + LT(R192G) and challenged with 10^5 viable *C. albicans*. Sera obtained 100 days post-challenge. Lanes 10–15—sera from mice immunized with HK-CA alone.

protected against colonization of the kidney and lethal i.v. challenge. Animals immunized with HK-CA alone (Lanes 10–15), adjuvant alone (not shown), or saline (not shown) prior to i.v. challenge developed no antibody responses to the cytoplasmic extract, as detected by Western blot (Fig. 5) and were not protected against colonization following i.v. challenge.

To summarize, it is clear that i.n. immunization with killed *C. albicans* in conjunction with LT(R192G) afforded significant levels of protection. This novel approach offers new possibilities for the development of an effective, inexpensive and easy to administer vaccine against fungal pathogens.

4.3. Vaccines against Viral Pathogens

Efforts are now being made to develop safe, and effective mucosal vaccines against viral pathogens such as rotavirus. Viral gastroenteritis caused by rotavirus cause more than 500,000 deaths annually. In a study conducted by O'neal et al. (O'Neal et al., 1998) the immunogenicity and efficacy of a potential vaccine composed of virus-like particles (VLPs) and LT(R192G) was examined in an animal model. VLPs are made by coinfecting insect cells with baculovirus recombinants expressing rotavirus structural proteins. These structural proteins self-assemble into VLP's. Adult female CD-1 mice were vaccinated intranasally with VLP's in combination with either CT, LT or LT(R192G). All vaccinated animals developed high serum antibody titers, which were not different between groups. The intestinal rotavirus specific IgA responses were higher in animals given VLPs plus LT or LT(R192G) than in animals receiving CT or antigen alone. To determine the efficacy of the vaccine, immunized animals were challenged orally with wild-type murine virus, and protection was determined as percent reduction in viral shedding. All mice vaccinated intranasally with VLPs in conjunction with LT or LT(R192G) were solidly protected from challenge, while animals given CT as an adjuvant exhibited a reduction in viral shedding that ranged form 66–100%. These results illustrate the benefit of using an effective nontoxic mucosal adjuvant to induce protection against a viral disease that causes significant mortality and morbidity in humans.

Recent efforts in our laboratory (unpublished results) focus on the feasibility to enhance the immune responses against HIV antigens after mucosal immunization with purified HIV glycoproteins (gp160 and gp120) administered in combination with LT(R192G). Experiments aimed to optimize the parameters of immunization demonstrated that after three intranasal immunizations with 10 µg of gp120 combined with

LT(R192G), vaccinated mice mounted a significant anti-gp120 serum IgG response as well as significantly elevated levels of gp120-induced IFN- gamma and IL-10. Further studies are on the way to investigate the effect of this vaccination protocol in the generation of HIV-specific secretory IgA and CTL responses.

5. CONCLUSIONS

Vaccination as a means of preventing infection has had a great impact on human health in this century. The success of mucosally administered vaccines is best exemplified by the polio vaccine, which is responsible for the near worldwide eradication of this devastating disease. Mucosal vaccines are easy to administered and in general are safer and less costly than parenterally administered vaccines. The development of novel methods of mucosal immunization offers many exciting possibilities. In particular, the use of detoxified mucosal adjuvants that induce effective immune responses when administered with inactivated microbial pathogens or with purified protein subunits holds great promise for the development of a new generation of vaccines. Our laboratory is currently focusing in the practical use of genetically detoxified LT mutants in potential vaccines against infectious diseases. One such mutant, LT(R192G), has been shown to be safe and effective in animals and humans and there is mounting evidence demonstrating the efficacy of LT(R192G)-containing vaccines in several animal models and with a variety of antigens of diverse microbial origin.

ACKNOWLEDGMENTS

The authors are especially indebted to Dr. John D. Clements for his guidance, direction, and friendship. Presented investigation was supported by Public Health Service grants AI12806 and AI42777 from the National Institutes of Health and by a grant from SmithKline Beecham Biologics awarded to J.D. Clements.

REFERENCES

Belyakov, I.M., Ahlers, J.D., Brandwein, B.Y., Earl, P., Kelsall, B.L., Moss, B., Strober, W., and Berzofsky, J.A., 1998, The importance of local mucosal HIV-specific CD8(+) cytotoxic T lymphocytes for resistance to mucosal viral transmission in mice and enhancement of resistance by local administration of IL-12, J Clin Invest. 102(12):2072–81.

Boyaka, P.N., Marinaro, M., Jackson, R.J., Menon, S., Kiyono, H., Jirillo, E., and McGhee, J.R., 1999, IL-12 is an effective adjuvant for induction of mucosal immunity, J Immunol. 162(1):122–8.

Bruhl, P., Kerschbaum, A., Eibl, M.M., and Mannhalter, J.W., 1998, An experimental prime-boost regimen leading to HIV type 1-specific mucosal and systemic immunity in BALB/c mice, AIDS Res Hum Retroviruses. 14(5):401–7.

Buge, S.L., Richardson, E., Alipanah, S., Markham, P., Cheng, S., Kalyan, N., Miller, C.J., Lubeck, M., Udem, S., and Eldridge, J., et al., 1997, An adenovirus-simian immunodeficiency virus env vaccine elicits humoral, cellular, and mucosal immune responses in rhesus macaques and decreases viral burden following vaginal challenge, J Virol. 71(11):8531–41.

Burnette, W.N., Mar, V.L., Platler, B.W., Schlotterbeck, J.D., McGinley, M.D., Stoney, K.S., Rhode, M.F., and Kaslow, H.R., 1991, Site-specific mutagenesis of the catalytic subunit of cholera toxin: substituting lysine for arginine 7 causes loss of activity, Infection and Immunity. 59:4266–4270.

Cardenas, L. and Clements, J.D., 1993, Development of mucosal protection against the heat-stable enterotoxin (ST) of *Escherichia coli* by oral immunization with a genetic fusion delivered by a bacterial vector, Infect Immun. 61(11):4629–36.

Cardenas-Freytag, L., Cheng, E., Mayeux, P., Domer, J.E., and Clements, J.D., 1999, Effectiveness of a vaccine composed of heat-killed *Candida albicans* and a novel mucosal adjuvant, LT(R192G), against systemic candidiasis [In Process Citation], Infect Immun. 67(2):826–33.

Cheng, E., Cardenas-Freytag, L., and Clements, J., 1999, The role of cAMP in mucosal adjuvanticity of *Escherichia coli* heat-labile enterotoxin (LT), Vaccine. In press.

Chong, C., Frieberg, M., and Clements, J.D., 1998, LT(R192G), a non-toxic mutant of the heat-labile enterotoxin of Escherichia coli elicits enhanced humoral and cellular immune responses associated with protection against lethal oral challenge with *Salmonella* spp., Vaccine. 16(7):732–740.

Clements, J.D., Hartzog, N.M., and Lyon, F.L., 1988, Adjuvant activity of *Escherichia coli* heat-labile enterotoxin and effect on the induction of oral tolerance in mice to unrelated protein antigens, Vaccine. 6:269–277.

de Haan, L., Verweij, W.R., Feil, I.K., Holtrop, M., Hol, W.G., Agsteribbe, E., and Wilschut, J., 1998, Role of GM1 binding in the mucosal immunogenicity and adjuvant activity of the *Escherichia coli* heat-labile enterotoxin and its B subunit, Immunology. 94(3):424–30.

Di Tommaso, A., Saletti, G., Pizza, M., Rappuoli, R., Dougan, G., Abrignani, S., Douce, G., and De Magistris, M.T., 1996, Induction of antigen-specific antibodies in vaginal secretions by using a nontoxic mutant of heat-labile enterotoxin as a mucosal adjuvant, Infect Immun. 64(3):974–9.

Dickinson, B.L. and Clements, J.D., 1995, Dissociation of *Escherichia coli* heat-labile enterotoxin adjuvanticity from ADP-ribosyltransferase activity, Infection and Immunity. 63:1617–1623.

Dickinson, B.L. and Clements, J.D., 1996, Use of *Escherichia coli* Heat-labile Enterotoxin as an Oral Adjuvant. In: *Mucosal Vaccines*. H. Kiyono, P.L. Ogra, and J.R. McGhee. San Diego, Academic Press: 73–87.

Dietrich, G., Bubert, A., Gentschev, I., Sokolovic, Z., Simm, A., Catic, A., Kaufmann, S.H., Hess, J., Szalay, A.A., and Goebel, W., 1998, Delivery of antigen-encoding plasmid DNA into the cytosol of macrophages by attenuated suicide *Listeria monocytogenes*, Nat Biotechnol. 16(2):181–5.

Domenighini, M.C.M., Pizza, M., and Rappuoli, R., 1994, Common features of the NAD-binding and catalytic site of ADP-ribosylating toxins, Molecular Microbiology. 14:41–50.

Duncan, J.D., Gilley, R.M., Schafer, D.P., Moldoveanu, Z., and Mestecky, J.F., 1996, Poly(lactide-co-glycolide) microencapsulation of vaccines for mucosal immunization. In: *Mucosal vaccines*. K. Hiroshi, P.L. Ogra, and J.R. McGhee. New York, Academic Press: 159–173.

Elson, C.O., 1989, Cholera toxin and its subunits as potential oral adjuvants, Immunology Today. 146:29–33.

Field, M., 1980, Regulation of small intestinal ion transport by cyclic nucleotides and calcium. In: *Secretory diarrhea*. M. Field, J.S. Fordtran, and S.G. Schultz. Baltimore, Md., Waverly Press: 21–30.

Fischetti, V.A., Medaglini, D., and Pozzi, G., 1996, Gram-positive commensal bacteria for mucosal vaccine delivery, Curr Opin Biotechnol. 7(6):659–66.

Fontana, M.R., Manetti, R., Giannelli, V., Magagnoli, C., Marchini, A., Olivieri, R., Domenighini, M., Rappuoli, R., and Pizza, M., 1995, Construction of nontoxic derivatives of cholera toxin and characterization of the immunological response against the A subunit, Infection and Immunity. 63:2356–2360.

Freytag, L.C. and Clements, J.D., 1999, Bacterial toxins as mucosal adjuvants, Curr Top Microbiol Immunol. 236:215–36.

Ghazi, H.O., Potter, C.W., Smith, T.L., and Jennings, R., 1995, Comparative antibody responses and protection in mice immunized by oral or parenteral routes with influenza virus subunit antigens in aqueous form or incorporated into ISCOMs, J Med Microbiol. 42(1):53–61.

Giuliani, M.M., Del Giudice, G., Giannelli, V., Dougan, G., Douce, G., Rappuoli, R., and Pizza, M., 1998, Mucosal adjuvanticity and immunogenicity of LTR72, a novel mutant of *Escherichia coli* heat-labile enterotoxin with partial knockout of ADP-ribosyltransferase activity, J Exp Med. 187(7):1123–32.

Haq, T.A., Mason, H.S., Clements, J.D., and Arntzen, C.J., 1995, Oral immunization with a recombinant bacterial antigen produced in transgenic plants [see comments], Science. 268(5211):714–6.

Harford, S., Dykes, C.W., Hobden, A.N., Read, M.J., and Halliday, I.J., 1989, Inactivation of the *Escherichia coli* heat-labile enterotoxin by *in vitro* mutagenesis of the A-subunit gene, European Journal of Biochemistry. 183:311–316.

Häse, C.C., Thai, L.S., Boesman-Finkelstein, M., Mar, V.L., Burnette, W.N., Kaslow, H.R., Stevens, L.A., Moss, J., and Finkelstein, R.A., 1994, Construction and characterization of recombinant *Vibrio_cholerae* strains producing inactive cholera toxin analogs, Infection and Immunity. 62:3051–3057.

Hashigucci, K., Ogawa, H., Ishidate, T., Yamashita, R., Kamiya, H., Watanabe, K., Hattori, N., Sato, T., Suzuki, Y., and Nagamine, T., et al., 1996, Antibody responses in volunteers induced by nasal influenza vaccine combined with *Escherichia coli* heat-labile enterotoxin B subunit containing a trace amount of the holotoxin, Vaccine. 14(2):113–9.

Hathaway, L.J., Partidos, C.D., Vohra, P., and Steward, M.W., 1995, Induction of systemic immune responses to measles virus synthetic peptides administered intranasally, Vaccine. 13(16):1495–500.

Katz, J.M., Lu, X., Galphin, J.C., and Clements, J.D., 1996, Heat-labile enterotoxin from *E. coli* as an adjuvant for oral influenza vaccination. In: *Options for the Control of Influenza III*. L.E. Brown, A.W. Hampson, and R.G. Webster. New York, Elsevier Science: 292–297.

Katz, J.M., Lu, X., Young, S.A., and Galphin, J.C., 1997, Adjuvant activity of the heat-labile enterotoxin from enterotoxigenic *Escherichia coli* for oral administration of inactivated influenza virus vaccine, J Infect Dis. 175(2):352–63.

Komase, K., Tamura, S.-I., Matsuo, K., Watanabe, K., Hattori, N., Odaka, A., Suzuki, Y., Kurata, T., and Aizawa, C., 1998, Mutants of *Escherichia coli* heat-labile enterotoxin as an adjuvant for nasal influenza vaccine, Vaccine. 16(2/3):248–254.

Langermann, S., Palaszynski, S., Sadziene, A., Stover, C.K., and Koenig, S., 1994, Systemic and mucosal immunity induced by BCG vector expressing outer-surface protein A of *Borrelia burgdorferi*, Nature. 372(6506):552–5.

Lee, C.K., Weltzin, R., Thomas, W.D., Jr., Kleanthous, H., Ermak, T.H., Soman, G., Hill, J.E., Ackerman, S.K., and Monath, T.P., 1995, Oral immunization with recombinant *Helicobacter pylori* urease induces secretory IgA antibodies and protects mice from challenge with *Helicobacter felis*, J Infect Dis. 172(1):161–72.

Levi, R., Aboud-Pirak, E., Leclerc, C., Lowell, G.H., and Arnon, R., 1995, Intranasal immunization of mice against influenza with synthetic peptides anchored to proteosomes, Vaccine. 13(14):1353–9.

Levine, M.M., Kaper, J.B., Black, R.E., and Clements, M.L., 1983, New knowledge on pathogenesis of bacterial enteric infections as applied to vaccine development, Mircobiological Reviews. 47:510–550.

Lillard, J.W., Jr., Boyaka, P.N., Hedrick, J.A., Zlotnik, A., and McGhee, J.R., 1999, Lymphotactin acts as an innate mucosal adjuvant, J Immunol. 162(4):1959–65.

Lobet, Y., Cluff, C.W., and W. Cieplak, J., 1991, Effect of site-directed mutagenic alterations on ADP-ribosyltransferase activity of the A subunit of *Escherichia coli* heat-labile enterotoxin, Infection and Immunity. 59:2870–2879.

Lowell, G.H., Colleton, C., Frost, D., Kaminski, R.W., Hughes, M., Hatch, J., Hooper, C., Estep, J., Pitt, L., and Topper, M., et al., 1996, Immunogenicity and efficacy against lethal aerosol staphylococcal enterotoxin B challenge in monkeys by intramuscular and respiratory delivery of proteosome-toxoid vaccines, Infect Immun. 64(11):4686–93.

Lowell, G.H., Kaminski, R.W., VanCott, T.C., Slike, B., Kersey, K., Zawoznik, E., Loomis-Price, L., Smith, G., Redfield, R.R., and Amselem, S., et al., 1997, Proteosomes, emulsomes, and cholera toxin B improve nasal immunogenicity of human immunodeficiency virus gp160 in mice: induction of serum, intestinal, vaginal, and lung IgA and IgG, J Infect Dis. 175(2):292–301.

Lycke, N., Tsuji, T., and Holmgren, J., 1992, The adjuvant effect of *Vibrio cholerae* and *Escherichia coli* heat-labile enterotoxins is linked to their ADP-ribosyltransferase activity, European Journal of Immunology. 22:2277–2281.

Mason, H.S., Ball, J.M., Shi, J.J., Jiang, X., Estes, M.K., and Arntzen, C.J., 1996, Expression of Norwalk virus capsid protein in transgenic tobacco and potato and its oral immunogenicity in mice, Proc Natl Acad Sci U S A. 93(11):5335–40.

Merritt, E.A., Sarfaty, S., Pizza, M., Domenighini, M., Rappuoli, R., and Hol, W.G., 1995, Mutation of a buried residue causes loss of activity but no conformational change in the heat-labile enterotoxin of *Escherichia coli*, Nature Structural Biology. 2:269–272.

Michalek, S.M., Childers, N.K., Katz, J., Dertzbaugh, M., Zhang, S., Russell, M.W., Macrina, F.L., Jackson, S., and Mestecky, J., 1992, Liposomes and conjugate vaccines for antigen delivery and induction of mucosal immune responses, Adv Exp Med Biol. 327:191–8.

Moldoveanu, Z., Porter, D.C., Lu, A., McPherson, S., and Morrow, C.D., 1995, Immune responses induced by administration of encapsidated poliovirus replicons which express HIV-1 gag and envelope proteins, Vaccine. 13(11):1013–22.

Morrow, C.D., Moldovenu, Z., Anderson, M.J., and Porter, D.C., 1996, Poliovirus replicons as a vector for mucosal vaccines. In: *Mucosal vaccines*. K. Hiroshi, P.L. Ogra, and J.R. McGhee. New York, Academic Press: 137–146.

Morrow, C.D., Novak, M.J., Ansardi, D.C., Porter, D.C., and Moldoveanu, Z., 1999, Recombinant viruses as vectors for mucosal immunity, Curr Top Microbiol Immunol. 236:255–73.

Moss, J., Stanley, S.J., Vaughan, M., and Tsuji, T., 1993, Interaction of ADP-ribosylation factor with *Escherichia coli* enterotoxin that contains an inactivating lysine 112 substitution, Journal of Biological Chemistry. 268:6383–6387.

Mrsny, R.J., Daugherty, A.L., Fryling, C.M., and FitzGerald, D.J., 1999, Mucosal administration of a chimera composed of *Pseudomonas* exotoxin and the gp120 V3 loop sequence of HIV-1 induces both salivary and serum antibody responses [In Process Citation], Vaccine. 17(11–12):1425–33.

Muster, T., Ferko, B., Klima, A., Purtscher, M., Trkola, A., Schulz, P., Grassauer, A., Engelhardt, O.G., Garcia-Sastre, A., and Palese, P., et al., 1995, Mucosal model of immunization against human immunodeficiency virus type 1 with a chimeric influenza virus, J Virol. 69(11):6678–86.

O'Neal, C.M., Clements, J.D., Estes, M.K., and Conner, M.E., 1998, Rotavirus 2/6 viruslike particles administered intranasally with cholera toxin, *Escherichia coli* heat-labile toxin (LT), and LT-R192G induce protection from rotavirus challenge, J Virol. 72(4):3390–3.

Oplinger, M.L., Bakar, S., Trofa, A.F., Clements, J.D., Gibbs, P., Pazzaglia, G., Bourgeouis, A.L., and Scott, D.A., 1997, Safety and immunogenicity in volunteers of a new candidate mucosal adjuvant, LT(R192G). Program and abstracts of the 37th Interscience Conference on Antimicrobial Agents and Chemotherapy, Washington, D.C., American Society for Microbiology.

Partidos, C.D., Pizza, M., Rappuoli, R., and Steward, M.W., 1996, The adjuvant effect of a non-toxic mutant of heat-labile enterotoxin of *Escherichia coli* for the induction of measles virus-specific CTL responses after intranasal co-immunization with a synthetic peptide, Immunology. 89(4):483–7.

Pizza, M., Domenighini, M., Hol, W., Giannelli, V., Fontana, M.R., Giuliani, M.M., Magagnoli, C., Peppoloni, S., Manetti, R., and Rappuoli, R., 1994, Probing the structure-activity relationship of *Escherichia coli* LT-A by site-directed mutagenesis, Molecular Microbiology. 14:51–60.

Roberts, M., Bacon, A., Rappuoli, R., Pizza, M., Cropley, I., Douce, G., Dougan, G., Marinaro, M., McGhee, J., and Chatfield, S., 1995, A mutant pertussis toxin molecule that lacks ADP-ribosyltransferase activity, PT-9K/129G, is an effective mucosal adjuvant for intranasally delivered proteins, Infect Immun. 63(6):2100–8.

Rosenthal, K.L., Copeland, K.F.T., and Gallichan, W.S., 1996, Recombinant adenoviruses as vectors for mucosal immunity. In: *Mucosal vaccines*. K. Hiroshi, P.L. Ogra, and J.R. McGhee. New York, Academic Press.

Schodel, F. and Curtiss, R., 3rd, 1995, *Salmonellae* as oral vaccine carriers, Dev Biol Stand. 84:245–53.

Sixma, T.K., Kalk, K.H., Vanzanten, B.A.M., Dauter, Z., Kingma, J., Witholt, B., and Hol, W.G.J., 1993, Refined structure of *Escherichia coli* heat-labile enterotoxin, a close relative of cholera toxin, Journal of Molecular Biology. 230:890–918.

Sixma, T.K., Pronk, S.E., Kalk, K.H., Wartna, E.S., vanZanten, B.A.M., Witholt, B., and Hol, W.G.J., 1991, Crystal structure of a cholera toxin-related heat-labile enterotoxin from *E. coli*, Nature (London). 351:371–377.

Smith, R.E., Donachie, A.M., and Mowat, A.M., 1998, Immune stimulating complexes as mucosal vaccines, Immunol Cell Biol. 76(3):263–9.

Staats, H.F., Nichols, W.G., and Palker, T.J., 1996, Mucosal immunity to HIV-1: systemic and vaginal antibody responses after intranasal immunization with the HIV-1 C4/V3 peptide T1SP10 MN(A), J Immunol. 157(1):462–72.

Tacket, C.O., Mason, H.S., Losonsky, G., Clements, J.D., Levine, M.M., and Arntzen, C.J., 1998, Immunogenicity in humans of a recombinant bacterial antigen delivered in a transgenic potato, Nat Med. 4(5):607–9.

Tribble, D.R., Bakar, S., Oplinger, M.L., Bourgeouis, A.L., Clements, J.D., Trofa, A.F., Pazzaglia, G., Pace, J., Walker, R.I., and Gibbs, P., et al. 1997, Safety and enhanced immunogenicity in volunteers of an oral, inactivated, whole cell *Campylobacter* vaccine co-administered with a modified *E. coli* heat-labile enterotoxin adjuvant, LT (R192G). Program and abstracts of the 37th Interscience Conference on Antimicrobial Agents and Chemotherapy, Washington, D.C., American Society for Microbiology.

Tsuji, T., Inoue, T., Miyama, A., Okamoto, K., Honda, T., and Miwatani, T., 1990, A single amino acid substitution in the A subunit of *Escherichia coli* enterotoxin results in loss of its toxic activitiy, Journal of Biological Chemistry. 265:22520–22525.

Weltzin, R., Kleanthous, H., Guirakhoo, F., Monath, T.P., and Lee, C.K., 1997, Novel intranasal immunization techniques for antibody induction and protection of mice against gastric *Helicobacter felis* infection, Vaccine. 15(4):370–6.

Wu, H.Y., Nahm, M.H., Guo, Y., Russell, M.W., and Briles, D.E., 1997, Intranasal immunization of mice with PspA (pneumococcal surface protein A) can prevent intranasal carriage, pulmonary infection, and sepsis with *Streptococcus pneumoniae*, J Infect Dis. 175(4):839–46.

Xu-Amano, J., Jackson, R.J., Fujihashi, K., Kiyono, H., Staats, H.F., and McGhee, J.R., 1994, Helper Th1 and Th2 cell responses following mucosal or systemic immunization with cholera toxin, Vaccine. 12(10):903–11.

Xu-Amano, J., Kiyono, H., Jackson, R.J., Staats, H.F., Fujihashi, K., Burrows, P.D., Elson, C.O., Pillai, S., and McGhee, J.R., 1993, Helper T cell subsets for immunoglobulin A responses: oral immunization with tetanus toxoid and cholera toxin as adjuvant selectively induces Th2 cells in mucosal associated tissues, Journal of Experimental Medicine. 178:1309–1320.

Yamamoto, M., Vancott, J.L., Okahashi, N., Marinaro, M., Kiyono, H., Fujihashi, K., Jackson, R.J., Chatfield, S.N., Bluethmann, H., and McGhee, J.R., 1996, The role of Th1 and Th2 cells for mucosal IgA responses, Ann N Y Acad Sci. 778:64–71.

Yamamoto, S., Kiyono, H., Yamamoto, M., Imaoka, K., Fujihashi, K., Van Ginkel, F.W., Noda, M., Takeda, Y., and McGhee, J.R., 1997a, A nontoxic mutant of cholera toxin elicits Th2-type responses for enhanced mucosal immunity, Proc Natl Acad Sci U S A. 94(10):5267–72.

Yamamoto, S., Takeda, Y., Yamamoto, M., Kurazono, H., Imaoka, K., Yamamoto, M., Fujihashi, K., Noda, M., Kiyono, H., and McGhee, J.R., 1997b, Mutants in the ADP-ribosyltransferase cleft of cholera toxin lack diarrheagenicity but retain adjuvanticity, Journal of Experimental Medicine. 185:1203–1210.

INDEX